VOLUME TWO

Current concepts in radiology

VOLUME TWO

Current concepts in
RADIOLOGY

Edited by

E. James Potchen, M.D.

Professor, Department of Radiology
The Johns Hopkins Medical Institutions
Baltimore, Maryland

With 354 illustrations

SAINT LOUIS

The C. V. Mosby Company

1975

Library of Congress Cataloging in Publication Data (Revised)

Potchen, E   James.
   Current concepts in radiology.

   Includes bibliographies.
   1. Radiography. I. Title. [DNLM: 1. Radiography.
2. Radiology.   WN100 P859c]
RC78.P667   616.07′57   72-83971
ISBN 0-8016-3986-7

GW/CB/B 9 8 7 6 5 4 3 2 1

Contributors

RALPH E. COLEMAN, M.D.

Fellow in Nuclear Medicine, Mallinckrodt Institute of Radiology, Washington University School of Medicine, St. Louis, Missouri

MARTIN W. DONNER, M.D.

Professor and Chairman, Department of Radiology and Radiological Science, The Johns Hopkins Medical Institutions, Baltimore, Maryland

WARD EDWARDS, Ph.D.

Director, Social Science Research Institute, University of Southern California, Los Angeles, California

JOHN V. FORREST, M.D.

Associate Professor, Department of Radiology, Washington University School of Medicine, St. Louis, Missouri

DENNIS G. FRYBACK

Doctoral Candidate, Department of Psychology, University of Michigan, Ann Arbor, Michigan

BOB W. GAYLER, M.D.

Associate Professor, Department of Radiology and Radiological Science, The Johns Hopkins Medical Institutions, Baltimore, Maryland

E. RALPH HEINZ, M.D.

Professor and Chairman, Department of Radiology, University of Pittsburgh School of Medicine, Pittsburgh, Pennsylvania

ATSUKO HESHIKI, M.D.

Assistant Professor of Radiology, The Johns Hopkins Medical Institutions, Baltimore, Maryland

A. EVERETTE JAMES, Jr., Sc.M., M.D.

Associate Professor of Radiology, Director of Diagnostic Radiological Research, The Johns Hopkins Medical Institutions, Baltimore, Maryland

BENJAMIN LEV, Ph.D.

Associate Professor of Operations Research, School of Business Administration, Temple University, Philadelphia, Pennsylvania

LEE B. LUSTED, M.D.

Professor, Department of Radiology, University of Chicago Medical School, Chicago, Illinois

HEBER MacMAHON, M.B.

Resident in Diagnostic Radiology, Department of Radiology, Washington University School of Medicine, St. Louis, Missouri

E. JAMES POTCHEN, M.D.

Professor, Department of Radiology, The Johns Hopkins Medical Institutions, Baltimore, Maryland

DONALD SASHIN, Ph.D.

Assistant Professor of Radiology and Scientific Director, Radiological Imaging Group, Department of Radiology, University of Pittsburgh School of Medicine, Pittsburgh, Pennsylvania

WILLIAM R. SCHONBEIN, S.M.

Director, Management Information Systems, The Johns Hopkins Medical Institutions, Baltimore, Maryland

STUART S. SAGEL, M.D.

Associate Professor, Department of Radiology, Washington University School of Medicine, St. Louis, Missouri

FRANCIS J. SHEA, M.D.

Associate Professor, Department of Radiology, School of Medicine, Temple University, Philadelphia, Pennsylvania

BARRY A. SIEGEL, M.D.

Associate Professor of Radiology and Director, Division of Nuclear Medicine, Mallinckrodt Institute of Radiology, Washington University School of Medicine, St. Louis, Missouri

ERNEST J. STERNGLASS, Ph.D.

Professor of Radiology and Consultant, Radiological Imaging Group, Department of Radiology, University of Pittsburgh School of Medicine, Pittsburgh, Pennsylvania

JOHN R. THORNBURY, M.D.

Professor, Department of Radiology, University of Michigan Medical School, Ann Arbor, Michigan

Dedicated to

RADIOLOGISTS OF THE FUTURE

Preface

The second volume of *Current Concepts in Radiology* is designed in keeping with our original premise "to bring together selected aspects considered important to the practicing radiologist and radiologist in training for optimal application of current information to patient care." During the past two years, the practice of radiology has seen increasing attention directed toward its role in effective patient management. With constraints on resources available for health care, the physician is faced with an increasing need to select among alternative choices in his diagnostic armamentarium. Thus there is an ever-increasing need for the referring physician and his radiologist consultant to develop an appreciation of efficient resource allocation to complement the art and science of medical practice. Diagnostic radiology has significantly decreased the cost of health care by providing more efficient and effective management of patients. It seems timely to compile some available information on the subject of patient management in a format conducive to implementing these concepts in the practice of radiology. Admittedly, some of this material, when presented in a structured form, may seem foreign to the practicing radiologist. However, it is fair to say that unstructured consideration of these concepts are everyday components of radiologic practice.

The first four chapters are designed to provide a foundation for understanding how one might study more effective and efficient uses of radiology. Admittedly, some of the mathematical background may not be appealing to my fellow clinicians. However, for those interested it does provide a more formal basis for appreciating the concepts discussed. Diagnostic efficacy is becoming an everyday concern. These chapters are designed in part to provide appreciation for its implications and application.

The middle three chapters were selected in an effort to present some developments in our understanding of the radiologic image and the effect of its characteristics on the interpretation of radiographs.

The last four chapters were chosen to address specific areas in which clinical radiology has been making significant strides in the past few years. Admittedly, others may have chosen different topics from among the advances we have seen in clinical radiology. My recognition of the potential contributions of transverse axial tomography and diagnostic ultrasound came too late for inclusion in this volume. However, these subjects will continue to be developed and thus be more appropriate for a subsequent volume in this series.

I would like to acknowledge my appreciation to the many contributors who have so freely taken time from their busy schedules to assist in the preparation of this volume. I also appreciate the efforts of my able associates, especially Janet Evans and Gail Pecci, who are largely responsible for the ultimate completion of this task.

E. James Potchen

Contents

1 Operations management in radiology

Benjamin Lev and Francis J. Shea

Operations management in radiology may be defined as the management of all the operational systems in the radiology department that transform inputs into outputs.[21] The most familiar system is that which transforms an x-ray request slip into a diagnostic report through multiple subsystems. The modern radiology department functions in many areas in addition to performing and reading x-ray studies. This chapter is a partial discussion of the activities that have evolved to permit the orderly function of a typical department.

Scheduling system. Patient scheduling can be broken down into outpatient scheduling, which requires advanced scheduling for up to a week or more in the future, and inpatient scheduling, which as a rule requires scheduling the patient within the next 2 days.

Personnel scheduling includes assignment of technicians to the various examination rooms and assignment of radiologists to various locations (examination rooms, reading films, special studies, etc.).

Patient identification system. The patient identification system assigns each patient a number that is also used for film identification and retrieval. The identification system may be a manual one in which the patient number is given by a numbers clerk when the patient is registered. It may be semiautomated, in which the information is stored on a semiautomated card access system, or it may be fully automated, involving a terminal that is connected to a computer where all patient identification data are stored.

Patient flow system. The patient flow system includes the close supervision of patients from the time at which they are sent from their floor or the outpatient reception desk until the time they leave the department. The goal here is to achieve a smooth flow of patients and to avoid situations in which patients wait for excessive lengths of time.[11,20] This system is dependent upon the availability of escort personnel and elevators when needed.

Film reporting system. The time elapsed from the end of the x-ray examination to the time at which the referring physician receives the radiologist's report can vary from minutes at one extreme to a week or more at the other. This span

Supported by Grant GM 14548-08, National Institute of General Medical Sciences.

1

of time can be especially important when a delay in reporting results in a delay in treatment. Reporting systems can be either manual or automated.[13] One measure of the effectiveness of a radiology department is the time required to transmit diagnostic information to the referring physician.

File room management system. Typically a department has an active file room that holds new films for the first several weeks; these files are then transferred to the inactive file room. Inactive file rooms hold films for variable periods of time, depending upon local preference and regulations. Some departments store films indefinitely. A large department may accumulate several million films within a few years, and in such cases a reliable system is needed to identify and retrieve inactive films.

Cost accounting and billing system. The radiology department should be capable of determining the cost of performing each x-ray examination and giving a breakdown of the annual budget into personnel and supply categories. The final billing charge will be based upon examination costs as well as the costs of the billing process and a surcharge for bills that are uncollectable.

Equipment selection and replacement policy. The equipment selection and replacement policy is the basis for determining when to replace existing equipment or purchase additional equipment. The reason for replacement might be obsolescence or high maintenance costs. A study of the entire department is needed at the time of replacement to determine the type of equipment that will add most to the overall efficiency of the entire department.[18]

•   •   •

Radiology departments vary considerably, and to some extent their management systems and decision criteria must also vary. The following are some of the factors that influence the operation of the department:

> Volume of cases (patients per year)
> Type of cases (examination mix)
> Inpatient/outpatient ratio
> Socioeconomic composition of patients
> > Likelihood of showing up on time for scheduled appointment
> > Likelihood of collecting bill
> Type of practice
> > Private office
> > Nonteaching hospital
> > Teaching hospital
> > Clinic
> Mode of patient arrival (walk, wheelchair, stretcher)
> Location of practice
> > Ability to recruit staff, technicians, and nontechnical personnel
> > Cost of living index

This long list of variables makes it impossible to come up with one plan for an "ideal" department or with a predetermined set of rules detailing how to efficiently run radiology departments. In the next few pages we would like to discuss specific factors that we feel are important to take into consideration in planning the operation of a radiology department.

HUMAN FACTORS

Any system that is not fully automated and that requires human intervention in its operation must deal with human factors. A radiology department is a system in which man and machine are working together and depend upon each other. The usual bottleneck in a radiology department is that part related to personnel. In order to increase capacity, obtain higher productivity, and lower costs, one must increase personnel output.

At the turn of the century Frederick Taylor[24] published *Principles of Scientific Management,* in which he emphasized the conditions required to increase worker productivity. Standard equipment, push-button operation, and wage incentives based on production rate encourage and help individuals to increase their productivity.

The next phase of improving performance is in group performance. It has been found that group productivity and satisfactory human relationships within the group motivate each member to contribute his share toward higher and better performance. It is important that each member in the department understand his part in the total operation and the fact that the department must function well as a unit. Setting group goals will encourage each individual to contribute more in this social environment.

A third aspect of the evolution of modern management is the emphasis on job enlargement and satisfaction.[4,6,7] The technician and radiologist as individuals would like to advance themselves. If a technician performs only one type of examination for a long period of time, he becomes an expert in that specific examination, but within the radiology department there are many different examinations performed; by rotating staff from one to the other it is possible to introduce variety and prevent boredom. Similarly one would like to rotate the assignments of radiologists and avoid repetitive work. Greater variation will increase job satisfaction, which is a basic human need. Specialization is good momentarily, but repetition creates the risk of dissatisfaction and lack of motivation, which in turn may produce a high rate of absenteeism, turnover, low quality, low awareness, higher accident rates, etc. Too frequent rotation for technicians is also disadvantageous, since approximately a month is required for an individual to reach a high level of proficiency in a given area.

Human needs may be ranked in an hierarchical order.[14] Each time one level is satisfied, man tries to satisfy the next level. After meeting such basic needs as food and clothing, he progresses to job satisfaction and group productivity. When these needs are met he moves to job security and job participation, levels at which he tries to make changes and improvements in the environment in which he works. Again, it is important to encourage personnel

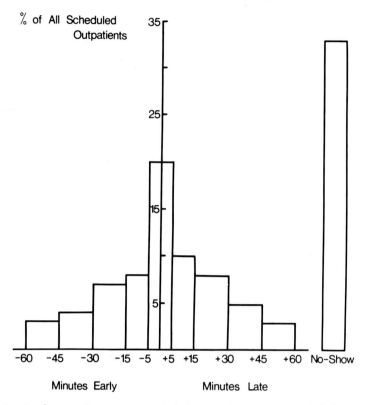

Fig. 1-1. Distribution of outpatient arrival time as a function of scheduled appointment time.

to participate in improving the operation; otherwise, as before, when needs are not satisfied the result may be lower levels of performance and disassociation from the group.

When dealing with human factors we must not forget patients. One of the big difficulties in developing a good patient scheduling program is the fact that patients do not show up at the appointment time. Revesz and Shea[19] have shown that outpatient arrival time at Temple University Hospital is almost a gaussian distribution, with the average occurring at the appointment time and with a third of the patients not coming at all (Fig. 1-1). This distribution is specific for Temple University. Each department has its own population and the distribution will vary from one place to another. When designing a patient scheduling system, however, this factor must be considered.

Another patient-related aspect is the fact that the diagnostic department is a service department, and in order to maintain referrals of outpatients it is important that patients not have to wait for long periods of time at the risk of losing referrals in the future.

DEPARTMENT LAYOUT

The objectives in designing department layout may be divided into two main categories: (1) location of the department with respect to other facilities in the hospital and (2) layout within the department itself.[25]

In choosing an area for the department the objectives include minimizing inpatient and outpatient travel distances, minimizing the time required for orderlies to transport inpatients, minimizing elevator usage, and excluding nonradiology traffic from the department.

The layout within the department should result in minimized patient travel within the department and avoidance of the use of patient corridors and holding areas by radiology personnel. Related activities performed by such personnel as reception clerks, scheduling clerks, patient number identification clerks, and record clerks should be grouped in contiguous space to minimize the need for carriers and communications equipment. The design should also be based upon minimizing construction costs and operating costs.

Department design is a one-shot operation, and considerable thought should be given to obtaining the optimal configuration so as to ensure smooth operation for the expected life of the department. In addition, clearly identifiable expansion space should be available.

It has been shown that patient congestion in corridors is minimized by having those studies that require the shortest examination time performed in examination rooms nearest the patient entrances to the department. By similar logic, angiographic examination rooms should be furthest from the patient entrances. It is also important that the mammography thermography suite be in a quiet area of the department, removed from stretcher patients and hospital personnel. Women scheduled for breast examination are, as a rule, more apprehensive than the average patient and require a relaxed environment.

Patient holding areas and personnel work areas should not be mixed, to minimize congestion and to permit personnel to discuss a case without being overheard by patients. The simplest floor arrangement for accomplishing this objective is a three-layered arrangement, as shown schematically in Fig. 1-2. There are many variations of the three-layered department, and these may be adapted for departments of varying sizes and to construction constraints.

If a department is large, it may not be possible to keep the entire department together as one large unit. If decentralization becomes necessary, there are several possible approaches that have varying effects on construction and operating costs. These include the following options:

1. The department may be divided into self-sufficient suites—general radiographic suite, fluoroscopic suite, angiographic suite, intravenous pyelography suite, and ultrasound, mammography, and thermography (UMT) suite. These suites must be linked to the department control center and to the file room by communications equipment that could increase operating costs, but the total number of rooms required should not increase.

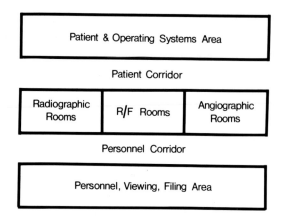

Fig. 1-2. Three-layered department arrangement. Patients and personnel enter from left.

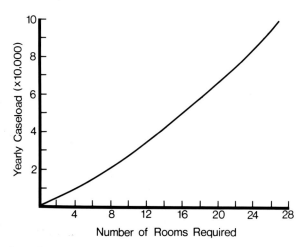

Fig. 1-3. Number of x-ray rooms required as a function of caseload. (Modified from Naylor, A. F.: Radiology department planning seminar reference material, New Orleans, 1973, American College of Radiology.)

2. The department may be divided into inpatient and outpatient sections. Such an arrangement can be made for large departments but it is necessary to duplicate some equipment. Based on Naylor's data[16] relating caseload to department size (number of examination rooms), we have constructed a curve for predicting room requirements as a function of caseload (Fig. 1-3). A department that performs 70,000 examinations per year operating in one location that would require 21 examination rooms, whereas the same department, split into two sections each doing 35,000 examinations yearly, would require 24 examina-

tion rooms (12 rooms for each section). These figures assume that all rooms have a yearly throughput close to the average for the department. This assumption is valid only if the department, when split, provides all services to patients in each subdepartment. Specifically, the division of the department into self-sufficient suites does *not* increase the number of rooms required, whereas division into an inpatient and outpatient section does. Again, any form of splitting will probably necessitate increased expenditures for communication and control equipment.

3. The most severe form of splitting is that necessitated by a hospital built on a program floor concept, in which each floor of the hospital is devoted to a specific area such as cardiopulmonary or neurosensory medicine. Under the program floor concept,[9] the radiology department is required to provide all general radiographic and fluoroscopic studies on each floor as well as special procedures related to the program of the floor in question. Such a concept poses severe problems in communications and control and requires considerable duplication of personnel and equipment. We recently evaluated a proposed program floor hospital that would have required operating the diagnostic radiology department on seven floors; we estimated operating costs for the diagnostic radiology department to be a minimum of 30% greater than the operating costs for a one-floor centralized department.

The advantage of the program floor concept is that most x-ray studies can be done on the patients' floor, decreasing patient travel time, orderly time, and travel time of the referring physician. In addition, there is lower utilization of elevators.

RESOURCE UTILIZATION

Most of the operating systems of a radiology department are dependent upon the resources available and the utilization factors attached to these resources. More sophisticated operating systems such as computer-based dynamic scheduling systems can conversely influence resource utilization.

Room utilization

A typical large general diagnostic radiology department performs about 10,000 examinations per year in each unit of three rooms (3333 examinations per room per year). Analysis of data published by Revesz et al.[20] has shown that the above figure corresponds to about 40% room utilization during the routine 8-hour working day. Room utilization is defined as the average number of minutes spent by patients in each examination room divided by the time the room was available for use—420 minutes (8 hours less 1 hour closed during lunch). A scheduling system that could increase examination room throughput could potentially cut department equipment costs significantly. We have estimated that an angiographic room can be used for as many as 1000 cases per year at present.

Technician utilization

An x-ray technician can handle approximately 3333 routine examinations per year (10,000 examinations by three technicians) or 500 angiographic examinations per year. These numbers vary considerably, however, depending upon the mix of examinations performed. For the general diagnostic work load these figures represent only about 40% utilization of technicians as radiographers (time spent in the examination room).[20] A similar figure is reported by Shuman and Wolfe.[22] In the design of operating systems, thought should be given to methods of increasing technician productivity, for example, having lower paid, less skilled personnel transport patients, move patients on and off tables, and find films for the radiologist. An arrangement whereby a technician and a technician's helper jointly operate two examination rooms with the technician doing only radiography could conceivably lower operating costs.

Radiologist utilization

A radiologist's output, measured in terms of number of cases per year, is a highly variable and highly individualistic parameter, as indeed it is for all physicians. In setting up operating systems it is necessary to know what the average output will be and then give reasonable compensation for that output (see the discussion of operating costs later in this chapter). By training clerical personnel to prehang all films read by the radiologist and to take them down later, it is possible to significantly increase the number of films that a radiologist can read per hour. Unpublished reports by radiologists who have clerks prehang films show up to a 40% increase in the radiologist's output.

Nontechnical personnel

The estimated number of nontechnical personnel required to staff a department is based upon experience with several hospital practices and is fairly similar to the figures cited by Donaldson.[5] We have found that cutting nontechnical personnel below the figures cited results in complaints regarding service by radiologists, referring physicians, and patients. Much of the operation of a radiology department can be automated, and this can reduce the number of clerks and typists required. Automation, however, requires a large initial financial outlay and continuing costs for personnel, software development, added terminals, etc.

We are always facing the trade-off between staff utilization and faster service to patients, which to some extent are competing factors. We have to compromise between an acceptable waiting time for patients and an acceptable level of staff utilization.

OPERATING COSTS

Operating costs of the department should represent actual costs as determined by a cost accounting survey. Shuman and Wolfe[22] have done a detailed cost accounting of the radiographic examinations at the Presbyterian-University Hospital in Pittsburgh in order to come up with the true cost of each study. Today, however, most departments estimate costs using a relative cost table such as that prepared by the American College of Radiology.[2] In our experience operating costs can usually be adequately met in a nonacademic department by using ACR relative total cost values multiplied by $6. The billing charge would of course be higher to compensate for uncollectable bills.

Operating costs for routine caseload

As noted previously, there are many factors that influence operating costs. Tables 1-1 and 1-2 represent estimates that reflect the experience of one of the authors (F. J. S.) with the hospital practice of radiology predicted at fiscal 1973-1974 dollar values and should be readjusted annually to reflect changes in the cost of living index. These tables may not be acceptable for nonhospital prac-

Table 1-1. Operating cost breakdown for each unit of $240,000 yearly receipts from routine examinations

Dollar amount	Fund	Total (%)
80,000	Professional fund	33.33
36,000	Technician fund*	15.00
28,000	Nontechnical personnel fund†	11.67
40,000	Film chemical, and supplies fund .	16.67
32,000	Equipment fund‡	13.33
24,000	Floor rent§	10.00
240,000		100.00

*Salaries for three technicians, including overtime and fringe benefits.
†Salaries for nontechnical personnel including overtime and fringe benefits.
‡Includes one radiographic fluoroscopy (RF) room and two radiographic rooms.
§Assumes 4000 ft² gross space.

Table 1-2. Operating cost breakdown for each unit of $240,000 yearly receipts from angiographic examinations

Dollar amount	Fund	Total (%)
80,000	Professional fund	33.33
24,000	Technician fund*	10.00
21,000	Nontechnical personnel fund†	8.75
46,000	Film, chemical, and supplies fund	19.17
60,000	Equipment fund‡	25.00
9,000	Floor rent§	3.75
240,000		100.00

*Salary for two technicians.
†Salary for three nontechnical personnel.
‡Costs for one angiographic room.
§Assumes 1500 ft² gross space.

tices or for all areas of the country. Billing charges include operating costs and a surcharge to cover uncollected bills. All personnel costs are gross costs, including salary, fringe benefits, and malpractice insurance. Nontechnical personnel include administrative, secretarial, clerical, and darkroom personnel. The equipment fund covers the purchase and maintenance of major radiographic equipment. Floor rent represents compensation for space and the following services: janitorial, billing, payroll, inpatient escort, and patient number identification.

In attempting to estimate operating costs we have found it more valuable to use expected income rather than case volume as a criterion, since there is considerable variation in case mix from institution to institution. If one uses the ACR total fee value multiplied by $6, then we can talk of an operating cost unit of $240,000 as the basis for estimating personnel and supply costs. This figure would correspond to from 8000 to 15,000 general cases per year, depending upon the nature of the practice. Again, it is assumed that operating costs exactly equal gross receipts from billing.

Operating costs for angiographic caseload

Operating costs for the angiographic caseload are much higher per case due to the increased cost of equipment and to the relatively long period of time required to perform these studies. The data in Table 1-2 are based on the assumption that all of the studies are performed by the radiologist.

Operating costs for teaching programs

A school for x-ray technicians can usually be operated on a cost-effective basis, for the costs incurred in running the school are offset by the need for fewer staff technicians to operate the department. In the first year of operation a school will require an additional outlay of funds, but by the second year it should be self-supporting.

A radiology residency training program can also be run on a cost-effective basis. A routine residency program, in which the resident spends the vast majority of his time doing general radiology, can be set up so that the expenses of the residency program (chiefly residents' salaries) are offset by the need for fewer staff radiologists. An enriched radiology residency training program, in which up to half of the residency period is spent in nonincome-producing activities such as angiography, neuroradiology, and electives, can still be cost effective if the staff radiologists are willing to accept academic rather than professional salaries for the time spent in resident supervision. In order to maintain a balance within an academic department, we suggest that roughly half of each staff members' time should be spent as a professional radiologist and the other half in academic pursuits such as radiology resident teaching, medical student and nonradiology resident teaching, and research.

A major addition to the operating costs of a department occurs if there is an active teaching program for medical students and nonradiology residents. There is of course a need for additional staff radiologists for teaching and conference participation, but a more subtle need is that for markedly increased numbers of nontechnical personnel, primarily because of the increased demands on the x-ray file room and also because of the need to maintain services at times other than during the routine working day. Depending upon the institution and its programs, these costs as well as the costs of funding a research program will add significantly to the operating costs of the department. At Temple University these costs amount to approximately a third of the hospital operating costs. The costs described previously are not part of the true hospital operating costs of the department but are rather academic costs borne by the sponsoring institution and outside funding sources rather than by the hospital through patient billing.

PLANNING FOR A NEW DEPARTMENT

At the present time the average number of medical radiographic examinations per person per year is about 0.56.[15] Based solely on this criterion, a three-room routine radiology suite would require a population of about 18,000 people to support it (10,000 cases per year). Knowles[8] has estimated that one radiologist is required for about each 23,000 people in the area. Another useful figure for estimating is that each hospital bed will generate approximately 50 examinations per year. If the practice is such that outpatient volume is equal to inpatient volume, then one would estimate that hospital practice will have 100 examinations per year for each hospital bed. As an example a planned 200-bed hospital will generate approximately 10,000 inpatient routine examinations and 10,000 outpatient routine examinations per year. These methods for planning the size of a radiologic facility are rough estimates at best but do provide a starting point from which more refined estimates can be made.

A teaching hospital may generate more cases per patient than a nonteaching hospital, depending upon the degree of need for radiographic confirmation expressed by physicians requesting examinations. A clinical practice in which the patient will probably be seen by the same physician for his medical care is likely to generate fewer radiologic cases than a clinical practice that does not involve a continuing doctor-patient relationship.

Forecasting future needs for existing departments

In attempting to forecast a future radiologic work load it is necessary to predict the population to be served in the foreseeable future (a somewhat nebulous phrase, but here we arbitrarily define foreseeable future to mean within the next 5 years). One means of doing this is by extrapolation; the number of cases performed during the past few years is plotted on graph paper and then a curve is drawn through these points and extended for the next 5 years.

When such a method is used, the prediction is most reliable for the first year but becomes progressively less reliable for succeeding years.

The most significant single determinant of the future radiologic caseload will be the impact of national health insurance, if enacted. Depending upon the scope of the coverage provided, the radiologic caseload could increase by as much as 20% nationally and by an even higher figure in those areas in which the health needs of the community have been largely neglected to date.

Space requirements

Various rules for estimating space requirements have been developed. All measurements to be given are in gross space, which includes all floor space designated as being in the department, including corridors. Donaldson[5] has stated that 100 ft² per patient per day is desirable; this translates into 3880 ft² to handle 10,000 routine cases a year. Analysis of Terry and McLaren's data[25] shows that they estimate 2920 ft² to handle 10,000 cases per year in a non-teaching hospital and 4090 ft² to handle 10,000 cases per year in a teaching hospital. In computing floor rent we estimate 4000 ft² for 10,000 routine cases and 1500 ft² for 1000 angiographic cases. Naylor[16] has presented data showing the number of cases per year per room that can be handled, depending upon the size of the department (Table 1-3). He has also broken down space requirements into functional groups, as shown in Table 1-4.

As an example based on Naylor's data (Table 1-4 and Fig. 1-3), a department performing 70,000 examinations per year would require 21 rooms, and the total

Table 1-3. Examinations per year per room based on department size*

Very large (more than 23 rooms)	4200
Large (12-23 rooms)	3160
Medium (4-11 rooms)	2600
Small (1-3 rooms)	1880

*Based on data from Naylor, A. F.: Radiology department planning seminar reference material, New Orleans, 1973, American College of Radiology.

Table 1-4. Space distribution based on 300 ft² for examination room*

Patient-related space	350 ft²
Examination room	300 ft²
Technician and aides	300 ft²
Film files	150 ft²
Professional	200 ft²
Total (nonteaching dept.)	1300 ft²
Teaching	200 ft²
Total (teaching dept.)	1500 ft²

*Based on data from Naylor, A. F.: Radiology department planning seminar reference material, New Orleans, 1973, American College of Radiology.

gross space required would be 27,300 ft² in a nonteaching hospital and 31,500 ft² in a teaching hospital.

MANAGEMENT INFORMATION SYSTEMS

A quarter of a century ago few people envisioned a wide variety of applications for the computer, which had then just been invented. Very few people could then predict the dimension and impact that computers would have on our lives. Computer penetration into new fields and applications is daily becoming deeper. We are all familiar with the role of computers in medical research. The nature of modern research methodologies is such that the use of the computer is required in one way or another in a high percentage of current investigations. The low cost of minicomputers and time-shared larger computer systems makes it possible for even a small department to afford the use of computer time for its research. What we would like to emphasize here is another view of the use of the computer, that is, in management information systems (MIS). MIS has been used for a long time by top management in large organizations and it is now possible to apply the same techniques to lower levels of the organization, at the departmental level, for example.

Radiology departments that employ 50 people and have an annual budget of more than $1,000,000 and a volume of over 50,000 cases per year can very easily apply and use MIS. The main purpose of MIS is to help run the daily operation of the department. Many data collections, manipulations, and simple decisions that are now done manually can be done by machine.[3,23] The savings in terms of money, accuracy, and efficiency can be considerable.

The decision maker, from the chairman of the department down to the clerk who answers the phone and makes patient appointments, needs data in order to make correct decisions. We have to furnish the relevant data within a reasonable period of time to aid in the decision-making process. Lack of the appropriate information may result in an arbitrary decision. On the other hand, piles of irrelevant data can also disturb the decision-making process and the smooth operation of the department. We have to watch for these dangerous extreme situations: too little data that results in an arbitrary decision and too much data that is overwhelming and difficult to absorb and analyze and that consequently results in wrong decisions.[1]

It is important that there also be a mechanism built into the MIS that will simplify the execution of decisions. For example, suppose we have an automated scheduling system, and a decision has been made to schedule a patient's appointment for 9:27 A.M. Any deviation from this time will cause delays in other parts of the system. Obviously it is difficult if not impossible to execute that decision, for patients will not be able to come exactly at 9:27, and a delay in their arrival time might disturb the operation of other subsystems.

Before going into the details of what MIS can do, we would like to say that the success of any system depends very much upon the role its users play in building it. If a decision maker does not participate in building the system he probably does not understand its operation and will avoid using it. On the other hand, if he takes part in putting it together, then he will use it. It is also important to periodically reevaluate and update the MIS.

Next, let us discuss some problem areas in which MIS can be helpful. The easiest place to start is with the accounting department. Bills are sent to the patients, and this is a function of the type of radiographic examination performed. Also employee salaries are based upon the number of hours worked, regular time, and overtime. A more sophisticated example of MIS in a radiology department can be a scheduling system. A patient calls and would like to have an appointment. We can build a system (like an airline ticket information system) in which the clerk will feed the necessary information into a terminal linked to a computer; while the patient is on the phone, a list of potential openings for his examination will show up on a screen, and the clerk will pick a time convenient for the patient. This is only one example of a scheduling system. We can have a MIS, part of which will include statistics on the department—volume per day, week, month, and year; cases broken down by radiographic examinations; utilization figures for employees, examination rooms, and equipment; generation of income; and breakdown of expenses. In fact, any information concerning the department can be stored in the computer and can be made available to the decision maker. MIS can generate information that will help in arriving at decisions such as the following:

1. *Forecasting: short-range and long-range planning.* By furnishing information on the past and the trend of changes, MIS can help to predict the future. Information on changes in the pattern of patient mix or case volume, for example, are good indicators of future demands and requirements.

2. *Cash flow: gives status of the cash balance in a department.* Data on uncollected bills, outstanding debts, etc. will assist administrators in making their financial decisions.

3. *Staff assignment.* Scheduling technicians to examination rooms as well as assignments for radiologists and other staff can be done with MIS. MIS can compile all of the necessary information and make up the schedule.

4. *Department layout.* Changes in patient mix and the inpatient/outpatient ratio might be a reason for changing department layout. New examination rooms and equipment will improve patient flow and the level of service provided by the department. Top management must be aware of such changes and respond appropriately.

5. *Inventory control.* An automated system can record inventory levels of film, chemicals, and other necessary materials and prepare orders for supplies as needed.

6. *Quality control.* One means of determining the quality of a technician's work is to record the number of repetitions needed in the examination

room staffed by that technician. A high percentage of repeated films would indicate a problem either with the work of that technician or with the equipment itself.

This is only a partial list of the types of decisions to which MIS can contribute. We recommend that a department start with less critical and complex areas in which the expectations are not too high. Only gradually should other aspects be added to the MIS.

OTHER COMPUTER USES
Simulation studies

Industry had been using the computer for the last 20 years as a laboratory for new experiments. We are referring to simulation techniques, in which a model of the department is built on the computer, using either a standard computer language such as Fortran or a special simulation language such as General Purpose Simulation Systems (GPSS), Simscrip, or Codanet. Once we have a computer model we can verify its replication of the actual process by "running" the model and comparing its results to the actual performance of the department. Only after the model is accurate enough for our purposes in replicating the actual system can we test various operating policies and observe performance under the different input variables. This is a laboratory in which a manager can test his new ideas without interfering with the current operation of his department. He can try changing his staff, rooms, caseload, scheduling procedures, patient mix, etc. These are very inexpensive experiments once the computer simulation model is built. Only after the performance of the model satisfies our demand do we proceed to implement changes in the department. Simulation technique is a very powerful tool, especially when dealing with complex systems such as a radiology department.

Patient scheduling system

Earlier we mentioned scheduling algorithms as one of the uses of MIS. We would like to elaborate on this here and show how it can be used. A main computer stores information on what is happening to patients in the department. There are several terminals spread over the department at such key points as the control desk, reception desk, and advanced scheduling desk. Each terminal will feed information on new arriving patients to the main computer. The computer itself will make decisions (based on given algorithms) concerning room assignments, advance appointments, examination times, etc. Our version of this system (TEMPLX) has been implemented at Temple University Hospital.[10]

Reporting systems

Several film reporting systems now exist at varying stages of development. These have been reviewed by Mani and Jones.[13] One system, the RAPORT system marketed by the General Electric Company, is now commercially available. In addition to rapid, semiautomated, multicopy report typing based on a mark sense card input, the RAPORT system now has a storage capacity of 2500 cases with report on disk that is accessible from a remote terminal, a statistical data package, a label printer to print labels for marking card, film jacket, and file card, and a file room control package for keeping track of film location. The system is being expanded to allow for the generation of a punch card for patient billing. The punch cards would have to be processed in batch mode on a large computer outside the radiology department.

Patient identification systems

Traditionally each department in the hospital has maintained its own patient identification system, often with its own numbering system. We feel the maintenance of multiple identification systems in a hospital is wasteful in terms of manpower, space, and time and therefore ultimately wasteful in terms of dollars. Hospitals should provide a unique number for each patient who comes to the hospital, including private outpatients. This number should be permanent and easily retrievable, either by a phone call to a central operator or directly from the hospital computer via a remote terminal. This hospital system should be operative at all times.

Film storage and retrieval systems

A typical radiology department maintains an active film file of the most recent cases plus any older studies done on those patients for several days. In addition, there should be an inactive file in a reasonable proximity to the current file. We do not recommend computer control of the inactive file.

Automated retrieval systems for film jackets require additional space in addition to capital investment and operating costs for maintenance. We feel that a current and remote file area can be operated by clerks at less cost than the cost of retrieval equipment and maintenance plus the additional floor rent for the required extra space.

There are now several film miniaturization systems commercially available; these convert full-size x-ray films to microfilm. The main advantages of such a system are that it requires less space (lower floor rent) and the microfilm can be retrieved via computer control very rapidly. For microfilming systems to be of value they must be cost effective, and the microfilm and viewing equipment must be of diagnostic quality. To fulfill the first condition requires that the cost of microfilming, microfilm storage, and microfilm projection equipment be less than the floor rent paid for space in the inactive file room.

The quality of the entire microfilm process is currently being studied by several institutions, and there is reason to believe the microfilm copies will be of diagnostic quality. A major problem that is still unsolved is the necessity of being able to view multiple films from the same study almost simultaneously, as is done with the view box mode of presentation.

References

1. Ackoff, R. L.: Management misinformation systems, Mgmt. Sci. **14:**4, 1967.
2. American College of Radiology: A reference for radiology relative values, Chicago, 1973, American College of Radiology.
3. Amstutz, A. E.: Information systems in management science, Mgmt. Sci. **15:**2, 1968.
4. Brayfield, A. H., and Crockett, W. H.: Employee attitude and employee performance, Psychol. Bull. **52:**396, 1955.
5. Donaldson, S. W.: The practice of radiology in the United States: facts and figures, Am. J. Roetgenol. Radium Ther. **66:**945, 1951.
6. Herzberg, F.: Work and the nature of man, Cleveland, 1966, World Publishing Co.
7. Herzberg, F.: One more time—how do you motivate employees? Harvard Bus. Rev. **46:**53, 1968.
8. Knowles, J. H.: Radiology—a case study in technology and manpower, N. Engl. J. Med. **280:**1271, 1969.
9. Lapayowker, M. S., Kundel, H. L., and Shea, F. J.: Planning of a vertically oriented radiology department in a program floor hospital. In Proceedings of the international symposium on the planning of radiological departments, Dipohi, Otaniemi, Finland, August, 1972.
10. Lev, B., and Caltagirone, R. J.: Evaluation of various scheduling disciplines by computer simulation, Paper presented at the Winter simulation conference, Washington, D. C., 1974.
11. Lev, B., Caltagirone, R. J., and Shea, F. J.: Patient flow and utilization of resources in a diagnostic radiology department: analysis by simulation techniques, Invest. Radiol. **7:**517, 1972.
12. Madrick, R., and Ross, J.: Information systems for modern management, Englewood Cliffs, N. J., 1971, Prentice-Hall, Inc.
13. Mani, R. L., and Jones, M. D.: MSF: a computer-assisted radiologic reporting system, Radiology **108:**587, 1973.
14. Maslow, A.: Motivation and personality, New York, 1954, Harper & Row, Publisher.
15. National Academy of Sciences: The effects on population of exposure to low levels of ionizing radiation, Washington, D. C., 1972, National Academy of Sciences.
16. Naylor, A. F.: Radiology department planning seminar reference material, New Orleans, 1973, American College of Radiology.
17. Patchen, M.: Supervisory methods and group performance norms, Admin. Sci. Q. **7:**275, 1962.
18. Reisman, A.: Managerial and engineering economics: a unified approach, Boston, 1971, Allyn & Bacon Publishing Co., Inc.
19. Revesz, G., and Shea, F. J.: Reducing patient delays in a diagnostic radiology department, Invest. Radiol. **8:**396, 1973.
20. Revesz, G., Shea, F. J., and Ziskin, M. C.: Patient flow and utilization of resources in a diagnostic radiology department, Radiology **104:**21, 1972.
21. Shore, B.: Operations management, New York, 1973, McGraw-Hill Book Co.
22. Shuman, L., and Wolfe, H.: A computerized cost allocation system for hospital use, Pittsburgh, 1972, University of Pittsburgh Press.
23. Stern, H.: Information systems in management science, Mgmt. Sci. **17:**2, 1970.
24. Taylor, F. W.: Principles of scientific management, New York, 1919, Harper & Row, Publishers.
25. Terry, W. G., and McLaren, J. W.: Planning a diagnostic radiology department, Philadelphia, 1973, W. B. Saunders Co.

2 Study on the use of diagnostic radiology

E. James Potchen

Most physicians agree that diagnostic radiology has made significant contributions to the advancement of medicine over the past quarter century. This presumption is based upon the experience of individual physicians in the care of their patients and is supported by the marked increase in the number of radiologists training in response to the demand for more comprehensive diagnostic radiologic services. Conclusive data on the growing number of radiologic services is difficult to compile. However, the growth in supporting industries (x-ray film, equipment, etc.) and two surveys done by the Bureau of Radiologic Health confirm that approximately 6% of the total health expenditures in this country is devoted to diagnostic radiology.

The use of a diagnostic procedure is considered by many to be an adequate indication that it is useful. However, this argument is no longer sufficient when society is seeking alternative ways of redistributing health care resources in order to improve their yield without further increasing expenditures. To quote Louis Lasagna in a review of Morton Mintz's *The Therapeutic Nightmare:* "If survival (of a procedure) alone is to be considered a measure of goodness, then we must all pay homage to the oyster which has survived unchanged for over 300 million years."*

Society's concern over rising health care costs can best be appreciated by looking at some of the available data. The portion of the gross national product (GNP) allocated for health expenditures increased from 4.6% to 7% between 1950 and 1970. No other segment of the economy consumed a greater percentage increase in the allocation of the consumer dollar. How much has society benefited from this redistribution of expenditures?

It is difficult if not impossible to evaluate the influence of this increased allocation for health care. The measurable parameters of resource redistribution toward health expenditures suggest that it has little if any impact on society. The annual death rate remained essentially unchanged between 1950 and 1970 (9.6 versus 9.4/1000 people). Some physicians attribute the increased

---

*From The New York Times Book Review, Nov. 28, 1965.

cost of health care to federal programs such as Medicare. However, when the data is analyzed, of the 2.4% increased allocation of the GNP to health expenditures, only 0.6% can reasonably be said to be due to the enactment of Medicare.

Medicine has made remarkable contributions toward erasing some diseases and effects of injuries that were considered hopeless only 20 years ago. The transition of medicine from the office of the primary care physician to the modern medical center with its advanced technology has resulted in a redistribution of resources allocated to fund medicine, which is currently out of proportion to the actual increase in today's life span. The mission of medicine is changing from "saving lives" to improving the quality of life. Increasing health expenditures may relate to an improvement of the quality of life and the effects are therefore not evident in statistics on the death rate. Since the quality of life has not been measured and improvement is not self-evident, it remains appropriate to examine other grounds for resource redistribution. If inappropriate bases can be identified, it seems reasonable to study them in depth to clarify the issues and to suggest alternatives to current trends.

According to the Bureau of Radiologic Health's data, the cost of diagnostic radiology has increased by about $1 billion between 1964 and 1970; that is, 100 million examinations as opposed to 142 million examinations were performed. The increasing use of diagnostic radiology represents an important component of rising health expenditures. Since the benefits of this increased use are not detectable in any health statistics, it seems appropriate for radiologists to devote some effort to studying the process of medical diagnosis to best clarify the role of diagnostic procedures in patient management.

It is far easier to estimate the cost of diagnostic radiology than to document its benefits. Although most physicians intuitively feel the benefit of diagnostic radiology, in the eyes of many this intuition alone is insufficient grounds for increasing expenditures without a firmer scientific foundation. With this background in mind, the use of diagnostic radiology should be studied. We seek to develop a quantitative appreciation of the merits of alternative diagnostic approaches. These studies are designed not only to measure the benefit of diagnostic radiology but hopefully to point to a more rational and efficient use of resources in caring for patients. Faced with a finite limitation on total health expenditures, we must now seek the most appropriate distribution of these expenditures to maximize the contribution of medical care. It is time for research in diagnostic radiology to go beyond the development of new diagnostic techniques; it is time for research to develop tools in order to better study the use of radiology and what it means to patients.

Systems modeling is a technique by which we formalize and communicate our thinking on the components of a complex process. The process of medical diagnosis is especially suited to analysis by modeling techniques. Therefore we seek to develop a model of the diagnostic process that will allow the physician to make a quantitative assessment of the potential yield of a diagnostic x-ray film when he is faced with a choice among alternatives.

ENTROPY MINIMAX ANALYSIS AND DIAGNOSTIC EFFICACY

When a physician sees a patient, he is assaulted with a mass of information from which he must pick and choose salient features that will enable him to devise a diagnostic strategy. The information concerning a patient can be broken down into a number of attributes (signs, symptoms, history, results of prior diagnostic tests, etc.), each of which has its own unit of measure. One cannot simplify the information as to whether the patient has a headache or a sore throat into a single common denominator, to say nothing of the information concerning the results of urinalysis or a family's history of myocardial infarction. The presence, absence, or magnitude (severity) of each attribute is assessed independently, and a pattern is sought in the constellation of attributes. From this pattern the physician estimates the probability that a specific therapeutic maneuver will benefit the patient. The patterns are classified in medical training and are referred to as diseases or syndromes (Fig. 2-1).

The information that a patient presents to his physician can be looked upon as a number of attributes. The attributes compose a pattern from which the physician uses his training and experience to devise a diagnostic strategy. This strategy will hopefully provide additional information, thereby sharpening the pattern to a point at which a therapeutic manuever could beneficially affect the course of a patient's disease.

This model of the diagnostic process is suited to quantitative analysis in terms of information theory. Attribute-outcome analysis can be used to measure the effect of each attribute on some specified outcome state. Each component of diagnostic information (attribute) can be normalized to a common denominator in terms of information. Information theorists define information as a change in randomness. For example, a series of totally random words contains no information. As in thermodynamics, a totally random situation has maximal entropy. Maximum information minimizes entropy. Thus if one could measure the contribution of each attribute to the entropy of a pattern, one could measure the

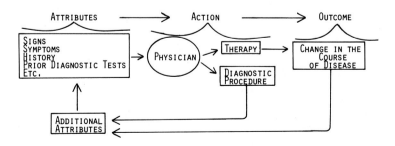

Fig. 2-1. Description of diagnostic process.

amount of information contained in each attribute in relation to all other attributes that may or may not contribute to the pattern. The amount of information contained in each attribute in relation to a specified outcome then becomes the common denominator whereby the relative importance of the diagnostic procedure in relation to other sources of information can be compared. For example, despite the fact that each attribute is evaluated in entirely different units by measuring the amount of information in relation to some outcome, the relative contribution can assess the knowledge of the severity of headaches, the results of a skull x-ray film, the results of a brain scan, or the results of a family history to the probability that a patient has a treatable brain tumor.

It is important to appreciate that this information theory approach to the diagnostic process is not the same as a simple two-dimensional correlation of a diagnostic observation with some outcome. Simply correlating the incidence of abnormal brain scans with treatable brain tumors does not yield identical data, nor is it an appropriate model for what happens in the diagnostic process. Although in some instances a single diagnostic observation becomes dominant in determining the physician's actions in regard to a patient, more often the physician is faced with a number of observations (attributes) to which he gives varying weight in devising a therapeutic strategy.

The important point to bear in mind is that observations (attributes) interact with each other in the physician's thought processes regarding a patient; thus no simple two-dimensional correlation properly describes the information used by the physician in formulating a clinical judgment. Rather, the simultaneous correlation of a number of attributes with a specified outcome requires the physician to go beyond the two-dimensional matrix and traditional correlation coefficients to a matrix that allows as many dimensions as he has observations (attributes)—an n-dimensional matrix, where n is the number of attributes that contain information relevant to the outcome state.

Techniques recently developed in multivariate analysis allow for the discovery of patterns in data consisting of various attributes, where the contribution of each attribute to the pattern and to the probability of some outcome can be evaluated in terms of a change in the entropy of the system, that is, in terms of the information contained within each attribute in relation to all other attributes within the system and in relation to a specified outcome. Entropy minimax is such a technique.

The principles of entropy minimax, in correlation with various approaches in the study of medical decision making, are described by Schonbein in Chapter 3. However, there are precise analytic tools that allow the physician to analyze the relative amount of information contained in each diagnostic observation (attribute) that will bear on a specific outcome state of the patient. Through the use of these tools it will be possible to analyze prospectively the relative amount of information that a diagnostic x-ray examination can be expected to yield in a given symptom complex (that is, attributes the patient presents to a physician). Although pilot projects have demonstrated the feasibility of this approach to measuring the relative contribution of various pieces of diagnostic information to a specific outcome, further work is necessary before we have sufficient quantitative data on the merits of diagnostic x-ray examinations.

Bell and Loop use a questionnaire to assess the attributes that physicians use in ordering a skull film in children with head injuries. The physician was asked to check off the various signs, symptoms, historical data, etc. that would contribute to his decision to order a skull x-ray film. Faced with these attributes, he was then asked to predict the probability of whether or not the patient actually had a skull fracture, which would then be demonstrated on the skull x-ray film.

Schonbein used Bell and Loop's original data to determine the relative amount of information contained in each attribute in correlation to two specific

---

Attributes affecting physician's subjective probability including physician's estimate of severity of injury
Attributes having significant effect (approximate order of importance)

 1. Evaluation of injury
 2. Drowziness
 3. Conscious/unconscious
 4. Consciousness scale
 5. Breathing
 6. Sensory abnormality
 7. Ear discharge
 8. Eardrum discoloration
 9. Nose discharge
 10. Headache
 11. Palpable bony malalignment
 12. Swelling
 13. Hematoma
 14. Retrograde amnesia

Attributes not appearing in cell definitions

 1. Vomiting
 2. Seizure
 3. Other reflex abnormalities
 4. Anisocoria

outcome states of the patient. The initial outcome would determine the physician's a priori prediction as to whether or not a fracture would be demonstrated. The second outcome would determine the possibility of a fracture being seen on the x-ray film.

Lists are compiled in accordance with the relative amount of information each attribute contains in predicting the outcome state of the patient when all the attributes are seen together. By comparing the hierarchical list of attributes that the physician uses in making his clinical judgment with the second list of attributes that correlates with the presence of a fracture on the skull x-ray film, as shown below, the physician is then able to discover the discrepancies between clinical judgment and diagnostic reality.

These lists detail for the physician the relative importance of each piece of information he has available in determining the specific outcome state of the presence or absence of a fracture on the skull x-ray film. Therefore it is possible to add or subtract an attribute in order to see the effect of this change on the

---

Correlation of attributes with x-ray outcomes including physician's estimate of severity of injury
Attributes appearing in cell definitions (approximate order of importance)

1. Evaluation of injury
2. Consciousness scale
3. Conscious/unconscious
4. Sensory abnormality
5. Ear discharge
6. Other reflex abnormality
7. Palpable bony malalignment
8. Headache
9. Nose discharge
10. Vomiting
11. Anisocoria
12. Hematoma
13. Drowziness
14. Retrograde amnesia
15. Swelling

Attributes not associated with cell definitions

1. Seizure
2. Eardrum discoloration
3. Breathing

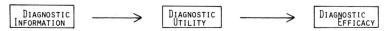

Fig. 2-2. Description of diagnostic efficacy.

amount of information each attribute contains in correlation with each other. These studies can be developed in order to determine the importance of specific diagnostic tests as compared to other clinical information with regard to their impact on specific outcome states. For example, the outcome state would appropriately be commensurate with "what the physician did for the patient." By employing these techniques, it is possible to develop data on the relative merits of alternative diagnostic tests, for example, skull x-ray films, brain scans, arteriography, or any other appropriate diagnostic test that will have an effect on what the physician can do for his patient (Fig. 2-2).

Admittedly, this does not address the issues of efficacy. Merely knowing what the physician does for his patient will not explain the effect of what he did during the course of his patient's disease. But here again, one could use an additional outcome state, that is, what happened to the patient as a relative measure of meaningful information contained in each diagnostic attribute. I would suggest that by this systematic attack on the issue of efficacy, we may eventually be able to obtain a more quantitative appreciation of the benefits to be obtained by the use of diagnostic x-ray examinations. Once these benefits are more effectively quantified, one could more easily identify the motivational factors other than efficacy.

It appears that this could be a long and arduous research task, but the amount of information or case material required for this type of data analysis is considerably less than the information needed for the more standard Baysian or even Bollerian approach previously advocated by other investigators (Lusted, Jaquey, etc.). By using entropy minimax in skull x-ray study, it has been possible to obtain a statistically valid sample using 200 patients, as it was by using 2000 standard cases in data analysis methods. Therefore the task of obtaining additional quantitative information on diagnostic efficacy and the use of radiology is considerably less when the statistical force of entropy minimax analysis is employed.

DEFENSIVE MEDICINE AND USE OF DIAGNOSTIC RADIOLOGY

The most promising avenue of investigation relates to a better understanding of diagnostic efficacy in an effort to improve those clinical situations in which motivational factors other than efficacy predominate in the use of diagnostic x-ray examinations. Of the other motivational factors, it seems reasonable to first address the issue of defensive medicine. Many radiologists are aware that clinicians often order an x-ray study because if they feel that they did not they would be liable to accusations of malpractice or invoke the

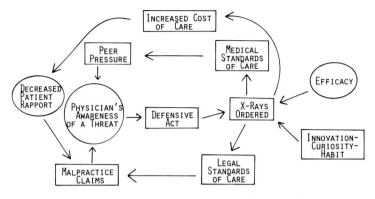

Fig. 2-3. System dynamic model of defensive medicine.

criticism of their peers, despite the fact that they did not personally feel that the x-ray would furnish relevant information. This practice is particularly evident in the emergency room and is best documented in the study of pediatric head injuries by Bell and Loop. Other studies have shown that this is perhaps a very significant motivational factor for many physicians.

The definition of defensive medicine in diagnostic radiology is that the use of a diagnostic test by the physician is not intended to help him in making a diagnosis and determining a course of therapy; rather, it is an effort to protect himself from his perceived legal responsibilities or potential incrimination by his peers. In the Duke University Law School study, the law students ascertained that approximately 7% of diagnostic studies are ordered by physicians with the dominant motivation of defense. Other studies have shown a considerably higher incidence of defensive use of diagnostic x-ray studies.

The American College of Surgeons' survey reveals that 72% of the surgeons interviewed admit that they use some x-ray procedures with the primary motivation of defense. By taking into account the previous studies, it can be inferred that a significant percentage of the total use of diagnostic x-ray examinations is based on the motivation of defensive practice. Using diagnostic radiology as a model for further analysis of the system of defensive medicine would be most appropriate.

Systems analysis is a modeling tool that permits discrete appreciation of the factors that influence each other in a complex system. While it does not necessarily provide new data, it does necessitate a highly disciplined, intellectual effort in an attempt to ascertain, on a more quantitative basis, those factors that lead to such complex processes as the defensive use of diagnostic radiology.

Fig. 2-3 is a summary model of our efforts to effect a dynamic systems analysis of defensive medicine, it is based upon data obtained from interviews of a number of physicians, lawyers, and insurance companies in addition to extensive materials available through the President's Commission on Medical

Malpractice. The commission's data was obtained through surveys, consumers, patients, lawyers, insurance companies, and physicians as well as from extensive hearings, specific research, hospital records, etc. Interesting material relevant to the issue of defensive medicine has evolved from the work of the commission.

The physician's awareness of a threat is antecedent to his defensive use of a diagnostic procedure. The use of a procedure in this way is not clearly separated from other motivational bases when standards are set for either the legal responsibilities to provide medical services equivalent to the standards of normal practice or for the perceived peer responsibility to practice medicine as others do in a similar situation. Both legal and medical issues define the standards of care against which the physician feels he is measured when requesting a diagnostic procedure. Both legal and medical standards are ideally based upon clinical efficacy. However, no effort has been made to clearly separate diagnostic efficacy from other factors that initiated the development of the diagnostic procedure as a standard approach to a clinical situation and to established standards of care. Many diagnostic procedures originate when a physician is curious about the possible outcome of a procedure; if he has a favorable experience, the use of the procedure may become a habit, and a standard of care is thus established. It is not necessarily a prerequisite that this standard benefits the patient.

In assessing the system further, while many patients perceive a medical experience as negative, very few proceed to a state of litigation. In almost every medical malpractice case, particularly in those that are classed in the nuisance category, there is a breakdown in rapport between patient and physician.

Using this as a model, diagnostic radiology, in which the primary objective of care is to change the course of the patient's disease, would be used less in defense by those physicians who have established a close rapport with their patients than by those physicians (for example, physicians in large urban emergency rooms) who have less opportunity to establish mutual understanding with their patients. It is this rapport between the patient and his physician that is primarily responsible for the very low incidence of medical malpractice suits in relationship to the number of negative medical experiences perceived by patients.

Approximately 45% of the patients interviewed in a consumer survey felt that either they or a member of their family had a negative medical experience at some time in their lives. However, considerably less than 1% of these experiences results in a malpractice suit, since in most instances the patient wishes to protect his physician. This finding may be somewhat surprising to the many physicians who practice medicine in constant fear of malpractice litigation. Realistically, however, this information verifies that their most effective defense is not necessarily to order additional diagnostic tests but rather to increase their efforts to establish a more effective communication with their patients.

The magnitude of the problem of the defensive use of diagnostic radiology can perhaps best be appreciated by looking at the most conclusive data available in order to see the relationship of the magnitude of radiology used in defense as compared to the number of malpractice suits that actually occur. In 1972 insurance companies reported approximately $50 million in claims filed in malpractice suits. Of this total, approximately 90% of the claims were related to overt negative experiences such as removal of the wrong kidney or leaving a sponge in at surgery. Approximately 10% could appropriately be included in the "nuisance" category. It is from claims in this nuisance category that the physician primarily attempts to protect himself by ordering additional diagnostic procedures not necessarily felt to be of benefit to the patient. Thus the dollar value of the type of claim from which the physician seeks protection by the use of defensive medicine is somewhere between $5 and $10 million a year in the United States. The total cost of the use of radiology in the United States in 1970 was approximately $4 billion; the motivation for examinations representing a figure of up to 25% of this total is a basis other than true efficacy. Therefore approximately $1 billion may be spent for protection against an actual threat of perhaps only $5 to $10 million.

I am not in a position to make a value judgment on this apparently wide discrepancy between the magnitude of the defensive use of radiology and the actual threat itself. Indeed, I do not even know whether a change in the usage would increase or decrease the threat. I can only point out that there is a significant discrepancy between the magnitude of monies used by the physician to defend himself against perceived liability as compared to the extent of the true liability itself.

The use of dynamic systems analysis to resolve some of the problems in the defensive use of diagnostic radiology might provide a clue as to the magnitude of the problem and the effect that continued defensive medicine has on the increasing use of defensive medicine, since these are positive feedback loops. It is therefore self-evident that the defensive use of medicine will continue to increase unless some mechanism can be found to break the continuing feedback system.

Further studies are being undertaken by other investigators in an effort to discover how changes in this complex system might be effected. This resumé is only a brief introduction to the total issue, which is dealt with more extensively by Twine and Potchen. I suggest that those interested in further studies of this subject avail themselves of that body of literature.

INNOVATION-CURIOSITY-HABIT AND USE OF DIAGNOSTIC RADIOLOGY

Finally, I would like to discuss the third factor that influences a physician's use of diagnostic x-ray examinations, namely, innovation-curiosity-habit. Essentially, this means that the physician requests the procedure because he is curious as to what the results will be, either because he has recently heard that it is a new and exciting approach that may or may not help his patient or that he has gotten into the habit of requesting a procedure despite the fact that the examination has no apparent relevance to the specific clinical situation he is facing. The relative significance of this motivational basis is difficult to estimate quantitatively since in many instances the clinical situation is at times so confusing that the physician ordering the procedure is not entirely aware of his own motivation.

The use of innovation-curiosity-habit is somewhat more common in academic institutions in which there is a greater degree of experiencial learning taking place than in institutions staffed by more experienced physicians. Indeed, one of the major problems in the use of diagnostic radiology in academic institutions has been the fact that many physicians feel that only through their own personal experience can they gain sufficient data as to the utility and efficacy of a diagnostic procedure in a specific symptom complex. Perhaps this is true. However, it could equally well be argued that, were quantitative data on the relative merits of alternative diagnostic procedures available, the need for personal experience on an ad hoc basis could be considerably diminished.

In order to study the problem of innovation-curiosity-habit we have chosen to use a rather standard approach called market analysis of product life cycles. A diagnostic procedure can be viewed as a product furnished by the radiologic community to aid in patient management. When a new procedure is "invented," colleagues of the inventor make increasing use of it first; subsequently others throughout the medical community employ it as they become aware of its potential benefit in the specific clinical situation they are facing. The use of the procedure therefore increases until a point in time, at which it is not felt to contribute meaningfully to patient care; the level of use then reaches an equilibrium.

This equilibrium value of use for a particular test may persist for long periods of time, particularly if there is no other diagnostic test appropriate to replace it or if physicians become increasingly aware that what they thought was going to be useful for patients has not as yet proved to be so; therefore there is an ultimate decrease in its usage. Interestingly, as one observes a decline in the use of a diagnostic procedure that was formerly popular, the level of use never quite seems to reach zero. Studies indicate that the number of physicians using a diagnostic procedure at the late phase of its product life cycle appears to be identical to the number who first were responsible for its adoption.

While I appreciate that the attempt to determine the value of a diagnostic procedure by observing its use over a period of time may be somewhat iconoclastic, I would suggest that this is a useful approach in an attempt to identify those procedures that are employed largely on the basis of innovation-curiosity-habit as opposed to those that are efficacious. In any event, with the frequent

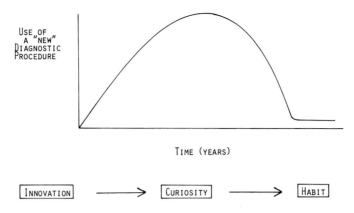

Fig. 2-4. Description of innovation-curiosity-habit.

development of new diagnostic techniques as in clinical nuclear medicine, it is theoretically possible to maintain a high use rate for an entire discipline without ever meeting the criterion that the discipline contribute significantly to patient care. It is reasonable to look at the use rate of diagnostic procedures in an attempt to assess changes over a period of time in an effort to better understand some of the motivational bases behind their ultimate application. Many new diagnostic procedures in series are constantly being developed and renewed. In view of this, one diagnostic procedure less in vogue than another could therefore easily be replaced by another procedure readily available to take its place, thus maintaining a constant high use rate (Fig. 2-4). The only area I know of in which this phenomenon has been specifically studied is the use of the renogram.

In the mid-1950s the use of the renogram became extremely popular as a technique in evaluating patients with essential hypertension. However, by the late 1960s the use of the renogram decreased markedly in comparison with its peak use in the early 1960s, not so much because it was replaced by other diagnostic tests that were more effective in providing additional units of information on the patient but rather because many physicians felt that the renogram did not contribute as much as they had hoped toward the management of a large population of patients. Thus the use of renograms provides a model for examining a product life cycle, and if we were to accumulate more accurate data on the relative use of various diagnostic procedures at this time, we might be able to develop a prospective analysis of the use rate in time to appreciate factors that affect the use of diagnostic x-ray examinations.

SUMMARY

A model of the factors that affect the use of diagnostic x-ray examinations is based on three significant yet not exclusive components. These are diagnostic efficacy, the defensive use of radiology, and innovation-curiosity-habit.

1. Diagnostic efficacy is the use of a diagnostic procedure that provides in-

formation to the physician and changes his behavior in the management of the patient such that it alters the course of the patient's disease.

2. The defensive use of radiology is the use of a diagnostic procedure not necessarily to benefit the patient but rather to protect the physician himself from his perception of either legal liability or peer incrimination.

3. Innovation-curiosity-habit is the use of a diagnostic procedure because the physician wants to see what the developments will be; the procedure may or may not benefit the patient.

In any clinical situation it is unlikely that any single motivational factor functions to the exclusion of others. However, in all probability the specific dominance of one motivational basis over another exists in most clinical situations. Based on preliminary data, it now seems appropriate to devise studies that will yield more quantitative information on the relative merits of alternative diagnostic procedures using the entropy minimax approach. Such studies could provide quantitative data on the relative amount of information produced by a diagnostic procedure in comparison to the amalgamation of attributes that a patient presents to his physician for evaluation. Once these studies are underway, I would be confident that we could sharpen our estimates of the merits of alternative diagnostic approaches and develop a more rational basis for the selection of diagnostic procedures that are designed to benefit the patient.

Selected readings

1. Bell, R. S., and Loop, J. W.: The utility and futility of radiographic skull examination for trauma, N. Engl. J. Med. **284:**236, 1971.
2. Christensen, R.: A general approach to pattern discovery, Technical Report No. 20, Berkeley, 1968, Department of Physics, University of California, Berkeley.
3. Christensen, R.: Entropy minimax method of pattern discovery and probability determination, Paper presented at Carnegie-Mellon University and The Massachusetts Institute of Technology, 1971.
4. Edwards, W., Lindman, H., and Phillips, L. D.: Personal communication, 1973.
5. Fano, R. M.: Transmission of information, Cambridge, Mass., 1961, The M.I.T. Press.
6. Feinstein, A. R., Clinical judgement, Baltimore, 1967, The Williams & Wilkins Co.
7. Good, I. J., and Card, W. I.: The diagnostic process with special reference to errors, Methods Inf. Med. **10:**176, 1971.
8. Lusted, L. B.: Introduction to medical decision-making, Springfield, Ill., 1968, Charles C Thomas, Publisher.
9. Lusted, L. B.: Decision-making studies in patient management, N. Engl. J. Med. **284:**416, 1971.
10. Potchen, E. J.: A strategy for the study of efficacy, Paper presented at the American College of Radiology meeting, San Francisco, April, 1973.
11. St. John, E. G.: The role of the emergency skull roentgenogram in head trauma, Am. J. Roetgenol. **76:**315, 1956.
12. Twine, E. H., and Potchen, E. J.: A dynamic systems analysis of defensive medicine, M. S. dissertation, The Massachusetts Institute of Technology, Boston, 1973.

3 Analysis of decisions and information in patient management

William R. Schonbein

Current activities in the field of decision theory are concerned with two topics. The first is the formulation of optimum decision strategies that are intended to tell the decision maker how he should make his decision; the second is the formulation of methodologies for determining how decision makers actually do make their decisions. In the case of the formulation of decision strategies, the objective is generally the maximization of some specific function that can be related to benefit returned to the decision maker when he makes correct or optimum decisions. In the case of the formulation of methodologies for the determination of how decisions are made, the objective is to determine which of the components of the data base that were available to the decision maker actually influenced his decision and, if possible, to determine the relative importance of the various data components that influenced his decision. This latter topic we shall call decision analysis in order to distinguish it from the classic topic of decision strategies.

Our interest in decision analysis is motivated by the fact that the critical component in the proposed definitions of efficacy is the relationship between diagnostic attributes and a physician's decisions or actions. Thus the development of methodologies appropriate to the study of the relation between diagnostic attributes and decision outcome is of the utmost importance in the analysis of efficacy. Specifically, we can conclude from the material presented in Chapter 2 that the determination of efficacy involves the solution of the following problem: Given a set of observed decision outcomes and a corresponding set of attributes that presumably affected the decisions, determine which attributes affected the decision outcomes and, if possible, determine the magnitude of each attribute's effect. We need to define, in a manner that can readily be quantified, the various terms used in the above problem statement, since the ultimate objective is a set of hard statistical data.

To accomplish this first step in the solution of the decision analysis problem, consider the simple model of the information transmission, processing, and decision sequence shown in Fig. 3-1. On the left-hand side of the diagram is shown a message source followed by a transmission channel to

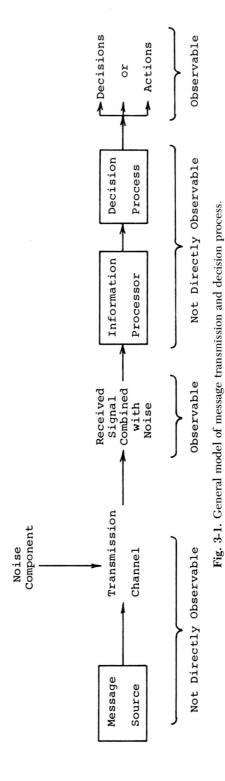

Fig. 3-1. General model of message transmission and decision process.

which a noise component has been appended. In the diagnostic problem the message source represents the patient's actual complex of symptoms, signs, historical data, etc. In other words, it represents the diagnosis of the patient's problems at a given point in time.

The transmission channel that follows the message source represents the mechanism by which information concerning the nature of the patient's ailment reaches the physician. An integral part of the transmission channel is a noise component, which we have shown interacting with the channel in an unspecified way. The noise component is meant to indicate in a general manner the fact that the transmission channel is not perfect. The noise component or the imperfection in the channel can take a number of forms. For example, the noise component could be an actual physical noise such as the poor quality of an x-ray film; alternatively, the noise component could represent the fact that in general the transmission channel represents a transformation of information that is not reversible. Irreversibility in the transmission channel would correspond to the objective answer that the patient might give to questions regarding localization or severity of pain.

Beneath the message source and the transmission channel is the indication that they are not directly physically observable. If in fact the source were directly observable, we would have essentially an ideal or perfect diagnostic procedure. However, since we do not have such perfect diagnostic procedures, we must deal only with those attributes that are directly observable for the purpose of decision analysis.

This brings us to the next item in Fig. 3-1, which we call the received signal. In communications terminology we would call this a vector signal, since it consists of components that contain the results of diagnostic tests, the data from the patient's history, and the various signs and symptoms. This signal is clearly time varying; moreover, it may have a very definite preferred time sequence structure. However, the principal property of importance for the purposes of decision analysis is that the signal is observable and in general reproducible. This vector signal then defines the attributes that we will assume form the basis for the physician's decisions and actions.

The next two items in Fig. 3-1 represent the processes that take place within the physician's mind. The first of these is the information processing of the attribute list that the physician has obtained. Information processing is extremely complex and clearly beyond the scope of the problem that concerns us. However, the one assumption we will make concerning information processing is that it produces some quantity upon which a decision can be based. We represent this by the inclusion in our model of an item labeled *decision process*. The assumption is that the information-processing activity yields a result that is delivered to the decision process and that the physician then proceeds to make his decision or order his actions based upon his decision process.

Again, we indicate by a bracket that the information processing and the decision process are not directly observable functions. Although some work has been done in the analysis of the manner in which individuals process information, this work has not progressed sufficiently for it to be useful in the solution of the decision analysis problem. On the other hand, a good deal of work has been done in investigating the manner in which individuals make decisions, and in fact, one of the principal methods of decision analysis is the direct outgrowth of a general model of the decision-making process.

Finally, the decisions or actions that the physician has taken are shown at the far right-hand side of the diagram. These decisions or actions are the observable outcomes of the diagnostic process and may include the choice of a specific therapy, the decision to request further diagnostic tests, or possibly the decision to take no further action.

Implicit in the model shown in Fig. 3-1 is the fact that the diagnostic process is dynamic. Thus both the attribute list that comprises the signal vector available to the physician at any time and the decisions or actions that follow from the study of those attributes are in themselves functions of time. To study the effect of various diagnostic attributes, the experimental plan must be carefully structured to ensure that the data obtained represents consistent points in time. Fortunately, for most cases of interest there are convenient points within the diagnostic process at which reliable data may be obtained. These points are generally the natural breaking points or the natural decision points in the flow of the diagnostic process.

In summary, the model in Fig. 3-1 implies that the only real observables are the diagnostic attributes and the actual decisions or actions of the physician. The basic assumptions are that we are not allowed to completely observe either the message source or the means by which that message is transformed into the list of attributes, nor are we allowed to observe either the information processing or the decision mechanism that the physician uses. Rather, we must infer the relationship of the attributes that exist at a given time in this diagnostic process to the decisions that presumably resulted from consideration of the attributes. Thus we are principally interested in investigating methods for inferring possible relationships in a quantitative fashion. The key to the decision analysis problem is a methodology that is capable of inferring causal relationships rather than attempting to model such relationships.

With these ideas as a background, we will next investigate a number of possible methodologies for performing decision analysis. Since a principal feature of this analysis is the requirement for quantitative results, these methodologies must necessarily involve a certain amount of mathematics. However, every effort has been made to minimize both the quantity and the complexity of the mathematical arguments. In addition, the discussion of the methodologies given below are arranged so that the essential nonmathematical aspects of the methods are given first, followed by the elementary mathematical developments. Thus the reader interested in gaining a basic knowledge of the various methods need not work his way through the mathematical details.

DECISION ANALYSIS METHODOLOGIES

In this section we will present three possible methods for the analysis of decisions. These methods differ primarily in two respects. First, they differ in the degree to which they deal with aggregate data obtained from many decision makers as opposed to studies of individual decision makers. Second, the methods differ in the degree to which they imply an a priori structure for the decision-making process. Fig. 3-2 summarizes the methods and the manner in which they differ.

In the upper left-hand corner of the matrix shown in Fig. 3-2, I indicate that the primary method for dealing with individual data using structured methods is by means of behavioral models derived from classic decision strategies. The method of derivation is very straightforward and involves manipulation of a classic decision strategy model. This is accomplished by using Bayes' theorem for inferring probabilities. An example of the formulation of this method is the first case considered below.

When dealing with aggregate data and using a structured approach, one basically has two choices. The first is the use of minimum variance techniques and the second is a statistical extention of the behavioral models just mentioned. The minimum variance approach will be discussed as the second case considered below. The extensions of the behavioral model are very straightforward statistical extensions of results obtained from individual case studies. The idea is simply to aggregate the results of individual studies and examine the results by the use of classic statistical methods. Since this extension is so simple and straightforward, it will not be given further consideration.

Degree of Structure Implied by the
Methodology

	Structured	Unstructured
Individual Data	Behavioral Models from Classical Decision Theory	?
Aggregate Data	a) Minimum Variance Approaches b) Extensions of Behavioral Models	Entropy Mimimax Pattern Discovery

(left axis: Degree of Data Aggregation)

Fig. 3-2. Methods available for analysis of decisions.

Within the category of unstructured approaches, there is at present no totally unstructured method for the examination of individual decision-making actions. However, given aggregate data there is at least one powerful unstructured approach known as the entropy minimax pattern discovery technique. This technique is unstructured in the sense that there are no a priori behavioral models implied by the methodology itself.

Likelihood ratio decision analysis

The first case for study is the behavioral model analysis of individual decisions. This model follows directly from classic decision theory and it is worth the effort to follow the development of classic theory to illustrate the assumptions inherent in this method of analysis. In classic decision theory the principal objective is to arrive at a mechanism or test by which one can make a decision that is in some sense optimum. Since classic decision theory is an attempt to build a model that will predict the behavior of the decision element, in a problem of this nature we are clearly considering one that rests in the box labeled *decision process* in Fig. 3-1. When we turn classic decision theory around to make it into decision analysis theory, it will be seen that this effort to model the decision element manifests itself in the form of a fundamental assumption that must be taken into account in the application of this method.

Perhaps the best means of obtaining a basic understanding of classic decision analysis is to study a simple hypothetical example involving the interpretation of a chest x-ray film. In this problem it is assumed that an individual physician examines a chest x-ray film and must make a decision as to whether or not he should recommend further diagnostic tests. For the sake of simplicity it is assumed that the principal determinant regarding further tests is dependent upon the patient having a small focal lesion. If the patient does indeed have such a lesion, then ordering the tests will result in a measurable benefit to the patient. If on the other hand the patient does not have a lesion, then refusal to order the tests results in no cost to the patient. However, there are two other alternatives. The first is that the physician assumes that the patient does have a lesion when in fact the patient does not, in which case the recommendation of tests results in a cost and no benefit to the patient. Alternatively, the physician may assume that the patient does not have a lesion, when in fact he does. In this case, not ordering the tests will result in substantial cost to the patient in terms of the progression of his disease. The various outcomes of this hypothetical example are shown in Fig. 3-3.

In classic decision theory the objective is to discover a mechanism by which the physician can make his decision between two hypotheses, namely H_1, the patient has a lesion, or H_0, the patient does not have a lesion, in such a way as to minimize the risk involved in ordering further tests. To accomplish this, classic theory requires that we construct a risk function that will include the costs involved and the related rates or probabilities of the events shown in Fig.

Actual State

	Lesion Present	Lesion Absent
X-ray Interpreted as Lesion Present	True Positive	False Positive
X-ray Interpreted as Lesion Absent	False Negative	True Negative

Interpretation

Fig. 3-3. Matrix of possible outcomes for classic decision theory example.

3-3 that would lead to incurring these costs. For our particular problem we may ignore without loss of generality the costs associated with correct decisions and concentrate only on the costs associated with false positive and false negative outcomes. In the first case, we can designate by C_{10} the cost associated with the false positive outcome of saying that a lesion exists when in fact there is none. Likewise we will call C_{01} the cost associated with the false negative outcome. Furthermore, we could indicate the rate or probability of an outcome, say false positive, as $P[\text{Say } H_1|H_0]P[H_0]$, where $P[H_0]$ is the a priori probability of no lesion and $P[\text{Say } H_1|H_0]$ is the conditional probability that the physician will say there is a lesion, given the condition that none is present. Using this notation, we can construct the following mathematical formulation of the risk:

$$\text{Risk} = C_{10}P[\text{Say } H_1|H_0]P[H_0] + C_{01}P[\text{Say } H_0|H_1]P[H_1] \tag{1}$$

A quantity in the form of equation 1 is generally referred to as an expectation, or an expected value of the cost involved. The objective of decision strategy will be to minimize the risk expressed by equation 1.

It is a general characteristic of classic decision theory that the minimization of a risk or cost function such as equation 1 involves the movement or adjustment of a boundary in a space; this is called decision space. The idea behind this boundary in decision space is simply that in order to make any decision, an individual gathers a certain amount of data or attributes and, in accordance with our earlier model, analyzes these attributes to form a quantity upon which he will base his decision. It is entirely feasible that this quantity be multidimensional, and therefore it is conceivable that this quantity could be represented as a vector in a multidimensional space. If in fact an individual will make his decision based upon this multidimensional vector, then a possible model as to the way in which that decision is made would be to assume that the decision is based upon the position of the vector in decision space. If this were the case, it could be assumed that certain regions of decision space are regions in which an individual would choose one hypothesis, whereas if the vector were to fall in another region of decision space, he would choose the alternate hypothesis.

In order to clarify this concept of decision space, the hypothetical example can be extended by assuming that the only factor that influences the physician's ability to detect the presence of a lesion image on the x-ray film is the difference in contrast between the lesion image and the background. In addition, it will be assumed that the distribution of differences in contrast for films in which lesions are present is known in advance. We designate this distribution by $p(x)$ and normalize the function $p(x)$ such that the probability of finding a difference in contrast of x' between two limits x_1 and x_2 is given by the integral of the function $p(x)$ between these two limits:

$$P[x_1 \text{ less than } x' \text{ less than or equal to } x_2] = \int_{x_1}^{x_2} p(x)dx \qquad (2)$$

A function $p(x)$, which is related to the probability of an event in the manner shown in equation 2, is called a probability density function. Fig. 3-4 is a plot of this hypothetical probability density function.

To complete this simple decision space, it is assumed that films containing no lesion images have distributions of contrast differences resembling the probability density function in Fig. 3-4, but shifted to the right by some amount. Mathematically, this results in the situation shown in Fig. 3-5, in which the conditional probability density function for films with lesion images is designated $p_1(x|H_1)$ and the conditional probability density function corresponding to films without lesion images is designated $p_0(x|H_0)$. Since it is assumed for the sake of this example that the contrast difference is the only attribute of importance in making the decision lesion present or not present, the problem could be reduced to the following form. The physician could, at least in principle, observe the area on the film that would encompass a suspected lesion and record the appropriate difference in contrast. This observed quantity, say x', would be plotted in the physician's decision space, which is just the horizontal axis of Fig. 3-5.

Fig. 3-5 shows a threshold value x_0 that will be used to partition the decision space into two decision regions. In order to make his decision, let it be assumed that the physician observes the region in which his observation x' falls and chooses accordingly. If x', the observed value of the contrast difference, is greater than x_0, the physician will assume that the patient has a lesion and will recommend further tests. If on the other hand the observed value of the contrast difference is less than x_0, he will assume that the patient does not have a lesion. Since the probability density functions for the two outcomes overlap, there is clearly a finite probability that the physician will make the wrong decision and consequently incur a cost. The objective is simply to find a position for the threshold x_0 that will minimize the risk involved in making the decision. This is accomplished mathematically by expressing the conditional probabilities

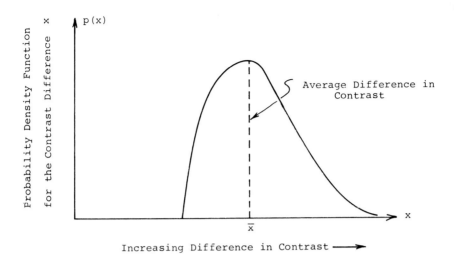

Fig. 3-4. Hypothetical distribution of difference in contrast between lesion images and background.

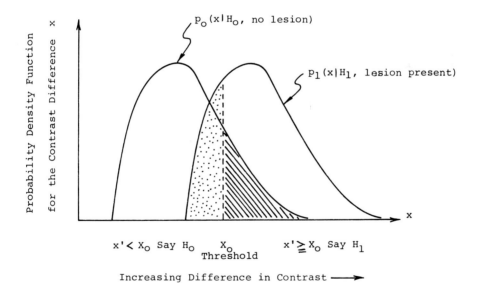

Fig. 3-5. Decision space resulting from juxtaposition of two probability density functions pertaining to hypothesis H_0 and H_1.

in equation 1 in the form of equation 2 and then performing the operation of differentiation. Following this operation, the result is set equal to zero and we obtain:

$$C_{10}P[H_1]p_1(x_0 | H_1) = C_{01}P[H_0]p_0(x_0 | H_0) \tag{3}$$

Equation 3 expresses in the form of an equality the relation that must exist between two probability density functions in order to achieve the minimum risk. This equation is often expressed in the form of the ratio:

$$\frac{p_1(x_0 | H_1)}{p_0(x_0 | H_0)} = \Lambda(x_0) = \frac{C_{10}P[H_0]}{C_{01}P[H_1]} \qquad (4)$$

This ratio of two probability density functions is generally referred to as a likelihood ratio and is represented by $\Lambda(x)$. We note that for our particular problem, the likelihood ratio evaluated at the threshold value is equal to a constant determined entirely by costs and a priori probabilities. If we knew the exact mathematical form of the probability density functions, we could then solve exactly for the value of the threshold, x_0. However, an alternative way of making our decision would be to calculate the likelihood ratio for the observed value of x' as shown in equation 5 and simply compare it to the value of the likelihood ratio evaluated at the threshold, x_0. This method is called a likelihood ratio test and equation 5 shows how to proceed in making our decision if we decided to utilize this method.

$$\frac{p_1(x' | H_1)}{p_0(x' | H_0)} = \Lambda(x') = \begin{array}{l} > \Lambda(x_0) \text{ Choose } H_1 \\ < \Lambda(x_0) \text{ Choose } H_0 \end{array} \qquad (5)$$

The principal results that follow from this analysis are that the minimization of the cost function can be achieved by use of a likelihood ratio test and that the likelihood ratio is completely determined by knowledge of two probability density functions that prevail under the two possible hypotheses. In addition, we have seen that a likelihood ratio test is exactly equivalent to the partitioning of decision space into a series of decision regions. This analysis can be extended and generalized to yield likelihood ratio tests that perform other functions such as minimizing the probability of making an error or alternatively, maximizing the probability of making a correct decision.[9,10] The next step in our analysis is to see how the above result can be reversed in order to provide a method for determining the attributes that contribute significantly to the formation of a decision.

The key to transforming the decision strategy developed earlier into a decision analysis tool is the application of Bayes' theorem, which is a method for inferring the probabilities of certain related events.[1] Since Bayes' theorem is central to the decision analysis method we are about to describe, we will digress momentarily to discuss the basis for Bayes' theorem and the assumptions necessary for its validity.

As an example of the simplest possible case of probability inference, let us assume that we have observed an event B that is related to an event A by a probability P[A,B] for the joint event A and B. The problem is to infer from knowledge of the occurrence of event B and the joint probability P[A,B] the conditional probability of the event A given B, P[A|B]. To do this, we first write a relation that contains the principal assumption implied by Bayes' theorem. This relation expresses the joint probability we are looking for as well as the probability of event B by itself. The relation is:

$$P[A,B] = P[A|B]P[B] \tag{6}$$

Equation 6 does not follow from an axiomatic development of the probability theory; rather, it constitutes an additional constraint that has the following implications. First, equation 6 requires that the probability measure be invariant with respect to partitioning of the sample space. This implication should be kept in mind, since we are dealing with a model that implies partitioning of decision space within which we have defined various outcome probabilities. Second, equation 6 implies that the probability measures remain consistent under conditions of variation in the number of data points included in the sample space. This consideration is not as important, since we are interested here in an analysis technique that relates to a single individual observation. It clearly becomes important when we move on to the consideration of aggregate data.

Once having written equation 6 and recognized its implications, Bayes' theorem follows by simple manipulation. We first rewrite equation 6 as:

$$P[A|B] = \frac{P[A,B]}{P[B]} \tag{7}$$

Next we recognize that if equation 6 is true, we may also express the joint probability in the numerator of equation 7 in a similar manner, so as to yield:

$$P[A|B] = \frac{P[B|A]P[A]}{P[B]} \tag{8}$$

Finally, using the theorem of total probability, we expand the denominator of equation 7 to give the form of Bayes' theorem normally quoted in elementary texts on probability and statistics.[11] This form is:

$$P[A|B] = \frac{P[B|A]P[A]}{P[B|A]P[A] + P[B|\bar{A}]P[\bar{A}]} \tag{9}$$

where $P[A]$ is the probability of the event A, and $\bar{A}$ represents all outcomes that are not A.

Once we have this result, we are in a position to derive a decision analysis technique from the minimum risk decision criteria. To do this, we first express the conditional probabilities for two possible outcomes, H_0 and H_1, in terms of the conditional probabilities and probability densities that we presumably already know. Thus by inserting the appropriate terms directly into equation 9, we obtain for the conditional probability of the outcome hypothesis H_1, given a particular value of x':

$$P[H_1|x'] = \frac{p_1(x'|H_1)P[H_1]}{p_1(x'|H_1)P[H_1] + p_0(x'|H_0)P[H_0]} \tag{10}$$

One can write a similar expression for the conditional probability for the outcome hypothesis, H_0. From an examination of equation 7 or equation 9, it is clear that this conditional probability will have the same denominator as equation 10 and that only the numerator will change. Thus if we form the ratio of the conditional probability for hypothesis H_1 to the conditional probability for hypothesis H_0, the denominator terms will cancel and we will have the following interesting result:

$$\frac{P[H_1|x']}{P[H_0|x']} \cdot \frac{P[H_0]}{P[H_1]} = \frac{\Omega_{x'}}{\Omega_0} = \Lambda(x') \tag{11}$$

Equation 11 contains the basis for the likelihood ratio method of decision analysis. The method is remarkably simple and straightforward and can be formulated as follows. To begin, we assume that the individual decision maker uses as decision criteria a method that leads to a likelihood ratio test. As we have noted, the likelihood ratio test can be applied to a wide variety of objectives and need not be limited to or even imply the minimization of risk as an objective. The next step is to note that equation 11 expresses the likelihood ratio in terms of two other ratios that correspond exactly to the classic definition of the odds in favor of an event. Thus we can rewrite equation 11 in the following form, where the notation $\Omega_{x'}$ designates the odds in favor of hypothesis H_1, given the attributes x' and Ω_0 represent the a priori odds in favor of the hypothesis H_1:

$$\Omega_{x'} = \Lambda(x')\Omega_0 \tag{12}$$

From equation 12 we see that in order to determine the effect of a given attribute on a decision outcome, it is only necessary to determine the decision maker's a priori odds in favor of a particular hypothesis and compare them with the same odds after the attribute is presented. If the odds are significantly changed, the implication from equation 12 is that the likelihood ratio must also be altered by the presence of the attribute x'. From our previous discussion this implies a relocation of a data point in decision space; therefore the attribute must have had an effect on the decision outcome.

The determination of the odds both a priori and a posteriori is done in practice by means of asking the decision maker directly for his subjective estimates of the odds at the time the attribute is presented. This technique requires some degree of skill on the part of the individual gathering the data in order to avoid introducing biases into the subjective probabilities as a result of the manner in which the question is phrased. Timeliness is also important in order to avoid subjective estimates that are biased by the appearance of additional or unwanted attributes before the subjective estimate is obtained. However, with sufficient care, experiments can be structured and executed so as to avoid these and other potential difficulties in obtaining reliable subjective data.[7]

Minimum variance decision analysis

Minimum variance techniques generally imply some degree of structure in the decision-making process. It is characteristic of these techniques that this structure must be specified prior to the data analysis, and with the possible exception of certain adaptive techniques, they cannot be inferred from the data. This structure is introduced by means of the specification of a mathematical function known as a discriminant function, which is in effect a model of the decision-making process. This function can assume a variety of forms, ranging from simple linear relationships that lead directly to the familiar concept of linear regression to the more complex nonlinear and binary coefficient discriminant functions.

The minimum variance procedure is relatively simple and can be summarized as follows. First, we assume we have a set of observed data vectors, x_{ij}, where the subscript "i" refers to the ith data vector and the subscript "j" refers to the jth component or attribute within the ith vector. For each data vector, we also have an observed outcome or action, which we designate by y_i. Next, we assume that we have a discriminate function for the ith data vector, which is a function of the components of that vector and a set $\{a_j\}$ of as yet unspecified coefficients. For simplicity we will indicate here a function $F[a_j x_{ij}]$, in which the number of coefficients equals the number of attributes in the data vector, and the functional form is simply a combination of coefficient products and vector components. Using this function, we form the difference e_i between the outcome of the ith data point and the value predicted by the discriminate function:

$$F[a_j x_{ij}] - y_i = e_i \tag{13}$$

Next, we approximate the variance in this difference by writing:

$$\frac{1}{N^2} \sum_{i=1}^{N} (F[a_j x_{ij}] - y_i)^2 = \frac{1}{N^2} \sum_{i=1}^{N} e_i^2 \tag{14}$$

in which N is the number of data vectors in our sample. Finally, in order to solve for the coefficients $\{a_j\}$, one would differentiate equation 14 with respect to each a_j to obtain a set of simultaneous equations that presumably can be evaluated to obtain the value of each a_j.

To use this technique as a decision analysis method, one would first obtain the coefficients $\{a_j\}$ for a particular discriminant function and data set and examine the values of the various a_j. Depending upon the relative significance of these values, one could infer the importance of the corresponding data vector components, or attributes, in determining a given outcome. Clearly, the validity of this approach is strongly dependent upon having selected an appropriate discriminant function, since the significance of the coefficient values is relative only to the specific discriminant function. To date the major effort in applying this technique has involved the use of mixed binary and analog discriminant functions in which the coefficients $\{a_j\}$ are either one or zero for data vector components that have binary values and are continuous variables for data components with scaler values. The results obtained with these techniques have led to the establishment of various profiles for the screening of events in order to detect or predict certain specific outcomes such as a bad credit risk in a collection of credit applications. The successes enjoyed by this technique have been commensurate with constructing such screening devices rather than in decision analysis per se. However, there is currently a significant amount of effort devoted to the search for "more efficient" discriminant functions that, in view of the above discussion, translates directly into better models of the decision process.

Entropy minimax pattern discovery *

In this section we will discuss a relatively new method of decision analysis that treats aggregate data in an unstructured manner.[3-6] The principal idea behind this method is the definition of attribute subsets that are capable of acting as predictors of various outcomes. Thus if the attributes pertinent to a new event were recorded, the probabilities associated with various possible outcomes for this event could be predicted by matching the attributes with previously defined subsets. Since a detailed description of this technique involves some notions and terminology not previously defined, we will initially consider a simple example of pattern discovery, primarily with the objective of defining the terms and concepts involved.

The example we will deal with has to do with a hypothetical experiment concerning the detection of a pattern on a checkerboard. In this experiment we use a common 64-square checkerboard consisting of 32 squares each of red and black arranged in alternating sequence. Each square is covered by a slip of white cardboard so that the color of the square is not visible. At this point we bring in an unbiased observer and we tell him that his objective is to predict, before the removal of each cardboard slip, the color of the square. Of course, he does not know that the board is only a common checkerboard. We advise him initially that he may assume there are as many red squares as black. In order to decide which cardboard slip is to be removed, we will use a random number generator to generate two random numbers between one and eight that will specify the row and the column of the square to be uncovered.

When the first square is selected, we ask the observer for his a priori estimation in regard to the probabilities of red and black. Assuming a rational observer, the answer will certainly be equal probabilities of one half. We then remove the cardboard and let the observer see the outcome. This process of randomly selecting a square, obtaining the observer's a priori probability, and

---

*The name given this technique follows the usage established by its principal developer, R. A. Christensen.

then observing the outcome is repeated several times until we arrive at a situation similar to that shown in Fig. 3-6. By the time the observer is this far advanced in our hypothetical experiment, we assume that he would be capable of predicting with a high degree of certainty the color of the next square to be uncovered.

If we studied the observer's a priori probabilities throughout the experiment, we might expect them to move from equally likely probabilities at the outset to values near unity and zero by the time the situation as shown in Fig. 3-6 is reached. If we were then to ask the observer how he was able to effect the change in his a priori probabilities, he would undoubtedly make reference to an emerging pattern within the data. Thus we arrive at a rather intuitive concept as to the significance of a pattern. The existence of a pattern, based upon an examination of available attributes, allows for a reduction in uncertainty concerning the outcome of future events. Moreover, we might hypothesize that the degree to which a pattern has reduced uncertainty could be expressed as a functional change in the a priori probabilities in regard to the various outcomes relative to identical probabilities having no data. Before considering a method of formalizing this concept of uncertainty reduction, we should relate this intuitive notion of a pattern to the problem of decision analysis.

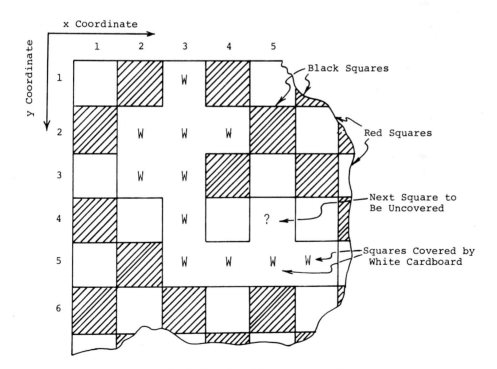

Fig. 3-6. Checkerboard problem in pattern discovery.

Using this intuitive notion of the significance of a pattern, we can advance the following methodology for the analysis of decisions. According to the model illustrated in Fig. 3-1, a physician is presented with a well-defined and observable set of attributes consisting of signs, symptoms, patient history, and the results of diagnostic tests. The outcomes that we want to relate to this attribute set are the observable decisions or actions that the physician takes. Ideally, this relation would take the form of a one-to-one correlation between the presence of a given attribute and the occurrence of a corresponding decision or action outcome. However, the real world is substantially more complex than this, and we recognize that it is far more likely that a particular outcome will be related to the simultaneous presence of an aggregate of attributes. Moreover, this relation is likely to be characterized not by the absolute certainty of occurrence of a given outcome but rather by the higher probability of the occurrence of the given outcome relative to the other outcomes being considered. Thus we are proposing a method of characterizing the relationship between attributes and outcomes to express the likelihood or probability of a given outcome in terms of the presence, absence, or magnitude of the attributes that the physician has observed. Clearly, if a given decision has a high probability of occurrence under the condition that a certain subset of attributes prevail, then we would say that these attributes affected the given decision. The measure of the effect's magnitude is defined by the change in the outcome probability after the examination of the attribute list relative to the a priori probability of the outcome.

In summary, the issue at question is the definition of a methodology that can identify attributes (that is, diagnostic tests) that substantially affect a physician's decisions. The answer proposed by the entropy minimax pattern detection methodology is that, if the presence or absence of an attribute contributes significantly to a change in the probability of a given outcome, it will be classed as a determinant of that outcome. At this point the principal ideas concerning the application of pattern detection to decision analysis have been presented, and the reader not wishing to follow the mathematics in the development given below may want to proceed directly to the summary section.

Returning now to the checkerboard problem, we consider one possible way in which our observer might choose to analyze the attributes associated with the outcomes red and black. The only attributes available to the observer are the numeric values of the x and y coordinates of the various squares that have been uncovered. He could arrange these attributes by using their actual scaler values, but there is a more compact representation for our purposes. Suppose the observer chooses to arrange the data according to the coordinates being odd or even numbers. If he makes this fortuitous choice, he could plot the results in the manner shown in Fig. 3-7. We refer to such an arrangement of attributes and outcomes as feature space. In this case the feature space is two-dimensional and the pattern is obvious.

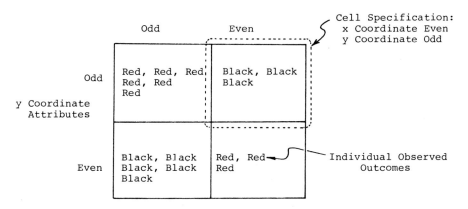

Fig. 3-7. Example of a feature space appropriate to checkerboard problem.

Fig. 3-7 also illustrates another important aspect of feature space, namely, the division of space into subspaces by the specification of one or more attributes. These subspaces are called cells. Each cell contains only those outcomes whose attributes exactly fit the attribute specifications that define the cell's boundaries. In addition, the cell definitions are such that the entire feature space is included in the set of cells and no two cells overlap. Thus an event consisting of a set of attributes and the corresponding outcome must be contained in one cell and one cell only. We will have more to say concerning cells and feature spaces, but the important points here are (1) that a feature space can be partitioned into cells by the specification of the presence or absence of one or more of the attributes and (2) that the boundaries of the cells and their number can be varied by changing the specification of the attributes.

At this point we have established two prerequisites to an analysis method. The first prerequisite is the use of a pattern as a mechanism for reducing uncertainty. The second prerequisite would be the concept of defining a pattern in terms of attributes in feature space. If we treat the reduction in uncertainty as the minimization of a dependent variable and if we treat the cell boundaries in feature space as the independent variables used to effect the minimization, we have a problem that is conceptually similar to the problem of minimizing Bayes' risk by means of suitably chosen boundaries in decision space.

Thus although decision analysis based upon pattern detection is dramatically different from decision analysis based upon likelihood ratios, the mechanism for developing these methodologies is strikingly similar.

The next developmental step of the pattern-detection algorithm is the specification of the measure of uncertainty that we will seek to minimize. Ideally, the measure of uncertainty should have the following properties:

First, it should be a continuous function of the probabilities only of the various possible outcomes. Second, it should give greater relative weight to the occurrence of rare events than to the occurrence of common events. This property will ensure that we have some mechanism for taking into account the intuitive notion that an event whose outcome in some sense surprises us conveys more information than an event whose outcome agrees with a previous prediction. The third and final property that we would like our measure to have is that of additivity in the algebraic sense. Specifically, the uncertainty associated with two independent sources of events should be just the algebraic sum of the uncertainty associated with each source taken separately. In addition, if the sources were related by some form of conditional probability, we would require that the additive property still holds with an appropriate weighting factor, which would be a function of the conditional probability.

There are a number of functions that fulfill the above requirements, but by far, the simplest of these is the measure of information advanced by Shannon and Weaver.[2,8,12] In its simplest form this measure states that given N possible outcomes, each with probability of occurrence P_n, the average information per outcome is given by:

$$H = - \sum_{n=1}^{N} P_n \log_2 P_n \tag{15}$$

Of course, the individual probabilities P_n must sum to unity:

$$\sum_{n=1}^{N} P_n = 1 \tag{16}$$

The use of a logarithm to base 2 has the advantage of expressing the information in units of bits per outcome, but any other base for the logarithm may be used without loss of generality.

The question could be asked as to why we would choose a measure of information as a measure of uncertainty. The answer is that they are for our purposes one and the same. We could argue this point intuitively by considering the extremes of the function defined by equation 15 and comparing the results with out intuitive notion of uncertainty. At one extreme we have the case of a single outcome that occurs with a probability of one. For this case the value of the information would be identically zero, which corresponds to our intuitive notion of the opposite of uncertainty being the occurrence of an event with absolute certainty. Somewhat more abstract is the case of one or more events with probability zero in combination with a certain event. Here again, the information is zero and likewise there is complete certainty regarding events that can never occur. On the other hand, if there were N possible outcomes, each with probability 1/N, we are inclined to think of this as a case

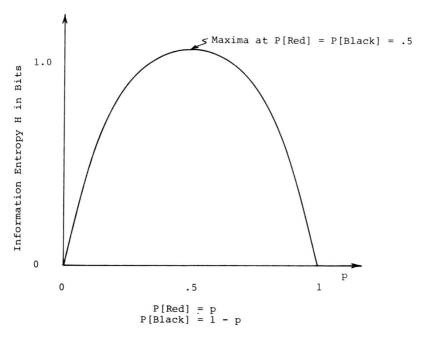

Fig. 3-8. Binary entropy function pertinent to checkerboard problem.

of maximum uncertainty, and indeed, the information measure is a maximum for equally likely events.

Returning briefly to the checkerboard example, we can now show graphically the information entropy function that is being minimized by the emergence of a pattern in the data. This function is illustrated in Fig. 3-8. Before any outcomes were available, the observer assumed equally likely probabilities that corresponded to maximum uncertainty and maximum entropy. As he obtained observations, he was able to differentiate the probability between the two possible outcomes of red and black. It is clear from Fig. 3-8 that any differentiation in probability in either direction will reduce the entropy function and that the greatest differentiation corresponding to the largest degree of certainty yields the minimum value for the entropy; hence the "mini" portion of the name "entropy minimax pattern discovery" given to this method.

In order to proceed with the development of this methodology, we need to answer two questions in detail. The first question pertains to the issue of probability estimation from experimental data. The second question is concerned with the method of partitioning feature space and the practical problems that evolve from such partitioning. We will consider the second problem first since there is still some terminology that must be developed.

The most convenient way of expressing both attributes and outcomes of a particular data base is by binary notation. Thus nonscaler attributes such as the patient's sex would be coded as either one or zero. Scaler or numeric attributes such as age can be coded with an appropriate number of binary digits. It is not necessary that scales of numeric variables be linear so long as the scaling remains consistent for all events in the data set. A sample of attributes, outcomes, and corresponding binary coding is shown in Fig. 3-9.

If we have the data to be analyzed in binary form as shown in Fig. 3-9, we can now define cells in feature space by specifying those attributes that must be ones, those that must be zero, or those that remain undefined. Fig. 3-10 shows a typical cell definition for a case in which there are only three attributes. We note that one of the three, attribute number 1, was left unspecified such that the cell includes events for which this attribute may be either a one or a zero. The largest cell that could be defined would be one for which no attributes were specified, such that the entire feature space was included. By specifying a single attribute the feature space is divided in half, while to specify all attributes creates the smallest possible cell.

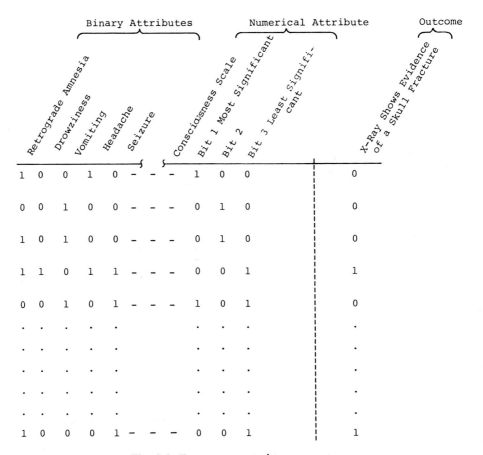

Fig. 3-9. Feature space in binary notation.

There are numerous ways in which a feature space can be partitioned into sets of disjoint cells whose union will completely fill the space. As a matter of convention, each distinct set of cells is called a screening. Fig. 3-11 shows three possible screenings for the case in which there are two binary attributes. The interested reader can quickly convince himself that there are twelve other screenings for the two-attribute case in addition to the three shown in Fig. 3-10. For the three binary–attribute case, the number of screenings is 4140, and if one has six binary attributes, the number of possible screenings increases to a number on the order of 10^{51}. Obviously some mechanism must be found for problems of real interest to limit the number of screenings that must be examined in order to obtain a reasonable approximation to the minimum entropy pattern.

Mechanisms for limiting the number of screenings required in a particular analysis have been developed and are in use. The principal method is to approach the minimum entropy screening by means of stepwise approximation. This method has been in use for some time and has given reasonably good results, although the method is still being developed. As is true with most

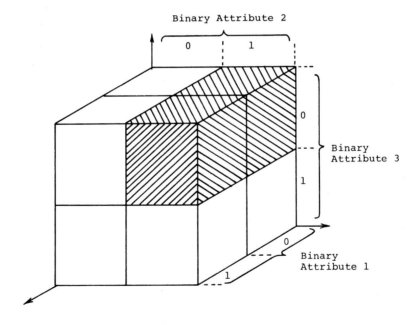

Cell Definition

    Binary Attribute 2 = 1

    Binary Attribute 3 = 0

Fig. 3-10. Three-dimensional binary attribute case showing possible cell definition.

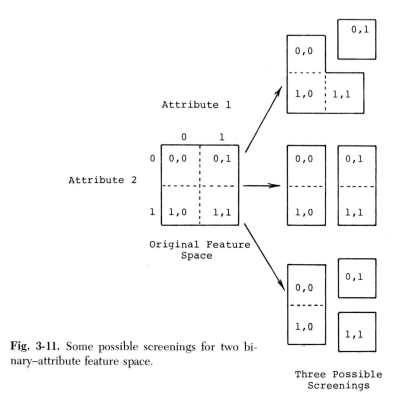

Fig. 3-11. Some possible screenings for two binary–attribute feature space.

approximation methods, one exchanges the completeness cost in the computation process for the effort on the investigator's part in analyzing intermediate results to ensure that the approximation is converging upon meaningful results. This approximation is no exception, and a fair degree of investigator intervention is required.

Assuming that we know at least in principle how to partition feature space into various screenings by means of attribute specification, we may now consider the second question concerning the actual information entropy calculation. The objective is to calculate a quantity similar to that defined by equation 15 and to structure the calculation such that the result will be a function of the various screenings as the independent variable. Since the fundamental element in a screening is the cell, we will first define the conditional probability of obtaining the kth outcome in the ith cell of the jth screening as:

$$\text{Probability } [k^{th} \text{ outcome} \mid i^{th} \text{ cell}, j^{th} \text{ screening}] = p_{k|ij} \tag{17}$$

Note that this is a conditional probability; we can therefore calculate a conditional entropy for the ith cell in the jth screening as follows:

$$H_{ij} = -\sum_{k=1}^{K} p_{k|ij} \log_2 p_{k|ij} \tag{18}$$

Now in order to construct the entropy associated with the jth screening, we need to form the weighted sum of the conditional entropies H_{ij} over the I cells in the jth screening. To do this, we define as the appropriate weighting factors the conditional probabilities of finding any of the k possible outcomes in the ith cell of the jth screening as:

$$P[\text{any outcome in } i^{th} \text{ cell of } j^{th} \text{ screening}] = p_{ij} \qquad (19)$$

Using this probability, we write for the entropy of the jth screening:

$$H_j = -\sum_{i=1}^{I} p_{ij} \sum_{k=1}^{K} p_{k|ij} \log_2 p_{k|ij} \qquad (20)$$

Finally, we need to define the method by which we will estimate the probabilities $p_{k|ij}$ and p_{ij}. The method itself is deceptively simple, and as is the case with many mathematical developments, the derivation of the method is not nearly so important as the assumptions upon which the derivation is based. Since the derivation of the probability estimation is covered by Christensen,[4] we will deal here with the assumptions and their implications. To form the probability estimation, we first assume that we can identify a total of t distinct ways in which an outcome T can occur and f distinct ways in which an alternative outcome F can occur. For instance, if T were the outcome of exactly two tails in three tosses of a fair coin, there would be a total of three ways in which this could happen, t = 3, and five ways it could fail to happen, f = 5. Moreover, if we had observed the outcome of T a total of x times in n trials, the unbiased probability estimate of T is given by:

$$P[T \text{ given x T's in n trials}] = \frac{x + t}{n + t + f} \qquad (21)$$

This estimate contains the following properties that are important in the entropy minimax pattern detection problem. First, the estimator is unbiased in that the estimate converges toward the relative frequency limit definition of probability as the number of trials increases. Second, the estimator has the property to maximize the entropy function as given in equation 20; hence the "max" portion of the term "entropy minimax pattern discovery." In other words, each entropy H_j, calculated for the jth screening by using the above estimator, will be in some sense an upper limit to the entropy of the jth screening. Consequently, when we select the nth screening as our pattern, based on the observation that H_n was the minimum entropy, we are selecting from a set of upper limits or maximum entropies. Finally, we note that in the event we should not have any data whatsoever in a particular cell, the probability estimates for that cell will reflect just our a priori knowledge. This follows from the fact that equation 21 reduces to the ratio t/(t + f) for the cell having no data, and this ratio reflects only the information that we possessed prior to observing any experimental events.

In the application of equation 21 to the evaluation of the entropy for the

j^{th} screening, we adopt the following notation. The conditional probability of the kth outcome in the ith cell is written as:

$$P_{k|ij} = \frac{n_{ijk} + w_{ijk}}{n_{ij} + w_{ij}} \qquad (22)$$

where n_{ijk} is the number of events with outcome k whose attribute values are such that they are contained in the ith cell of the jth screening. The total of all events, regardless of the outcome occurring in the ith cell, is designated as n_{ij}. The terms w_{ijk} and w_{ij} are the equivalents of the numbers t or f and the sum $t + f$, respectively, in equation 21. Thus the sum of the weighting factors w_{ijk} over all possible outcomes k is w_{ij} and the ratio w_{ijk}/w_{ij} is essentially the a priori probability of the kth outcome in the ith cell. Likewise, we define the probability of an event in the ith cell of the jth screening by:

$$P_{ij} = \frac{n_{ij} + u_{ij}}{n + u_j} \qquad (23)$$

Here the ratio of the weighting factors u_{ij}/u_j represents the a priori probability of finding any event in the ith cell, and n is just the total number of events in the sample.

The implication of equations 22 and 23 is that the weighting factors w_{ijk}, w_{ij}, u_{ij}, and u_j are in some sense dependent upon both the screening function and the cells within that screening. If in fact one had detailed a priori information concerning the relationship between attributes and outcomes such as previous pattern detection analysis, it would be possible to specify the weighting factors such that they did depend upon both the screening and the cell within that screening. However, one can show that in all cases u_j is independent of the screening and that if there is no a priori information, the factors w_{ij} and w_{ijk} are independent of both the screening and the cell within that screening. This result can also be used as a worst case assumption when we are unwilling to assume any significant a priori knowledge.

One interesting feature of equations 22 and 23 is that they specify a non-Baysian pair of probabilities. By this we mean that it is impossible to find a constant a_{ijk}, such that the joint probability of the kth outcome in the ith cell of the jth screening is given for all experimental values of n, n_{ij}, and n_{ijk} by:

$$P_{ijk} = P_{ij}P_{k|ij} = \frac{n_{ijk} + a_{ijk}}{n + u_j} = \frac{n_{ij} + u_{ij}}{n + u_j} \cdot \frac{n_{ijk} + w_{ijk}}{n_{ij} + w_{ij}} \qquad (24)$$

If it existed, the constant a_{ijk} would be in effect a joint a priori probability of the kth outcome in the ith cell of the jth screening. However, in order to exist, this joint a priori probability would require that the weighting factor u_{ij} be exactly equal to the weighting factor w_{ij}. To see why the equality cannot be required, we will consider the following example.

Suppose we had a case in which the attributes were physical measurements of three spatial coordinates. In addition, suppose the outcome set was completely unrelated to spatial position by any a prior knowledge. Moreover, we assume that we have no a priori knowledge concerning the distribution of events in the three-dimensional space, and we may therefore choose the weighting factors u_{ij} and u_j arbitrarily. One reasonable way of choosing these factors would be to make u_{ij} proportional to the volume occupied by the ith cell and to make u_j proportional to the total volume of feature space. The constant of proportionality would be an unrestricted parameter probably chosen by means of subjective considerations. On the other hand, the weighting factor w_{ij}, which is independent of both the cell and the screening by the above assumptions, relates only to the various outcome possibilities and is in no way determined by the spatial location of the events. Clearly, the two constants u_{ij} and w_{ij} must be independent, and therefore the probability estimates will be non-Baysian.

To this point, we have covered most of the significant aspects of the entropy minimax pattern discovery technique. The principal points in the application of this technique are the following. First, a data set is defined as having a number of attributes and outcomes. This data set is referred to as feature space. Attributes are defined as independent variables and, for the problem of evaluation of diagnostic efficacy, might consist of items such as signs, symptoms, patient history, and the results of various diagnostic tests. Outcomes could be defined as various physicians' actions that presumably were influenced by combinations of the presence, absence, or magnitude of various attributes. To determine what these combinations might be, we subject this data to an entropy minimax analysis. This analysis partitions the feature space into cells by specifying the presence or magnitude of some subset of attributes. Data events whose attributes match the cell definition are included in the cell, while those whose attributes do not match are included in other cells. Each distinct set of nonoverlapping cells spanning or covering the feature space is called a screening. For each screening, we construct a measure of the degree to which the screening has succeeded in separating the outcomes into individual cells in feature space. The measure used is the information entropy, which can be regarded as measuring the amount by which a particular screening has reduced the average uncertainty in predicting a physician's actions, given a particular set of attributes. In order to select the "best" screening we select that partitioning of the feature space that minimizes uncertainty or entropy.

The resulting pattern is expressed in two components. The first is a list of cell definitions in terms of the presence, absence, or magnitude of certain subsets of attributes. It is not necessary that all of the attributes appear in the cell definitions, as some attributes may be of no value in predicting outcomes and hence will not appear in any of the cell definitions. The second part of the pattern definition is a list of probabilities for the various outcomes in each cell. If a perfect screening could be found, the cell definitions would isolate and separate the outcomes completely and the probability of a particular outcome in each cell would be near unity, while all the others would have near zero probability of occurring in that particular cell. The results would never be identically one or zero because of the finite values of the a priori weights.

SUMMARY

A fundamental aspect of the efficacy study of diagnostic procedures is the relation of the results of these procedures to outcomes ranging in time sequence from a physician's decisions and actions during the diagnostic process to the final state of a particular patient's disease. Large-scale efforts to gather data appropriate to the determination of efficacy have only recently been undertaken; consequently, the methods of analysis appropriate to handling these data are still under development. In order to acquaint the reader with a basic understanding of the problems involved and the assumptions implied by the use of various methodologies, we have presented a detailed discussion of three approaches that roughly span the range of available methodologies. These approaches have been presented in the context of decision analysis as applied to the physician's diagnostic process, which constitutes the lowest echelon of the problems comprising the study of efficacy.

The first method discussed was a direct outgrowth of the likelihood ratio test for implementing optimum decision strategies. We saw that the use of a likelihood ratio model for the physician's decision-making process implied the partitioning of a decision space, the coordinates of which were just the diagnostic attributes, signs, symptoms, patient history, and diagnostic test results that the physician observed. We also saw that if the preceding model was in fact a valid representation of the physician's decision process and if the statistics of this process obeyed Bayes' theorem, then the process could be reversed to yield a method for the analysis of decisions. Specifically, the method relies on the ability of the data-gathering process to provide reliable measures of a physician's subjective probabilities concerning a given diagnostic outcome, both before and after having observed a given attribute. The ratio of these probabilities expressed as odds has been shown under the above assumptions to be equal to the physician's likelihood ratio. Thus a change in subjective probability following observation of a particular attribute can be interpreted as a change in the physician's likelihood ratio brought about by the observation of that particular attribute. The conclusion is that the attributes that affect that ratio must also affect the physician's decision, since the physician's decision is a function of his likelihood ratio.

While the results of the likelihood ratio method of decision analysis as applied to decisions by individual physicians can be extended by means of classic statistics to deal with aggregate data, we have also investigated an alternative method of dealing with aggregate data that was based on a minimum variance approach. In this approach we selected a function composed of the attributes that the physician observes, each multiplied by an unspecified coefficient. It was then hypothesized that the unspecified coefficients could be selected in a manner such that the function would predict the outcome or action that would follow from the observation of a specific set of attribute values. In practice we recognize that such a function would be highly unlikely to perform as a perfect predictor, but it would be reasonable to require that it predict within some optimized performance measure. The name of this technique suggests that the measure to be optimized is the variance between the actual and predicted outcomes. This technique is used as a decision analysis tool by noting the relative magnitudes, with appropriate consideration given to normalization of the results of the various coefficients. From such a comparison one can infer the relative importance of the various attributes that influence the physician's decision. The validity of the conclusions drawn from such an analysis are strongly dependent upon the type of function originally chosen, since this choice will necessarily imply a structure in the decision-making process. Although this technique has been used with some success in structured applications such as the screening of credit requests, the emphasis has been toward the development of predictor functions with minimal structure, which leads us logically to consider a decision analysis method that makes minimal structural assumptions.

Such a technique has been developed and depends for its validity upon the following assumption. In a set of observations of patient's attributes followed by the physician's decisions, the physician's objective was to use the information contained in the patient's attributes to influence his decision in a consistent and rational manner. In so doing the physician will create, within the sets of observed attributes, certain patterns consisting of collections or subsets of attributes that are associated with particular outcomes. The measure of the quality or goodness of association is the degree to which the various subsets of attributes can act as predictors to change the probability of a given outcome from what it would have been in the absence of knowledge of the attributes. In further studying this concept, we discovered that the classic definition of information entropy could be used as a basis for constructing an algorithm for the discovery of patterns in the set of attributes and outcomes. Once such a set of patterns has been established, we then say that these attributes, which act as predictors of the various outcomes, are determinants of the decisions that those outcomes represent.

References

1. Bayes, T.: An essay towards solving a problem in the doctrine of chances, Biometrika **45:**293, 1958.
2. Brillouin, L.: Science and information theory, New York, 1956, Academic Press, Inc.

3. Christensen, R. A.: Induction and the evolution of language, Berkeley, 1963, Department of Physics, University of California.

4. Christensen, R. A.: A general approach to pattern discovery, Technical Report No. 20, 1967, University of California, Berkeley, Computer Center.

5. Christensen, R. A.: Pattern discovery program for analyzing qualitative and quantitative data, Behav. Sci. **13**:423, 1968.

6. Christensen, R. A.: Entropy minimax, a non-Baysian approach to probability estimation from empirical data, Paper presented at the International conference on cybernetics and society, Boston, November, 1973.

7. Committee on Efficacy Studies, American College of Radiology: Efficacy study definitive study design, preliminary report, Chicago, 1973.

8. Fano, R. M.: Transmission of information, Cambridge, Mass., 1961, the M.I.T. Press.

9. Lusted, L. B.: Introduction to medical decision-making, Springfield, Ill. 1968, Charles C Thomas, Publisher.

10. Lusted, L. B.: Decision-making studies in patient management, N. Engl. J. Med. **284**:416, 1971.

11. Mendenhall, W., and Reinmath, J. E.: Statistics for management and economics, Belmont, Calif., 1971, Duxbury Press.

12. Shannon, C. E., and Weaver, W.: The mathematical theory of communication, Urbana, Ill., 1964, University of Illinois Press.

4 Studies on the use of the intravenous pyelogram

John R. Thornbury, Dennis G. Fryback, and Ward Edwards

This chapter describes a new method for measuring the diagnostic usefulness of radiologic information to physicians who request x-ray examinations of
their patients and presents the results of a pilot study. National studies based
on this method are in progress. The physician states his diagnosis and his
certainty about that diagnosis both before and after he receives the results
of the x-ray examination. Change in his diagnostic certainty, measured by a
number called the log likelihood ratio that is calculated from Bayes' theorem,
reflects the effect of the radiologic information.

DIAGNOSTIC USEFULNESS, BAYES' THEOREM, AND LOG LIKELIHOOD RATIOS

The usefulness of a radiograph may be defined in terms of three criteria:
1. Its effect on the ultimate well-being of the patient
2. Its effect on the attending physician's choice of therapy
3. Its effect on the attending physician's diagnostic thinking

Initially we intended to study all three criteria of usefulness, but we soon
found that the first two were unmeasurable with the tools at hand. Both require
an answer to the question "What would have happened if this x-ray film had
not been taken?" Our attending physician respondents could not answer this
question; therefore we focused on the third concept of usefulness.

Radiographs are information. The effect of information is to modify probabilities. Therefore we set out to measure the diagnostic impact of x-ray information by observing its effect on the probabilities physicians assigned to
diagnostic hypotheses. The mathematical tool we used is Bayes' theorem of
probability theory.

Bayes' theorem is well known because it is the formally optimal method
for revising probabilities in the light of new information. It can be illustrated

Supported in part by Contract HSM 110-72-293 between the American College of Radiology
and the Division of Regional Medical Programs, Health Resources Administration, Department
of Health, Education, and Welfare; and by a Traineeship Grant (GM-01231), National Institute
for General Medical Sciences.

59

by a simple example. Suppose a physician is attempting to determine whether or not his patient is in fact suffering from a certain pathologic condition. The condition may be described in terms of a diagnostic hypothesis; for example, this patient has metastatic hypernephroma.

Let us assume that on the basis of all information he has available at the moment, the physician is willing to estimate that the odds favoring this condition is a particular number, which we will symbolize as Ω. For example, Ω may be 4 or, in more familiar form, $4:1$. Assume further that some symptom is extremely likely to be present if the patient does indeed have the condition and extremely unlikely if he does not. If the physician now observes that the symptom is present, his revised odds favoring the diagnostic hypothesis should be very high; if he observes the absence of the symptom, his revised odds should be very low. If, on the other hand, some other symptom is *equally* likely whether or not the patient has the condition, then observing it should leave the odds unchanged. This intuitive argument practically defines Bayes' theorem, which is nothing more than the same argument in quantitative form. If the physician's odds favoring the diagnostic hypothesis H before the symptom is observed are Ω_0 and the odds after the observation are Ω_1, then Bayes' theorem states:

$$\Omega_1 = L \cdot \Omega_0 \tag{1}$$

where

$$L = \frac{P(S|H)}{P(S|\text{not } H)} \tag{2}$$

The quantity $P(S|H)$ is the probability that the symptom will be observed if H is true, that is, if the patient does indeed suffer from the condition. $P(S|\text{not } H)$ is the corresponding probability of observing S if the patient does *not* have the condition. The quantity L is known as the *likelihood ratio* for the observation and is formally a sufficient statistic describing the usefulness of the observation for distinguishing H from not H.*

Equation 2 suggests that the way to estimate L is to accumulate many instances in which S has been observed and estimate its relative frequency both when H is true and when H is false. This frequentistic approach, although often attempted in medical and other contexts, presents severe difficulties. Radiographs, diseases, and patients are to some extent unique, and therefore meaningful relative frequencies are difficult to accumulate, even when the record-keeping system permits.

Yet the numbers Ω, L, $P(S|H)$, and $P(S|\text{not } H)$ are meaningful independently of whether or not they refer to relative frequencies.[4] Often they can be well estimated, directly or indirectly, by expert judges—expert in the medical subject matter and at least somewhat trained in estimating such num-

---

*Further discussion of the properties of likelihood ratios may be found in Edwards et al.[4]

bers. A number of studies have shown that such estimates are effective sub-
stitutes for relative frequencies.*

A simple transformation of equation 1 gives:

$$L = \Omega_1/\Omega_0 \tag{3}$$

and taking logarithms (to the base 10) gives the final version of Bayes' theorem,
with which we actually worked.

$$\log L = \log \Omega_1 - \log \Omega_0 \tag{4}$$

To use equation 4, we ask the attending physician, before he receives the
x-ray information, what diagnosis he is considering and how sure he is that it is
correct. In this study we asked for that information in probability, not odds,
form. However, the transformation from probability to odds is simple:

$$\Omega = \frac{P}{1-P} \tag{5}$$

Therefore from equation 5 we calculate Ω_0. After the attending physician
receives the x-ray information, the same calculation gives Ω_1. Then, using
equation 4, we can calculate log L (or, more exactly, the absolute value of log
L, since information unfavorable to the hypothesis is just as useful as information favorable to it).

Our final definition of diagnostic usefulness of the x-ray information is thus
given quantitative form. The larger the log likelihood ratio, the greater the impact of the x-ray information. And the scale is linear; that is, an x-ray film with
a log likelihood ratio of 3 is twice as valuable as a film with a log likelihood ratio
of 1.5.

Significance of zero log likelihood ratios

A zero log likelihood ratio has a unique status. If the x-ray information yields
that diagnosticity, the x-ray information is irrelevant to patient management.
A zero log likelihood ratio is obtained whenever the physician's prior odds and
posterior odds are exactly the same. When this occurs, equation 4 yields a zero
for log L. The physician's problem after he receives such a piece of information
looks exactly as it did before he received the information (except that he can no
longer consider that information source as potentially useful in this case). Since
nothing has been modified by the information, the physician's treatment decisions cannot logically be affected by receiving that information.

It is important to realize that an x-ray film interpreted as normal does not
necessarily result in a zero log likelihood ratio. We are *not* saying that x-ray
films with normal results do not influence treatment decisions; of course they
often do. Normal results are themselves evidence and often change a set of
diagnostic probabilities, for example, a normal urogram in a case in which

---

*For medical examples, see references 1, 6, and 7 to 9; for nonmedical examples, see references
3, 5, and 11 to 13.

acute colicky flank pain initially raised the question of a ureteral calculus. A zero log likelihood ratio can occur only if the radiograph has *no* influence on the physician's diagnostic thinking; that is, it tells him nothing.

Retrospective discovery of a zero log likelihood ratio is interesting, but prospective prediction of it is more important. In retrospect a procedure that yields a zero log likelihood ratio (or, in qualitative language, that has no influence on the attending physician's thinking) has been a waste of time, money, and radiologic resources. In prospect a procedure that is likely to produce a zero log likelihood ratio under the circumstances in which it is used is likely to be a waste of time, money, and radiologic resources.

Seldom will a procedure yield a zero log likelihood ratio for all patients of a given description; if it did, physicians would be unlikely to consider ordering it. Whenever it yields a nonzero log likelihood ratio, then the questions we have bypassed in adopting the log likelihood ratio as a measure of diagnostic usefulness become relevant again. Whether or not the x-ray information was sufficiently useful to warrant its cost becomes, in this case, not only a matter of the magnitude of the log likelihood ratio (that is, how much it changed the physician's diagnostic thinking) but also a function of the relative risks and benefits of the physician's acting with as opposed to without the x-ray information.

We concentrate solely on change in diagnostic certainty effected by the x-ray result. We point out, however, that the expected change in diagnostic certainty resulting from obtaining the x-ray information is an important and necessary input to formal solution of the prospective decision problem concerning whether or not to obtain the x-ray information for a given patient.*

PRELIMINARY STUDY OF DIAGNOSTIC USEFULNESS OF INTRAVENOUS PYELOGRAMS

We present here the design and some results of a pilot study that was undertaken to determine whether the type of judgments required for application of the ideas we have discussed could be obtained and used. Our intent was to study intravenous pyelogram (IVP) information usefulness and to chart some of the pitfalls that would occur in applying our approach to studying the diagnostic usefulness of x-ray examination.

Methodology

We assessed the physician's diagnostic judgments at two points in the diagnostic process: (1) at the time the IVP was requested and (2) when the phy-

---

*For a simplified discussion of the mathematics involved in formal solution of such decision problems, see references 2 and 3. For more general discussions of decision theory applied to medical problems, see references 6, 8, and 9. Excellent discussions of general applied decision theory may be found in references 10 and 11.

sician received the IVP results. At each of these times the physicians were asked to complete a questionnaire.

In the first questionnaire, which replaced the usual x-ray request form, we asked for two types of information. The first was factual information (pertinent history, results of the physical examination, and laboratory findings) that the physician had when he ordered the IVP. This information served to classify the type of problem about which he expected the urogram to provide further information. The second type of information was judgmental and characterized the diagnostic thinking of the physician at the time he decided to order the IVP. This class of information was subdivided into two parts; one asked the physician's reason for ordering the IVP, and the other assessed aspects of his diagnostic certainty prior to the IVP. This latter class formed the heart of the questionnaire and measured the base diagnostic certainty from which later change was determined.

We asked for a global judgment of the physician's certainty about whether the IVP would be normal or abnormal. Subjective certainty estimates were asked in percentage probability format. This question appeared in the following form:

How certain are you that this IVP will be

Normal _____ %

Abnormal _____ %

TOTAL   100%

If a previous urogram had been done and the results were known to the physician, we asked if he expected the urogram that he was presently ordering to show a change. Next he was asked to assume that the present urogram would be *abnormal* and to indicate the type and location of the abnormality he expected to see. This indication was made by placing a check mark in a matrix listing major anatomic areas (for example, kidney, ureter, bladder, prostate) as columns and category of abnormality (for example, anomaly, vascular disease, calculus, neoplasm) as rows. Last, we asked the physician to state his current diagnosis and how certain he was that this was the true diagnosis. This question was asked in two parts:

1. If you had to make a diagnosis now upon which the patient's management would be based, what would it be? _____

2. If you saw 100 cases exactly like this one, in what percentage of them would you expect the above diagnosis to be the true diagnosis? _____ %

The second questionnaire, filled out when the physician received the results of the IVP, again collected judgments of certainty concerning whether the urogram was normal or abnormal, and whether or not this represented a change from the previous IVP (if any). The physician might read the films himself, read the radiologist's report, or do both. He indicated his own understanding of the IVP results by checking the type and location of the abnormality.

Calculation of log likelihood ratios

The probability that the physician gave on questionnaire No. 1 defined Ω_0; that which he gave on questionnaire No. 2 defined Ω_1. Then equation 4 gives the log likelihood ratio. (All logarithms were computed to the base 10.)

The only difficulty arises in the case in which the diagnosis that is given on questionnaire No. 2 is not the same one as that on questionnaire No. 1; here we used an approximation. We wanted to calculate the log likelihood ratio with respect to the second diagnosis given; therefore it was necessary to infer the probability that the physician would have assigned to that diagnosis if he had considered it when completing questionnaire No. 1.

Deriving at least a reasonable upper bound for this probability is not difficult. Suppose that P_1 is the probability the physician gave for the diagnosis stated on questionnaire No. 1. Since this was the diagnosis he considered most likely at that time, we know that the pre-IVP probability he would have given for the new diagnosis could have been no larger than either P_1 or $1 - P_1$, whichever is smaller. If it were larger than P_1, he would have reported it as the most likely diagnosis. Since P_1 is the probability of the diagnosis considered most likely, no other diagnosis can have more than probability $1 - P_1$, since the sum of these probabilities must be 1. We use, then, the smaller of the two quantitites as an upper bound for the unknown probability and proceed to calculate the log likelihood ratio as if this were the probability he would have given. The resulting log likelihood is then a *lower* bound for the true (absolute value of the) log likelihood ratio.

Since the IVP provided a new diagnosis, we know that it was of diagnostic value in any case, but we followed the outlined computational procedure to provide a quantitative index to show just how valuable the change in diagnosis was. An example of this sort of case is given in the discussion of results.

Clinical experiment

Two outpatient clinics were selected as sites for an informal investigation to see if physicians would participate in a study of the contribution of the IVP to the diagnostic process and whether or not they could supply numbers that reflected their diagnostic certainty. The primary goal was to see if diagnostic usefulness of urogram information could be measured by using the methodology we have proposed.

Physicians' judgments were collected in the General Medical Clinic and the Urology Outpatient Clinic at University of Michigan Hospital. The internists were surveyed in December of 1972 and January of 1973, for a total of

5 working weeks, excluding Christmas and New Year's Day. The urologists participated in February, 1973.

The physicians were approached informally by the investigators, initially through the chiefs-of-service. Both the internist and urologist were quite willing to cooperate and gave permission for the study, provided their residents and staff men were willing to take the time to complete the questionnaire in the midst of their usual daily chores in the clinics. These men were willing to participate after being informed of the project, its goals, and the time we estimated it would add to their already busy schedule (3 to 5 minutes per questionnaire).

The participating physicians were asked to answer the questions about percentage probabilities by giving percentages that best represented their true level of certainty but not to spend a long time worrying about the estimate. They were instructed that what was wanted was their *first*, intuitive, best estimate. All participants knew at the outset that there was an end date for the project in their clinic.

The paperwork was arranged so that questionnaire No. 1 was used as the x-ray request form. Questionnaire No. 2 was freely available in both clinics and in the uroradiology suite. In addition, copies of questionnaire No. 2 were attached to the patient's chart and to the radiology report when it was sent to the clinic. When the physician filled out questionnaire No. 2 he had a copy of his questionnaire No. 1 in hand, so that he knew what his original estimates were. Questionnaire No. 2 was to be filled out immediately upon viewing the films or seeing the report. If it were filled out some time after receipt of the urogram information, it is possible that the estimates might not represent *only* the effect of the x-ray information. The broad availability of the second questionnaire was to ensure its completion as closely as possible to the time at which the IVP result became known to the physician.

Following the completion of the study in the two clinics, a retrospective review of each patient's chart was carried out by one of us (J. R. T.) to determine the accuracy of the radiologic diagnoses. In addition, based on the chart information, the radiologist on the investigating team made a categorial judgment about the diagnostic usefulness of the IVP in each case by estimating the range in which the calculated log likelihood ratio fell: 0.0; greater than 0.0 but less than 1.0; greater than 1.0. This process was designed to determine whether log likelihood ratios obtained in the prospective study could be accurately determined from a retrospective chart review. The radiologist was not aware of the physician's actual estimates or the calculated log likelihood ratio in any of the cases.

A total of 26 physicians participated in the two clinics. In the medical clinic there were 3 staff internists and 17 residents. Six urologists took part in the study; 3 were staff physicians and 3 were urology residents. These 26 physicians returned the two questionnaires on 39 medical patients and 53 urologic patients. (One urology patient had two urograms during the experiment.)

Results

In certain carefully chosen ways, we conducted this study with an attitude of intentional neglect. We did not closely supervise the participating physicians as they performed the task of filling out questionnaires. We wanted to see how well they could make the estimates without someone looking over their shoulders. In addition, we wished to see what data collection problems would arise in this pilot project if no investigators reminded respondents regularly to complete the two forms and not leave anything out. Answers to these questions become important when it is realized that hundreds or even thousands of cases must be collected and analyzed to begin to get stable estimates of the average return in x-ray information for given classes of patients. Such an effort would necessarily involve many cooperating physicians, and this implies a relatively loose administrative control over them.

An example of one of the administrative problems to be faced is the attrition rate for the questionnaires. A total of 92 completed sets of questionnaires were returned to us. Our records show, however, that IVPs were initially requested for 157 patients using questionnaire No. 1. Fig. 4-1 shows the final dispensation of 157 cases. Questionnaire No. 2 was never returned for 65 of these cases, 47 of them for known reasons and 18 for unknown reasons. Of the 92 returned, 12 were missing one probability estimate or statement of diagnosis necessary for calculating likelihood ratios (apparently as oversight). Only 3 were missing *all* estimates. (One free spirit wrote, "I am not a soothsayer!") These attrition factors thus left us with 77 sets of questionnaires potentially useful for calculating likelihood ratios associated with the IVP information.

With tighter administrative control of the paperwork, most of the incomplete cases presumably could have been pushed to completion. However, for these to be valid data, the investigators would have to be certain the physician was reminded to fill out questionnaire No. 2 before he received additional non-radiologic information about the patient. Otherwise the assumption that any change in diagnostic certainty was due to the x-ray examination alone would be invalid. (In this and other such studies, this difficulty is inherent. The attending physician may well acquire more information or reflect more deeply about information already at hand between ordering an x-ray examination and seeing the result. In a hospital setting we have been unable to devise a means of circumventing this problem other than to try to keep track of all other information sources—a hideous task. The effect will be to bias some log likelihood ratios upward.)

Data quality on the 77 complete sets of questionnaires was good considering that the physicians were untrained in probability estimation and that the questionnaires were self-administered. However, two types of data deficiencies

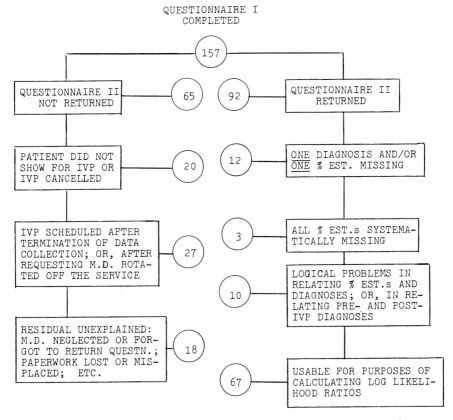

QUESTIONNAIRE I
COMPLETED

157

| QUESTIONNAIRE II NOT RETURNED | 65 | 92 | QUESTIONNAIRE II RETURNED |

| PATIENT DID NOT SHOW FOR IVP OR IVP CANCELLED | 20 | 12 | ONE DIAGNOSIS AND/OR ONE % EST. MISSING |

| IVP SCHEDULED AFTER TERMINATION OF DATA COLLECTION; OR, AFTER REQUESTING M.D. ROTATED OFF THE SERVICE | 27 | 3 | ALL % EST.s SYSTEMATICALLY MISSING |

10 — LOGICAL PROBLEMS IN RELATING % EST.s AND DIAGNOSES; OR, IN RELATING PRE- AND POST-IVP DIAGNOSES

| RESIDUAL UNEXPLAINED: M.D. NEGLECTED OR FORGOT TO RETURN QUESTN.; PAPERWORK LOST OR MISPLACED; ETC. | 18 | 67 | USABLE FOR PURPOSES OF CALCULATING LOG LIKELIHOOD RATIOS |

Fig. 4-1. Flow chart showing final dispensation of cases entering study.

were encountered. First, some of the physicians entered clinical findings (for example, hematuria or recurrent urinary tract infections) instead of diagnoses (for example, bladder tumor or chronic recurrent cystitis) when asked to state their diagnosis. They indicated that they were "100% sure" of these findings on the first questionnaire and equally sure on the second questionnaire, thus conveying no information about the effect of the IVP on *diagnostic* certainty. In some cases more than one diagnosis was stated and only one probability estimate was given. In cases of ambiguity such as these it was often possible to infer what diagnosis was being contemplated or what diagnosis the probability estimate corresponded to by critical evaluation of the accompanying probability estimates for normal versus abnormal and/or from the predictions of type and location of abnormality made on questionnaire No. 1. A second type of problem arose when a patient presented with a known chronic disease or known state (for example, postnephrectomy) and the physician entered that as his diagnosis. Properly, he should have written down a new acute problem diagnosis or complication and estimated his probability for that new diagnosis.

Deficiencies such as these prevented calculation of likelihood ratios in 10 cases. Thus a total of 67 cases were quantitatively analyzed. Table 4-1 gives the distribution of these 67 cases according to calculated log likelihood ratio. One of the advantages of the log likelihood ratio method as a measure of diagnostic usefulness as opposed to the proportion yield of abnormalities method is that the former allows the possibility of measuring the positive contribution to the diagnostic process from a normal or abnormal. Note that although the distribution for those that were normal is more skewed toward the zero end of the scale than is the distribution for the abnormal results, more than 50% of the IVPs that were interpreted as showing the patient to be normal would be judged as having made a positive diagnostic contribution. This is in direct contradiction to any standard of diagnostic usefulness based on normal studies as being of no diagnostic value.

Recall that a log likelihood ratio of zero was of special significance in terms of the diagnostic contribution of the x-ray film. Table 4-2 documents the diagnoses in cases in which the calculated log likelihood ratio was zero.

Of course, the calculation of the log likelihood ratios depends upon the numerical estimates of subjective certainty given by the physicians. There is a check upon the estimated probabilities that may be made. It is based upon the fact that if the physicians were indeed very good at assigning numerical probabilities to their subjective feeling of certainty, then in all those cases in which they stated that the probability was, say, 70%, the diagnosis stated should turn out to be the correct one in about 70% of the cases. At the time of this writing the final dispositions of too few cases are known to use this method of assessing the diagnostic probabilities.

However, the physicians were asked to state the probabilities that the IVP would show the patient to be normal versus abnormal. Using the radiologic report as a standard, we could calculate the percentage of times that the IVP was interpreted to be normal for those cases in which the physicians estimated the probability of normal in given ranges of probabilities. Strictly speaking,

Table 4-1. Distribution of log likelihood ratios for 67 cases

LLR	IVPs read as abnormal	IVPs read as normal	Total
0.0	5	15	20
0.1-0.5	7	8	15
0.6-1.0	9	5	14
1.1-1.5	7	3	10
1.6-2.0	0	3	3
2.1-2.5	2	0	2
2.6-3.0	2	0	2
3.1-3.5	1	0	1
Total	33	34	67

there are really too few cases for reliable calculations of this sort—any of the percentages are liable to large chance fluctuations. However, these figures are presented in Table 4-3 for the purpose of illustration.

Notice that we included all cases for which this specific information was available, regardless of whether it was one of the 67 cases about which we had sufficient information to calculate likelihood ratios. A total of 83 were sufficiently complete to be included. Because of the low number of cases, the percentages only roughly correspond to the estimates. In general, however, as the esti-

Table 4-2. Diagnoses for 0.0 log likelihood ratio cases*

Diagnosis	Number of cases
Essential hypertension	9
No recurrence of urethral lesion	1
Recurrent infection	1
UTI 2° infreq. voider	1
Rt. calculus—passed	1
Uninhibited neurogenic bladder	1
Benign prostatic hyperplasia	1
S/P rt. nephrectomy; inactive renal TB	1
S/P l. nephrectomy for CA kidney	1
S/P vesicopyelostomy	1
Essential hypertension/aortic aneurysm	1
IVP ordered because lab error raised question of azotemia; error discovered after IVP but before result was known to physician	1
Total	20

*In all cases the pre-IVP diagnosis and probability were the same as those given after the results of the IVP were known, except for the one case noted.

Table 4-3. Estimated probability of normal IVP result and actual outcome*

Estimated probability of normal result (%)	Result Normal	Result Abnormal	Normal result (%)
0.00-0.10	2	13	13
0.11-0.20	0	2	
0.21-0.30	0	1	33†
0.31-0.40	2	1	
0.41-0.50	4	6	
0.51-0.60	2	0	54†
0.61-0.70	1	0	
0.71-0.80	10	6	62
0.81-0.90	16	4	80
0.91-1.00	14	4	78

*Calculations were based on all nonpostoperative cases for which the necessary information was available, regardless of whether or not it was possible to calculate a likelihood ratio.
† Grouped to avoid zeros entering calculation of percentages when obviously due to low overall frequency.

Table 4-4. Correspondence between estimate of log likelihood ratio based on retrospective chart review versus that calculated from prospective information supplied by the physician

Estimated by chart reviewer	Calculated log likelihood ratio		
	0.0	Between 0.0 and 1.0	Greater than 1.0
0.0	10	5	1
Between 0.0 and 1.0	5	18	13
Greater than 1.0	0	2	1

mated probability of normal increased, so did the proportion of normal results. We consider the correspondence encouraging and feel that it shows that even busy physicians untrained in probability estimation can convey usable information with numerical estimates. (These data also suggest that too many estimates between 0% and 10% and between 90% and 100% were made. That could be a consequence of the severe distortion of the probability scale at both extremes. If so, an obvious remedy is to make all estimates in odds other than in probabilities.*)

Table 4-4 displays the results of the attempt to assess retrospectively the diagnostic contribution of the IVP based only on information contained in the medical chart. There seems to be some relation, but the precision of the categorization based on the medical record is not good overall. In fact, the radiologist was able to correctly classify according to usefulness only about 50% of the 55 cases for which classification was attempted.

Following are examples of data from three types of cases encountered in the experiment.

Case 1

Clinical problem. A 49-year-old male with recurrent left flank pain; previous IVP normal; previous transurethral resection for benign prostatic hypertrophy.

Survey data. Pre-IVP diagnosis, vesical neck contracture (20%; odds, 1:4); IVP result, left ureteropelvic junction obstruction; post-IVP diagnosis; ureteropelvic junction obstruction (99%; odds, 99:1).

Log likelihood ratio: $\log \dfrac{99}{1/4} = \log 396 = 2.60$

COMMENT: The log likelihood ratio of 2.60 is quite large and reflects the provision of an unexpected diagnosis by the IVP. At time of chart review, diagnosis (post left radical nephroureterectomy) was transitional cell carcinoma of left renal pelvis.

Case 2

Clinical problem. A 67-year-old male with urinary frequency, hesitancy, and nocturia.

Survey data. Pre-IVP diagnosis, prostatism with retention (70%; odds, 2.33:1);

---

*For more on this subject, see Edwards et al.[3]

IVP result, enlarged prostate, trabeculated bladder, PV residual, normal kidneys and ureters; post-IVP diagnosis, prostatism with retention (90%; odds, 9:1).

Log likelihood ratio: $\log \dfrac{9.00}{2.33} = \log 3.86 = 0.59$

COMMENT: The log likelihood ratio of 0.59 indicates that the IVP information had a moderate effect on certainty, although the diagnosis remained the same throughout. At time of chart review, patient was post-TUR, and diagnosis was benign prostatic hyperplasia with retention.

Case 3

Clinical problem. Asymptomatic 35-year-old female with hypertension recently discovered on routine physical examination.

Survey data. Pre-IVP diagnosis, essential hypertension (95%; odds, 19:1); IVP result, normal urinary tract; post-IVP diagnosis, essential hypertension (95%; odds, 19:1).

Log likelihood ratio: $\log \dfrac{19}{19} = \log 1 = 0.00$

COMMENT: The IVP information in the physician's judgment did not increase his already high certainty level that the true diagnosis was essential hypertension. This is quantitatively stated by the log likelihood ratio of 0.00. At chart review 6 months later, diagnosis was medically controlled essential hypertension.

Discussion

An especially practical result of this type of quantification of usefulness of information is that it readily identifies cases in which the urogram did not prove useful at all (that is, the 0.0 log likelihood ratio urograms). A zero log likelihood ratio means that the physician indicated exactly the same diagnostic certainty after the IVP that he did before the IVP. It is relatively safe to assume he would have done the same even if he were highly trained in making numerical estimates of subjective certainty. Interpretation of a 0.0 log likelihood ratio is thus much less dependent upon the quality of the numerical estimates than is interpretation of a nonzero log likelihood ratio. In addition, this method does not depend upon whether the urogram is normal or abnormal. In fact it permits the assignment of a numerical value to the usefulness of a normal urogram to the physician in his diagnostic assessment.

Identification of the zero log likelihood ratio cases makes possible another potentially useful analysis. In cases in which common denominators are identified, for example, the diagnosis of essential hypertension in patients with similar histories and physical and/or laboratory findings, a better understanding of the wisest indications for requesting excretory urograms could be developed. The goal would be to reduce the frequency of zero log likelihood ratio urograms by educating the practicing physicians in requesting urograms when they are most likely to be of diagnostic value. However, in order to produce statistically significant sign and symptom clusters, it would be necessary to study a much larger patient population.

We feel less confident of the numerical meaning on nonzero log likelihood ratios in this study. In principle, a simple linear relation exists between log likelihood ratios and diagnostic value. However, our respondents were untrained in estimating the relevant numbers, and a great deal of research on such estimates shows that their numerical meanings depend upon training. With better-trained respondents, perhaps a bit more time in which to respond, and perhaps a slightly different response mode (ideally, odds on a logarithmic scale), we believe that the full numerical properties of the log likelihood scale could be measured and exploited. For example, a ratio with log likelihood ratio in the numerator and some measure of cost of the procedure in the denominator would be a benefit-to-cost ratio of the kind familiar to management scientists and business executives. Such numbers, we believe, will some day have a role in medical decision making.

The attempt to estimate retrospectively the diagnostic contribution of the IVPs and the calculated log likelihood ratio in each case revealed that the chart information is a poor substitute for prospectively collected physicians' judgments (Table 4-4). As anyone who has reviewed medical records is well aware, the chart information really does not reflect what is going on in the physician's mind as far as diagnostic considerations and certainty are concerned. In addition, exactly when the physician received the x-ray information in the diagnostic process cannot be determined.

SUMMARY

1. The log likelihood ratio method of assessing physicians' diagnostic judgments makes it possible to measure the diagnostic usefulness of x-ray information (the urogram in our study). This method requires the collection of physicians' prior and subsequent diagnoses and the analysis of their certainty in relation to receipt of x-ray information. Logic is based on Bayes' theorem.

2. The log likelihood ratio method permits the measurement of diagnostic usefulness of *both* normal and abnormal x-ray examination results. Thus this methodology offers an alternative approach to that provided by other methods that are based on usefulness defined only in terms of abnormal x-ray results.

3. Retrospective chart review did not provide the same log likelihood results as those obtained from the prospective study; that is, the usefulness of urogram information as affecting the physician's diagnostic certainty could not be determined from review of the medical record.

4. Physicians in daily practice were able to provide diagnoses and assign a percentage number to their certainty. The quality of this data was satisfactory for log likelihood ratio calculation in 61% (67 out of 110) of urograms.

References

1. Betaque, N. E., and Gorry, G. A.: Automating judgmental decision making for a serious medical problem, Mgmt. Sci. **17**:B-421, 1971.
2. Edwards, W.: Optimal strategies for seeking information: models for statistics,

choice reaction times, and human information processing, J. Math. Psychol. **2:**312, 1965.

3. Edwards, W., Lindman, H., and Phillips, L. D.: Emerging technologies for making decisions. In New directions in psychology II, New York, 1965, Holt, Rinehart & Winston, Inc.

4. Edwards, W., Lindman, H., and Savage, L. J.: Bayesian statistical inference for psychological research, Psychol. Rev. **70:**193, 1963.

5. Edwards, W., Phillips, L. D., Hays, W. L., and Goodman, B. C.: Probabilistic information processing systems: design and evaluation, IEEE Trans. Biomed. Eng. **4:**248, 1968.

6. Ginsberg, A. S.: Decision analysis in clinical patient management with an application to the pleural-effusion syndrome, Report No. R-751-RC/NLM, Santa Monica, Calif., 1971, The Rand Corporation.

7. Gustafson, D. H.: Evaluation of probabilistic information processing in medical decision making, Org. Behav. Human Perform. **4:**20, 1969.

8. Gustafson, D. H., Kestly, J. J., Greist, J. H., and Jensen, N. M.: Initial evaluation of a subjective Bayesian diagnostic system, Health Serv. Res. **6:**204, 1971.

9. Lusted, L. B.: Introduction to medical decision making, Springfield, Ill., 1968, Charles C Thomas, Publisher.

10. Raiffa, H.: Decision analysis, Reading, Mass., 1968, Addison-Wesley Publishing Co., Inc.

11. Schlaifer, R.: Analysis of decisions under uncertainty, New York, 1968, McGraw-Hill Book Co.

12. Stäel von Holstein, C. A. S.: Assessment and evaluation of subjective probability distributions, Stockholm, 1970, The Economic Research Institute at the Stockholm School of Economics.

13. Winkler, R.: The assessment of prior distributions in Bayesian analysis, J. Am. Stat. Assoc. **62:**771, 1967.

5 Electronic imaging in diagnostic radiology

Ernest J. Sternglass, Donald Sashin, and E. Ralph Heinz

The development of high-resolution image intensifiers, television tubes, cameras, and electronic storage devices has introduced the possibility of significant advances in the techniques of diagnostic radiology by permitting electronic recording and instantaneous replay of radiographic images. Systems incorporating these components can increase diagnostic information, reduce procedure time, decrease patient trauma, reduce radiation dose, and permit new types of procedures that were previously not possible. These new electronic recording techniques have now been used in gastrointestinal examinations, selective catheterization, pediatric examinations, pelvimetry, tomography, orthopedic procedures, and neurosurgery as well as in the high-resolution transmission of radiographic film images.

CONCEPTUAL BASIS

Electronic radiography is a direct outgrowth of television fluoroscopy. By improving the image quality and providing electronic means of recording the final image, it has now become possible to eliminate some of the disadvantages of film radiography such as low sensitivity and chemical processing time, to provide instant replay, and to permit a reduction of radiation exposure to the absolute minimum.

Basically, electronic radiography is an x-ray recording technique that involves the substitution of the highly efficient photoelectric or photoconductive effect for the relatively inefficient photochemical effect that takes place in standard photographic film-screen combinations. In effect, it represents the application of the techniques of gamma-ray imaging developed in nuclear medicine to diagnostic radiology but with an order of magnitude improvement in spatial resolution.

Based in part on papers presented at the First Symposium on Electronic Imaging Techniques in Diagnostic Radiology, held at the University of Pittsburgh in April, 1973.

The work carried out at the University of Pittsburgh was supported in part by a grant from the Bureau of Radiation Health, Food and Drug Administration (1 R01 FD 00657-01), and a grant from the Pennsylvania Lions Sight Conservation and Eye Research Foundation, Inc.

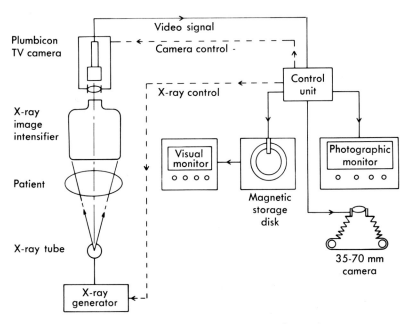

Fig. 5-1. Block diagram of typical electronic radiographic system.

This method of x-ray imaging may be understood with the aid of a schematic diagram (Fig. 5-1). X-rays produced in the usual manner are incident on the object, and those that penetrate are allowed to impinge upon the luminescent phosphor screen of an x-ray image intensifier that serves the same function as the scintillator in a scintillation counter or gamma camera. Light emitted by the phosphor screen releases photoclectrons from a thin photocathode in optical contact with the x-ray phosphor. The photoelectrons thus released are accelerated by some 30,000 volts and focused onto a small output phosphor, where they give rise to a greatly brightened image.

This intensified image is viewed by means of a television camera focused on the output phosphor of the intensifier. The optical image on the output phosphor of the intensifier is converted to an electronic charge pattern on the target of the camera tube. In effect, the camera tube target is the analog to photographic film, storing the pattern representing the spatial distribution of x-rays emerging from the object until it is read out or "developed" for further processing or viewing.

However, due to the greater quantum efficiency of the photoelectric effect as compared with the photochemical effect, this method is much more sensitive to the initial x-rays than the film technique by about a factor of 100 to 1000 times. The charge pattern produced on the camera-tube target is converted to a video signal by means of a scanning electron beam and can then be recorded by any one of the five methods discussed in the following paragraphs.

1. Historically, the first clinically successful method of recording the electrical signal produced on the television camera target involved recording on magnetic tape. However, the disadvantage of this technique lay in the fact that the image was not instantly available without rewinding the tape; thus a single frame could not be viewed for any length of time without serious deterioration. Furthermore, since only one of two interlaced fields making up a complete picture could be viewed in a static presentation and since the bandwidth of magnetic tape recorders was relatively low, the amount of detail in the image was considerably lower than could be achieved with conventional film systems. Therefore this technique was used primarily to replace spot filming in pediatric fluoroscopy.

2. The electrical signal may be recorded on a magnetic drum or on the more recently developed magnetic disk, which permits instantaneous display over a television monitor in a flicker-free manner that allows unhurried examination, exactly as does a radiograph. Aside from the great advantage of immediate availability, a modern disk recorder can store and display an image for long periods of time without significant deterioration. Furthermore, because it displays a full, interlaced picture and can be built with a bandwidth greater than that of tape recorders, the quality of the image is considerably better than that obtainable with television tape recorders. Because successive images can be precisely superimposed with each other or with a live television picture, the magnetic disk is a powerful radiographic tool that combines many of the advantages of x-ray film with the advantages of direct electrical recording, opening up a host of new clinical mapping, subtraction, and image-enhancement techniques whose clinical application has only just begun.

3. Alternatively, the electrical signal readout of the television tube may be recorded as an electrostatic charge pattern on one of the recently developed high-resolution semiconductor storage tubes for immediate examination. However, this image gradually deteriorates, and it is completely erased in a matter of 5 to 10 minutes of continuous viewing. Thus although it shares the advantage of instant availability with the magnetic disk, it lacks the permanence of a true radiographic image such as the disk can provide for later review. Furthermore, while a disk can store hundreds of images, a storage tube can handle only one or at the most four at a time. Nevertheless, it has already been applied clinically, and further developments are expected to improve both the life and quality of the image, which already exceeds that of the disk with respect to detail.

4. The electrical image stored on the target of the television camera may be recorded by photographing the screen of a high-resolution television monitor. This kinescopic technique was first successfully applied to the recording of spot films from a television tape produced during fluoroscopy in pediatric procedures. When used with the recently developed high-resolution

image intensifiers and television camera tubes, the detail that can be recorded is not limited by the bandwidth and noise characteristics of present disks and storage tubes, thus allowing the recording of electronic radiographs that equal or even exceed the image quality of typical film-screen combinations. Furthermore, it is a relatively low-cost technique and therefore lends itself potentially to mass screening procedures, with the final image recorded on 35 to 70 or 105 mm film.

5. The electrical signal from the television camera tube may also be converted to digital form with or without the aid of magnetic tapes or disks for automated analysis or processing in a digital computer. This method of electronic radiography has been made possible by the recent development of low-cost, high-speed, high-capacity digital memory units. It will clearly be of increasing value in the future in connection with the development of digital techniques of image enhancement, automated computer analysis, and the generation of quantitative information such as heart volume or calcium concentration. Furthermore, due to the great speed and flexibility of modern large-scale computer memories, the digital method of television image recording can be applied in the future to the generation of tomographic sections along the lines recently developed by British scientists, who have used a single scintillation crystal to intercept a scanning x-ray beam.

CLINICAL ADVANTAGES

As recently summarized by Lasser,[37] the following advantages of electronic recording techniques may be available to the practicing radiologist.
1. Dose reduction both to patient and staff
2. Increased speed of procedures
3. Improved tissue differentiation leading to better contrast and detail detectability
4. Saving of space if conventional large films can eventually be eliminated or greatly reduced
5. Simplified image storage and retrieval, made possible by either electronic or small format film storage
6. More rapid dissemination of the stored image through remote electronic transmission to permit faster access to present and past images
7. Potential reduction in medical costs through savings in time, space, and personnel needed for developing, filing, transporting, and retrieving diagnostic images
8. The application of on-line quantitative measurements of metabolic and physiologic events, including recording dynamic events at the microscopic level
9. Direct application to computer analysis of diagnostic images

PHYSICAL BASES FOR ADVANTAGES OF ELECTRONIC RADIOGRAPHY OVER FILM

Electronic techniques of recording an x-ray image possess fundamental physical advantages over film-screen systems in two important respects: (1) sensitivity or speed ꞏnd (2) ability to see small contrast.

Sensitivity

As first recognized in astronomy,[7] the photoelectric effect has a much higher quantum efficiency than even the fastest films available by about 100 times. Thus film-screen systems can at best record 1 out of 200 to 500 visible photons incident on an emulsion,[7] while modern photocathodes can convert typically 1 out of every 3 to 5 visible photons into photoelectrons independently of the rate at which the photons arrive or the total magnitude of the exposure.

Since with the aid of high-gain image intensifiers every photoelectron can be amplified sufficiently to be recorded as a distinct event, there is a fundamental advantage in sensitivity to the electronic method of recording images that leads to a series of indirect advantages. These are briefly summarized as follows:

1. Reduced exposure time with an attendant greater ability to stop motion
2. Reduction in focal spot size due to a reduced need for high x-ray intensity
3. Reduction in patient dose whenever this is an important consideration
4. Possibility of heavy selective filtration to produce quasi-monochromatic radiation with its greater inherent contrast
5. Use of larger geometric magnification to bring out fine detail
6. Greater use of air-gap techniques to reduce the effect of scattered radiation

Contrast detectability

As recognized during the early development of the x-ray image intensifier and in applications of image intensification in astronomy,[7,13,62,84] the ultimate limit to the ability to detect the small contrast differences encountered is set by the number of incident quanta or "events" that can be recorded per picture element, either before saturation takes place or before the film becomes too dark.

When the number of photons representing the original signal is too small, producing too weak a signal, then the detection of the signal against the background noise produced by the random variation in the number of recorded photons per picture element becomes impossible.

Thus, when only 100 x-ray photons are recorded, the normal statistical fluctuation of ± 100 or ± 10 makes it impossible to perceive a true patient contrast of less than $\pm 10\%$, or 10 out of 100 photons absorbed.

Typical x-ray film contains some 10,000 developable grains/mm². Thus even when nearly all the grains are sensitized and the film is almost saturated to its maximum useful density of 2.0 to 2.5, it is impossible to detect contrast differences smaller than those due to the normal statistical fluctuation of 100 out of 10,000, or less than 1%. When film is only lightly exposed, typically to densities of 0.20 to 0.25 just above the normal fog, there are 10 times fewer exposed grains per unit area, and the smallest detectable contrast is some three times larger, or about 3%.

In actual practice the eye requires about two to three times the minimum fluctuation or noise for positive recognition of a true density difference,[13,82] so that film-screen combinations limit the ability to see small contrast differences to the range of 2% to 5% in the actual clinical situation for an object size of about 1 mm and to even larger limiting contrasts for smaller object sizes.

In fact, since the image element area varies as the square of its diameter, a reduction in size of the detail desired leads to a quadratic increase in the number of quanta that must be recorded per unit area. Calling N the number of quanta that must be recorded per square millimeter, f the spatial frequency of the detail in line pairs per millimeter, and C the contrast (using $C = 1.0$ as 100%), one has the relation:

$$N = k(f^2/C^2) \qquad (1)$$

where k is an empirical constant measuring the number of statistical standard deviations in the random fluctuations required by the eye to detect a true "signal" or contrast difference, typically between 1 and 3.

Equation 1 can also be solved for the minimum contrast that can be detected, giving:

$$C = f\sqrt{k}/\sqrt{N} \qquad (2)$$

Thus in order to decrease the detectable contrast the number of recorded quanta N must be increased greatly; this can only be done by resorting to a recording medium other than x-ray film.

Electronic techniques can achieve this because the process of x-ray quantum interception or conversion to an electronic charge can be separated from the process of storing the charge. Unlike film, in which the grain of silver halide both intercepts the photon and stores the information as a black grain, electronic detectors can employ a separate storage medium, as first achieved in the gamma camera.[2]

In the simplest case one can use a photomultiplier to scan the image elements one by one, as in nuclear medicine, and register the photon counts in a mechanical register or digital computer memory of essentially unlimited storage capacity. This was in fact the approach used by Moon[46] in the early 1950s, and it is at the basis of the recently developed EMI transverse axial tomographic technique,[17a,51] which is able to visualize contrast differences of 0.1% to 0.3%, some 10 times smaller than can be visualized with x-ray film.

Alternatively, one can use television camera tubes with storage surfaces to accumulate the photoelectrons or photoconductive charges released as temporary or "buffer" storage elements before they are read out and permanently recorded on another medium.[82,89]

Typical camera tubes can record some 10^6 to 10^8 electronic charges/mm^2 of target area.[82,96] Thus even with a 10:1 reduction in size of the image, they can record 10^4 to 10^6 separate "events" for each square millimeter of patient area, assuming each absorbed x-ray quantum leads to about one "event" of an electron stored or to a minimum detectable contrast C of about 0.3% to 3.0%. Furthermore, by using repeated images and superimposing them on a storage tube or in a digital memory, as is now being done in applications in astronomy,[14,15,96] a further factor of 3 to 10 reductions in the minimum detectable contrast can be achieved with camera tubes, in effect further extending their dynamic range compared to film.

Such an enhancement of contrast detectability and dynamic range beyond that attainable with x-ray film is made possible without excessive patient dose due to the 100-fold greater sensitivity of the photoelectric process.

Thus it is clear that the electronic technique of recording a radiographic image opens up a new era in diagnostic radiology in which the detectable contrast for soft tissues and tumors can exceed by an order of magnitude what has been possible to visualize with x-ray film in the past.

Aside from these basic physical advantages, the electronic technique also possesses the practical advantages that arise from the direct production of image information in the form of electronic signals, which can be rapidly recorded, manipulated, and displayed for immediate examination. Thus, depending upon the particular application, either the improved image quality, the reduction in dose, or the greater convenience and saving of time may be of greatest practical value in the actual clinical use of electronic image recording.

TECHNICAL ASPECTS OF ELECTRONIC
PHOTOGRAPHY SYSTEMS

In order to achieve the ultimate aim of replacing x-ray film techniques with electronic recording, three different sets of technical problems must be solved. Briefly, they may be listed as follows:

1. The efficient conversion of x-rays to visible light photons at resolutions equaling or exceeding those obtained in actual screen-film combinations under clinical conditions
2. The production of an intermediate electrical image comparable to the photographic image in dynamic range and signal-to-noise ratio
3. The recording of the electrical image onto a storage medium of matching resolution and dynamic range from which single frames can be recalled nondestructively for immediate viewing and further processing

Conversion of x-ray to visible image

In the case of diagnostic x-ray imaging, three different avenues are open to accomplish the conversion of x-rays to a visible image; each approach possesses certain advantages, depending upon the application.

1. Imaging a large fluorescent screen onto an image intensifier of small cathode area by means of a high-efficiency optical system[47]
2. Use of an image intensifier with a diameter of 6 to 9 inches that has a very thin but highly efficient x-ray phosphor such as a thin CsI crystal inside the vacuum envelope[22,53,59]
3. Use of a special image intensifier* in which a vacuum-tight fiber optics faceplate replaces the front of the glass envelope, permitting the use of very thin but highly efficient x-ray phosphors on the outside surface of the tube

In all three approaches a very high x-ray absorption efficiency can be reached for the incident x-rays with phosphor thickness that will not limit the overall resolution to less than the desired values of 3 to 5 line pairs per millimeter (lp/mm) that are realized in most practical radiography today with typical x-ray focal spots. Thus a sheet of CsI only 0.1 mm thick will absorb close to 60% of all incident quanta at an average energy of 40 keV.[91,92] Such a thin receptor thickness is considerably smaller than the combined thickness of typical film-screen combinations, so that the inherent detail rendition capability of electronic techniques is greater than that of fast film-screen systems.

The major difference between the use of a large-area screen with mirror or lens imaging and the use of a somewhat smaller x-ray image intensifier is in the efficiency with which the emitted light is transferred to the photocathode of the device where the light is initially converted to photoelectrons. Geometric conditions are such that only a few percent of all the photons from each x-ray quantum can be collected from a large screen, while approximately 40% to 50% of all light quanta can be collected in the case of the x-ray image tubes in which the phosphor is in close proximity to the photo surface. Thus the latter approach will necessarily lead to a higher signal-to-noise ratio regardless of how much subsequent gain is introduced, since the initial collection efficiency will be the determining factor.

Accordingly, x-ray image intensifiers have been used as the x-ray conversion device in most early work, although the recent development of more efficient phosphors[10,19] and more sensitive camera tube cathodes may prove to make it possible to return to the use of an optical system focused directly onto a fluorescent phosphor screen,[3,63] thus avoiding the inevitable contrast loss of image intensifiers.

Initial experiments in this field were carried out with first-generation intensifiers, but in order to obtain the necessary resolution and conversion effi-

---

*Six-inch fiber optics faceplate image intensifier, The Aerojet-Delft Corp., Melville, N. Y.

ciency at high energies, special thin-screen CsI tubes now commercially available were used in most of the recent work.[53] A fiber optics faceplate intensifier was also successfully employed in early experiments since it provides a unique flexibility in optimizing the phosphor thickness for the requirements of maximum absorption and minimum thickness to attain the highest overall performance at various x-ray energies although at about twice the cost of standard intensifiers.

Visible to electrical charge image conversion

For the next stage in the system, it is necessary to utilize a television camera tube capable of accepting and storing a charge pattern over a wide dynamic range that can be read out as completely as possible in a single scan. Furthermore, the sensitivity must be such that the least number of photoelectrons released in the intensifier per x-ray photon absorbed will give rise to a signal in the camera tube output that is capable of overriding the amplifier noise. The first such camera tube,[25] originally developed for stellar photometry from an orbiting astronomic observatory under NASA sponsorship,[14] has more recently also found wide application in ground-based astronomy, as for example in the guidance of the 200-inch telescope of Mt. Palomar.[15]

This camera tube, known as the SEC camera tube (SEC is the abbreviation for secondary electron conduction), employs a very thin target of aluminum oxide coated with a conductive layer of aluminum onto the back of which a low-density layer of KC1 has been deposited.[25] Electrons from the photocathode are accelerated by some 8 to 10 keV so as to penetrate the target and produce secondary electrons in the low-density layer away from the photocathode. These secondary electrons are then rapidly drawn out of the layer by an electric field,[81] leaving behind a positive charge that represents the "latent image" equivalent to that stored in photographic film or xerography.

Due to the very high resistivity of this surface, the charge pattern can be stored for many minutes if desired, as is the case for the astronomic application[96] or the application to gamma-ray isotope imaging.[82] Also, the high energy of the incident photoelectrons leads to the production of up to 200 secondary electrons or stored charges per incident primary charge, thereby leading to a gain of up to 200 before any subsequent readout process with its inevitable introduction of noise.

As a result, this camera tube possesses characteristics strikingly similar to those of photographic film in terms of ability to store an image of wide dynamic range, but it has the advantage of direct electrical storage such that the charge stored is uniquely related to the number of photons incident. In effect, it can be shown that for stored charges close to 10^4 per picture element needed to attain a photon noise–limited signal-to-noise ratio of $\sqrt{10^4} = 100$, this device behaves like an ideal array of thousands of photomultipliers insofar as its approach to theoretical performance is concerned.[96]

The advantages over the earlier types of camera tubes may be summarized as follows:

1. Larger dynamic range than the image orthicon
2. Direct proportionality between incident photon flux and accumulated charge for quantitative measurements
3. Image storage without appreciable charge leakage before readout
4. Greatly reduced interference between adjacent picture elements as compared to the image orthicon
5. Essentially complete readout of the stored image in a single scan, unlike the case of the image orthicon or vidicon
6. Built-in image intensification up to approximately 200 as compared to the vidicon

Another camera tube possessing important advantages over the earlier vidicon and image orthicon is the image isocon.[48] It is closely related to the image orthicon in its general structure, but it differs in the method of readout of the stored charge pattern on its target. By arranging for the scanning electron beam to produce electrons that are scattered backward to the internal photomultiplier only in areas in which a signal is present, the high noise in the dark areas of pictures produced by the image orthicon is eliminated, resulting in a much "quieter" performance and therefore much higher contrast.

Therefore the following are the advantages of the isocon.

1. Excellent contrast rendition or image-transfer characteristics
2. High limiting spatial resolution or detail reproduction
3. Excellent dynamic range capability
4. Better contrast rendition at very low contrasts and light levels than the SEC vidicon
5. Availability in large photocathode sizes of 1.6 to 3.25 inches, thus providing many resolution elements across the image diameter

The major disadvantages of both of these new types of camera tubes are their higher cost and larger bulk compared with the vidicon and plumbicon tubes now most widely used in x-ray television systems. Therefore only in special applications is the cost of these tubes justified. In fact, for most fluoroscopic purposes and special applications requiring only moderate resolution, such as pelvimetry, for example, or the placement of catheters and needles during interventional procedures, present vidicons and plumbicons are more than adequate.

Thus the future of electronic radiography is no longer limited by the quality of the early television camera tubes on which the development of commercial television was based.

As to the spatial resolution presently available, vidicon tubes with target diameters of 16 to 18 mm have demonstrated limiting resolutions of about 40 lp/mm corresponding to 80 television lines/mm or 1200 television lines across the target raster. For a 6-inch or 150 mm diameter image tube, this represents a limiting resolution of some 12 television lines or 6 lp/mm, a level approaching or even exceeding the detail in typical radiographs using par-speed intensifying screens.

Final recording and visual display

The last major component in a completely electronic radiography system is represented by the final recording means, which must also provide a visual display on command without affecting in any way the original image needed for permanent storage.

Until a few years ago, the only available means of electrical storage for video signals did not lend themselves to the needs of clinically useful electronic radiography. These were rather low-quality electrostatic storage tubes or magnetic tape recorders that were unable to display a single image for any appreciable time without unacceptable levels of deterioration. New technical developments have now completely changed the situation both in magnetic and electrostatic recording, and in addition, there has been a breakthrough in the cost of large digital techniques of image storage.

Magnetic disks. A new method of analog information storage that has been developed in the last few years offers the necessary quality of picture information combined with rapid access and indefinitely long life. This is the magnetic disk storage system originally developed for digital information storage but now developed to store video television signals of a quality that is able to meet the requirements of electronic radiography.* In fact, these devices represent the practical realization of the potential first indicated by the magnetic drum recorder used for x-ray recording by Schut and Oosterkamp.[73]

The basic disk unit consists of an aluminum plate about the size of an ordinary phonograph record. It is coated with a thin layer of magnetic material and a protective coating that permits continuous reading of any given television frame over any desired time period without any detectable deterioration, since the magnetic reading head is physically separated from the disk surface by a thin layer of air. Each television frame is recorded on a single narrow track a few thousandths of an inch wide, so that 100 to 500 complete radiograms can be stored on one side of such a disk, which may store a total of 200 to 1000 pictures, depending upon the signal-to-noise ratio desired. A magnetic pickup head can be indexed to move rapidly to any one of the tracks in a matter of seconds, or multiple heads can be used to give access in as little as the television frame time of 1/30 second.

At the present time the frequency response of commercially available disks ranges from 4 megacycles to 6 mHz, and disks capable of handling even higher quality television images in the range of 10 to 12 mHz are now under development. A low-cost disk recorder unit that has become commercially available

---

*Videodisc recorder, model No. VDR 200MM, MVR Corp., Sunnyvale, Calif.

within the last year uses a removable plastic disk whose image quality approaches that of the metal disk units.

Most important is the fact that magnetic disks have demonstrated important capabilities of manipulating the images recorded so as to achieve precise subtraction, edge enhancement, and isodose contour plotting by simple analog techniques.[76,93]

Electrostatic storage tubes. Although the magnetic disk possesses the great advantages of being able to record many images of wide dynamic range for unlimited storage and replay, there are certain aspects of recently developed storage tubes that give them unique advantages for special purposes.

The early storage tubes, such as those used in the pioneering work of Wallman and Wickbom,[90] were of the direct viewing type and were not only poor in contrast rendition and resolution but also very costly. Within the last few years, a whole new family of low-cost storage tubes has been developed; these provide an electrical method of readout of a much higher picture quality that is comparable to what can be achieved with high-resolution camera tubes. These tubes have silicon storage targets capable of resolving 1000 to 2000 television lines and able to store an image for hours without appreciable loss of quality.[30,56] The image may be viewed for several minutes; the dynamic range or gray-scale rendition is far superior to that attainable with the early electrostatic storage devices and about the same as that obtained with magnetic disks.

The following are the principal advantages of these new tubes compared to disks.

1. They are small, compact, lightweight devices without any moving parts.
2. The cost of the tubes is only a few hundred dollars, although the associated circuitry brings the price into the range of a few thousand dollars.
3. The detail rendition or spatial resolution attainable is greater than for any disk unit presently available, equivalent to a bandwidth of the order of 30 mHz as compared to magnetic disks typically able to handle 4 to 6 mHz.
4. The storage tubes permit the summing or differencing of many separate television frames, and in general, they allow certain image enhancement operations to be carried out with greater ease than magnetic disks.

As a result of these characteristics, it appears that storage tubes will prove to be particularly useful in certain special applications such as the detection and measurement of very small density differences along the lines recently demonstrated by Mistretta et al.[44,45] at the University of Wisconsin.

Digital storage systems. In the last few years, rapid advances have also taken place in the techniques of converting the video signal produced in the readout of the stored charge image of television camera tube targets into digital form and storing it in digital memories, beginning with the application of television tubes in orbiting observatories.[14] The development of low-cost solid-state digital memories is progressing so rapidly that the cost of a memory to store the information contained in a single standard television frame, typically 1 to 2 million bits when 64 distinct gray levels are encoded, is expected to decline to some $20,000 in the near future, a cost comparable to that of high-quality magnetic disk recording systems.

Since in the application to single-frame electronic radiography there is no need to accomplish the readout at the high repetition rates of 30 frames/sec used in commercial television, there are no severe requirements on the speed of the analog-to-digital converter, although such high-speed converters are now available.

The following are the advantages of direct digital television readout and storage.

1. Compatibility with computer analysis of radiographs for quantitative measurements of organ volumes[94] and densities[11]
2. Ease of digital image quality enhancement[74,75] of the type originally developed for space applications
3. Compatibility with techniques of computer diagnosis presently under development[17]
4. No spatial distortion
5. Good signal-to-noise ratio
6. No moving parts
7. Accurate subtraction and addition of images
8. Essentially unlimited precision in the detection of small contrast differences well below the typical 1% to 2% discrimination capability of film and the unaided human eye, resulting from the large number of individual x-ray quantum events that can be stored per picture element

As computer technology advances and memory costs are further reduced, it is to be expected that direct digital recording of radiographic images will be increasingly used whenever quantitative information and complex image manipulations such as automated analysis or tomographic presentation are required.

Thus a whole new era of electronic image enhancement has been opened up by these new recording means, which seem to be ideally suited for the purposes of radiography when combined with the new high-resolution image intensifiers and camera tubes of the SEC and isocon type.

OVERALL IMAGING PERFORMANCE CAPABILITIES

The overall performance of an electronic radiography system is determined by the combined image-handling characteristics of all of its individual components as measured by the product of their respective modulation transfer function (MTF).[88]

The MTF of a given component is essentially nothing but a measure of the contrast reduction suffered by the image reproduced at different spatial frequencies or by features of different sizes measured in line pairs per millimeter.

The useful limiting resolution in an image reproduced by a given component is generally taken to be that detail size for which a 100% contrast in the input image is reduced to a barely discernible contrast of 5% in the output image.

Not only must the intensifier and TV camera chain MTF characteristics be considered in designing a complete system, but the equivalent MTF of the focal spot of the x-ray tube under the given geometric conditions must be taken into account.

Reduction in focal spot blurring by use of smaller focal spots

To illustrate the importance of the focal spot in limiting the overall performance of a radiographic system in actual clinical situations, Fig. 5-2 shows the MTF of a 0.3 and a 1.0 mm spot in the geometry used for gastrointestinal fluoroscopy and spot filming, respectively.[68] In the first case the limiting resolution is 5.0 lp/mm, while in the second case, normally used for taking the standard spot film, the limiting resolution is 1.5 lp/mm.

Thus no matter how well the other components perform, the focal spot can be the limiting factor in actual practice. This is illustrated in Fig. 5-3, which shows the overall performance of a standard spot film requiring the use of the 1.0 mm focal spot, and an electronically recorded spot film, for which the 0.3 mm spot may be used because of the much lower dose and thus lower x-ray

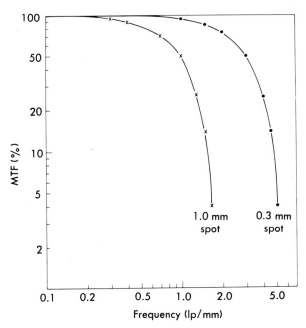

Fig. 5-2. Comparison of resolution and contrast performance of 0.3 and 1.0 mm focal spots used in electronic and standard spot films, respectively.

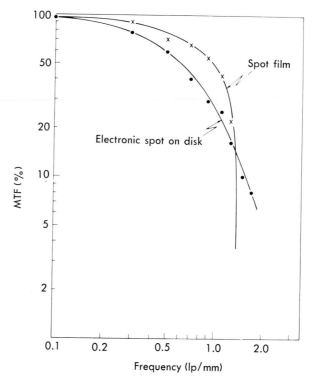

Fig. 5-3. Comparison of resolution of spot film and electronic radiographic image stored on disk recorder. Note that limiting resolution of standard spot films is determined by spot size.

tube current required when the photoelectric effect replaces chemical photography.

This example illustrates one of the important indirect advantages of electronic radiography, namely, the possibility of using much smaller focal spots than could be used with standard film, an advantage that follows from the greater efficiency with which x-ray quanta are utilized. Thus although standard film-screen combinations are in principle capable of achieving much higher spatial resolution than simple vidicon television camera and recording systems, in actual practice patient motion and the need to use large focal spots for spot filming so greatly limits the spatial resolution attainable that even a relatively low-cost television recording system can approach film with regard to resolution.

In general, the design of the system must be such that the performance of each component is arranged so as not to degrade significantly the image quality produced by the most critical components in the chain, generally the image intensifier and the disk recorder. Thus to achieve the highest possible spatial resolution, direct viewing of a thin x-ray phosphor screen by means of an optical system that focuses the image on a high-resolution camera tube must be utilized, the final image being recorded by photographing a cathode ray monitor capable of reproducing 3000 television lines.

Alternatively, the final image may be recorded on tape or in a digital memory using a slow-scan readout technique that permits a low bandwidth for the recording system.

Reduction in motion blurring by reduction in exposure length

The electronic technique of radiographic recording not only permits the use of finer focal spots as a result of its inherently greater efficiency but also offers the possibility of reducing the effects of object motion, which often limit the attainable resolution of radiographic systems in actual clinical situations by the use of shorter exposure times. Thus if object motion happens to be a limiting factor, exposure times one tenth to one hundredth of present values can typically be used before the ultimate limit set by quantum noise is reached.

Enhancement of inherent contrast by use of monochromatic radiation

When improved contrast rendition is of prime concern, electronic radiography allows the use of very heavy selective filtration to produce nearly monochromatic radiation from existing diagnostic x-ray tubes, as has recently been shown by Huen et al.[31,32,69] Since modern rotating anode tubes are capable of producing very high outputs so as to expose standard film adequately in a fraction of a second, it is possible to filter out 95% to 99% of the beam and still achieve adequately short exposures with the remaining narrow portion of the continuous spectrum when electronic means are used to record the image. Thus the development of high-resolution electronic imaging systems able to utilize x-ray quanta some 100 times more efficiently than film has opened the way to the practical realization of monochromatic x-ray techniques long recognized as possessing important advantages over the use of continuous spectrum radiation.[52,87]

The use of heavy selective filtration has therefore made it possible to produce quasi-monochromatic x-ray beams of small focal spot size designed to maximize the contrast for iodine and barium contrast media with an energy width of only about 12 keV, as illustrated in Fig. 5-4. This was achieved with a transmission of 5% of the original number of quanta through a filter consisting of a series of metals in the atomic number range $Z = 58$ to 64. Contrast improvements for low concentrations of contrast media of the order of 40% were obtainable relative to the normal x-ray beam.[31,32,69]

Further improvements in contrast detectability are possible with electronic recording through the use of K-edge subtraction when sufficiently intense monochromatic radiation can be obtained, as in the case of the multiple filtration technique. Thus very small density differences of contrast media in blood

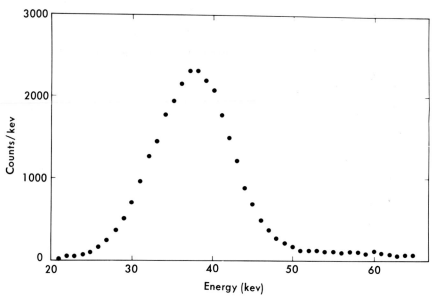

Fig. 5-4. A 65 kVp x-ray spectrum after beam has been filtered by composite filter.

vessels or even naturally occurring concentrations of various elements such as iodine in the thyroid can be visualized by using two sets of filters to reproduce images at two different photon wavelengths or energies, one located just above and one just below the absorption discontinuity at the K-edge of the element to be visualized, and subtracting the two images from each other.

The principle of this technique has long been recognized,[33,34,40] but only the great sensitivity of electronic recording and the resulting feasibility of the filtration technique to produce quasi-monochromatic beams combined with the possibility of electronically storing and superimposing successive images has brought this technique to the point where it has become clinically practicable.

By using two separate electronic storage devices, one for carrying out the initial subtraction and one for accumulating the small differences generated in a series of successive subtractions, the limits presently imposed by the saturation of the storage capacity of the recording means such as film can be overcome. As a result, the extremely small density differences that require the recording of millions of x-ray quanta per picture element, far in excess of the storage capacity of either film or television camera tube targets, can be visualized.

As an example, if one wishes to detect density differences as small as 0.1%, or 1 part in 1000, it is necessary to record 1 million separate events per picture element to sufficiently overcome the inherent statistical fluctuations, which are given by the square root of the number of independent events. This problem can be solved through the successive accumulation of the small difference signals in a series of subtraction processes by using a second electronic storage tube, as recently successfully demonstrated by Mistretta.[44,45]

As these results demonstrate, it may become possible to visualize various soft organs and tumors using external beams, either by virtue of the natural concentrations of certain elements or by the use of special contrast agents in a manner analogous to the use of radioisotopes but with much greater spatial resolution, shorter exposures, and lower doses to other parts of the body.

Increase in inherent object contrast through use of lower x-ray energies

The use of the more sensitive electronic techniques increase the ability to detect small contrast differences in the x-ray image, and these techniques also allow the use of lower x-ray photon energies for which the inherent contrast between tissues of different densities and chemical composition can be considerably greater but that can normally not be used because of insufficient penetration.

Again, it is the fact that the total number of quanta needed to produce an adequate image is much less when the more efficient photoelectric process is used, which makes it possible to utilize less penetrating radiation. This has important application to situations in which soft tissue contrast is of primary importance, as in mammography. This particular application of electronic techniques therefore shows special promise, not only because of the possibility of improving the chances of earlier diagnosis but also because of the significantly lower dose required to record the necessary number of x-ray photons when newly developed, highly efficient, thin x-ray phosphors can be combined with high-resolution television cameras.[63]

In fact, because of the relation between the number of quanta needed to detect a certain contrast difference at the quantum noise limit for a given spatial resolution (equation 1), it is clear that any improvement in the inherent contrast permits a sharp reduction in the number of quanta needed and therefore in the dose. Thus an increase of inherent contrast by a factor of two allows a reduction in dose by a factor of four when the system operates at the ultimate limit set by quantum noise, an important consideration when mass screening of many individuals in the population is contemplated.

Increase in contrast through reduction in scattered radiation reaching image plane

An additional advantage of being able to use lower x-ray beam energies is the fact that there is less Compton scattering relative to photoelectric absorption and thereby a further improvement in the contrast of the image due to a reduction in the fogging produced by the scattered radiation emerging from the patient.

The reduction in scattered radiation can be further enhanced by the use of the so-called air-gap technique, in which the distance between the patient and the image detector plant is increased so that the scattered radiation is distributed over a larger area.[88] Although this technique can be employed with film, it is limited both by the increased loss of spatial resolution when large focal spots must be employed to achieve adequate densities and by the reduction in primary beam intensity when the distance to the detector plane is increased. Since the electronic technique permits a smaller focal spot and needs fewer photons at the detector plane, the air-gap technique can be used to greater advantage in electronic radiography.

Finally, the amount of scattered radiation that reaches the image plane can be still further reduced through the use of a scanning x-ray beam whose motion is synchronized with that of a small detector, which intercepts only the direct primary radiation. This idea was first investigated by Moon,[46] who used a photoelectric detector, and it has more recently been applied in the EMI system for producing an axial tomogram by computer techniques.[17a]

The same principle can also be applied in the use of a thin, fan-shaped beam of x-rays scanning the object; a moving slit is used at the x-ray tube and a synchronously moving slit is used at the detector plant. This method of reducing the amount of scattered radiation recorded in the image dates back to the early years of radiology. It can be advantageously adapted to electronic radiography by substituting an electronic "gate" in the television camera system for the mechanical slit moving across the film, thus greatly reducing the loss of contrast from scattered radiation.

CLINICAL APPLICATIONS
Historical background and initial application in pediatrics

Historically, the first successful attempts to utilize electronic means of recording a static x-ray image[9] date back to the development of the x-ray image intensifier by Coltman[12] and his associates at the Westinghouse Research Laboratories and by the research group at the Philips Laboratories[86] in Eindhoven shortly after World War II.

The intensified image was photographed with either standard 35 mm or Polaroid film, thus providing a permanent record. However, the relatively low brightness gain of the early intensifiers, their small size, and their limited spatial resolution did not make a widespread replacement of standard films possible. This technique, however, was subsequently developed to permit both a practical method of cineradiography and 75 to 105 mm single-frame images whose quality has in recent years approached that of standard spot films[3] at doses typically some 5 to 10 times lower than those needed for standard x-ray film.

The next step in the development of electronic radiography was made possible by the application of television techniques to fluorescent screen intensification, beginning with the direct viewing system using an image orthicon focused on a large fluorescent screen that was developed by Morgan and Sturm at

Johns Hopkins University in 1951.[47] Shortly thereafter, television tubes were optically coupled to the x-ray image intensifier,[6,29] providing a further substantial gain in brightness close to the limit set by quantum noise considerations as worked out by Coltman[13] on the basis of analogous studies by Rose[60] for visible light.

These technical developments set the stage for the first clinically applied electronic systems for displaying single images in 1958 and 1959, when magnetic tape,[23,36] magnetic drums,[73] and electrostatic storage tubes[90] were first employed to present instantaneously available static images for clinical examination. However, the limitations of these early storage devices, discussed previously, prevented their widespread use for recording permanent images.

The major exception appears to have been in the application of video recording to spot filming in pediatric applications, developed by Girdany at Children's Hospital in Pittsburgh beginning in 1960.[23,24] Girdany was able to obtain satisfactory spot films for all his fluoroscopic procedures in children by kinescopically recording single images from a television monitor at x-ray tube currents of only 0.01 to 0.10 mA compared with the 1 to 10 mA needed for adults. This corresponds to dose rates of as little as 0.01 rad/min at the tabletop or to doses per frame of less than one millionth of a rad, very close to the ultimate limit expected on the basis of quantum noise limitations for a resolution of 1 mm.

Using the best available magnetic tape recorders and television cameras developed during the 1960s, Girdany has been able to routinely demonstrate esophageal varices and pyloric stenosis, the most demanding images that the pediatric radiologist has to deal with. Thus it has been possible to take a series of 20 to 30 electronic spot films during cystography without any additional radiation beyond the small amount needed for the 3-minute fluoroscopic procedure itself, or well below 0.1 rad total dose in the typical pediatric situation.

The next steps toward a clinically useful electronic radiography technique were made possible by the development of the high-resolution magnetic disk* in the mid-1960s.[93] For the first time, hundreds of truly permanent, flicker-free, low-noise images could be obtained for instantaneous presentation and unhurried examination by the fluoroscopist, in effect permitting a return to direct diagnosis from a fluoroscopic image as in the early days of radiology but without the presence of x-rays during image examination.

This potential was recognized independently by two groups, one at Emory University[42] and the other at Westinghouse[76]; it led to the development of the first commercially available electronic disk storage unit for the display of individual images capable of precision subtraction and arterial mapping, which was demonstrated at the 1968 Radiological Society of North America meeting in Chicago.

---

*Videodisc recorder model No. VDR 200MM, MVR Corp., Sunnyvale, Calif.

Initial applications in the departments of radiology at Emory University[42] and the University of Pittsburgh[18,67] were to "intermittent fluoroscopy" to achieve dose reduction, primarily in connection with gastrointestinal studies and the catheterization of the heart and great vessels.[42,64]

Single electronic radiographs were recorded by momentarily increasing the x-ray tube current by 5 to 10 times so as to present an image more nearly equivalent in quantum noise to that seen by the human eye, which integrates about 5 television frames in 0.2 second. Disks, storage tubes, and direct photography from a monitor were used in this way to record single images in pediatric and obstetric radiology.

As will be described, these initial clinical trials were followed by the extensive application of disk systems to arterial mapping; the maps were subsequently used to guide catheters and needles during interventional procedures, opening the way for the kind of new surgical and biopsy techniques anticipated in the late 1950s.

With the availability of high-resolution CsI tubes, the quality of the images improved significantly, so that spot films recorded electronically on a disk have been found to provide essentially the same diagnostic quality as 105 mm films without the need to wait for chemical development and at doses some 10 to 30 times lower than standard gastrointestinal spot films.

Obstetric applications

Electronic pelvimetry. The standard technique of film radiography for pelvimetry necessitates irradiating the fetus to levels that appear to carry a significant risk.[26,83] The amount of radiation necessary to achieve adequate film density is much greater than that required by quantum noise considerations alone.

With electronic radiography the radiation exposure in the direct beam is about one hundredth that required with film, and by adapting the method to orthopelvimetry[50] and exposing only a small field at each extremity of the diameter to be measured, the total fetal exposure is reduced by factors of 1000 to 10,000 and direct irradiation of maternal ovaries is avoided (Fig. 5-5).[65,72]

Two methods of recording the image for pelvimetry have been evaluated; these are the Polaroid television technique and electronic radiography using a silicon storage tube.

Polaroid television technique. The Polaroid television technique is the simplest and least expensive method. It involves directly photographing the image on the television monitor with a Polaroid camera.[71] Most television fluoroscopic units can be modified at the relatively low cost of about $500. Image quality has been adequate for accurate measurements. Radiation exposure in the direct beam has been measured as 3 mr, about 1/100 that encountered in standard film pelvimetry. Fetal exposure from scattered radiation is estimated to have been between 0.03 and 0.3 mr, or less than the daily dose from normal background radiation.

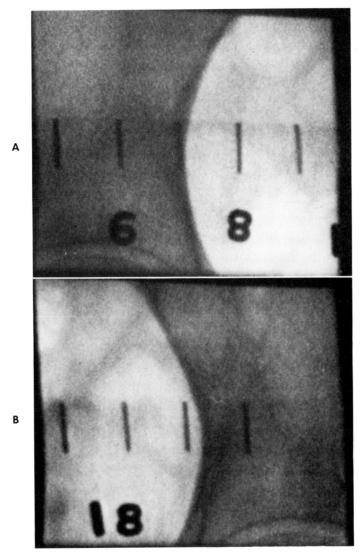

Fig. 5-5. A, Polaroid fluoroscopic image, taken of right edge of pelvic inlet, and ruler permitted measurement of pelvis in anteroposterior view. **B,** Polaroid fluoroscopic image of left edge of pelvic inlet has detail adequate to permit determination of crossing point of ruler and pelvic bone.

In summary, electronic Polaroid pelvimetry gives adequate clinical information with negligible fetal and maternal exposure to radiation. It can be adapted inexpensively to most television fluoroscopic systems and can be operated by one person without special training.

Electronic radiography using silicon storage tube. Electronic radiography using a silicon storage tube does not necessarily require photographing the monitor. A silicon storage tube is coupled to the fluoroscopic television chain.[72] The fluoroscopic television image is stored in the storage tube and instantly replayed on the monitor with the x-rays off. This image has less contrast than that obtained with the Polaroid technique, but it is adequate for its purpose. It can be viewed continuously for about 5 minutes before it decays, which is ample time to read the measurements.

Radiation dosages were found to be about half those encountered with the Polaroid technique.

Intrauterine fetal transfusion. Conventional methods of controlling catheter placement for intrauterine fetal transfusion using film radiograph or fluoroscopy involve a high fetal and maternal radiation dosage, thus presenting a possible risk.[26,83] With film radiography, handling and processing time prolong the examination, increasing the risk of trauma due to fetal movement and displacement of the needle. The principle and basic apparatus used for intrauterine transfusion are the same as for electronic Polaroid pelvimetry.[70-72]

Contrast and resolution are adequate to identify the fetal spine, the needle, the catheter, and the pattern of contrast material in the fetal peritoneal cavity. With this system, radiation to the fetus is reduced by a factor of about 100. Processing time for Polaroid films is about 15 seconds, greatly reducing the time for the procedure. The costs of adapting a standard television fluoroscopic system are low, and film costs are reduced.

Stereotaxic treatment of intracranial aneurysms

In order to reduce the operative morbidity and mortality in the treatment of intracranial aneurysms, researchers at a number of institutions have been investigating treatment techniques using transarterial and stereotaxic approaches.[1,49] The clinical application of these new procedures, which require the exact positioning of probes, has been limited by the need to use standard film radiography. Electronic radiography eliminates many of the disadvantages of ordinary film radiography in the placement of stereotaxic needles for the treatment of aneurysms and has now been developed to the point where it can be operated by the neurosurgeon himself.

The system of electronic radiography for neurosurgical procedures developed at the University of Pittsburgh[65,66,72] is composed of a two-track magnetic disk recorder (Westinghouse Videodisc recorder VDRX-200) coupled to a Siremobile television fluoroscopic unit of the C-arm type. The system is provided with four modes: map, stored + map, fluoro, and fluoro + map, which are selected by a four-position switch and controlled by a foot switch as follows:

1. Map: By stepping on the foot pedal as contrast is injected into the artery, the operator produces an electronic angiogram, or "map," which is stored on track A of the magnetic disk.
2. Stored + map: When the pedal is depressed, a new fluoroscopic image

is recorded and stored on track B, and both tracks are instantly replayed on the monitor with the x-rays off; a combined image results.

3. Fluoro: The pedal activates the fluoroscopic unit, which displays the live image on the monitor.

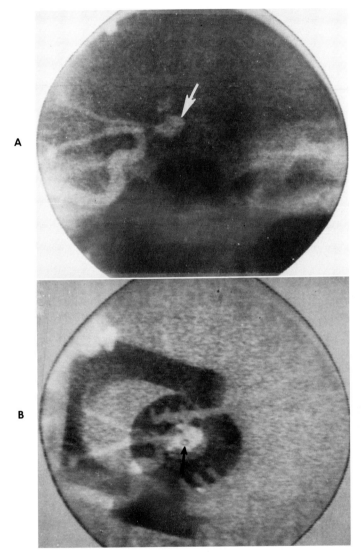

Fig. 5-6. A, Electronic angiogram showing aneurysm (arrow) of anterior communicating artery. **B,** Stereotaxic needle guide superimposed with angiogram of aneurysm displayed on television monitor. Drill guide appears as circle (arrow) centered in angiogram of aneurysm when positioning is completed.

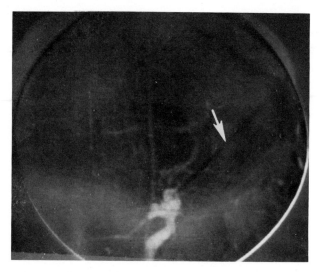

Fig. 5-7. Lateral view; blunt stilette (arrow) is advanced proximal to aneurysm. This electronic image shows blunt stilette prior to its replacement by stereotaxic needle for puncture of aneurysm.

4. Fluoro + map: Depressing the foot pedal produces a live television fluoroscopic image superimposed upon track A on the monitor.

The skull is fixed relative to the stereotaxic apparatus and the x-ray tube is centered over the aneurysm in the anteroposterior position. The map mode is selected and an electronic arteriogram showing the aneurysm is made (Fig. 5-6, *A*). Mode stored + map is then selected and images showing the needle guide superimposed upon the frozen image of the aneurysm are made as necessary, until the guide is satisfactorily placed over the aneurysm (Fig. 5-6, *B*).

The x-ray tube is then placed lateral to the aneurysm, an arteriogram is made in the map mode to show its position, and a needle is advanced through the guide using the fluoro + map mode until the tip reaches the aneurysm (Fig. 5-7). After injection of tissue adhesive, contrast is injected, and the fluoro mode is used to evaluate occlusion.

This technique has permitted the localization and treatment of an intracranial aneurysm with tissue adhesive injected through a transcerebral needle. The time required was approximately 1 hour, much less than with the standard attack by craniotomy. The neurosurgeon operates the electronic radiographic apparatus himself and has the simple mode switch and foot pedal under his own control.

In summary, a technique of electronic radiography has been developed that can be easily operated by a single person in the operating room. The system, which makes possible the rapid and accurate placement of a transcerebral needle, was successfully used for treatment of an aneurysm. This new procedure may permit earlier intervention with lower mortality and morbidity in the treatment of intracranial aneurysms, and it may be applicable to other interventional techniques.

Selective catheterization

The catheterization techniques presently used in most angiographic procedures place a premium on experience and necessitate extensive training. They often require prolonged examination times and the injection of large quantities of radiopaque contrast. These factors increase both the chance of mechanical trauma to the vessel and the possibility of a contrast reaction. In addition, both patient and personnel are exposed to significant radiation levels, especially when multiple organ studies must be carried out.

Electronic radiography provides a potential means of reducing procedure time, radiation exposure, and the volume of injected radiopaque contrast material. There are three levels of refinement of electronic storage techniques that can be applied, depending upon the degree of difficulty encountered in the catheterization of a particular vessel in vascular or neuroradiology.

Single image. The single-image method presents individual "frozen" electronic radiographs that substitute for live fluoroscopy.[42,70] These images display the location of the catheter relative to bony landmarks such as vertebrae and ribs. The angiographer can study these frozen images at leisure, with the x-rays off, before manipulating the catheter further. The progress of this manipulation can be recorded on successive electronic radiographs. To confirm that the branch vessel has been catheterized, a test injection of contrast is made and recorded on an additional similar electronic radiograph.

Arterial map with electronic image superimposition. The method utilizing an arterial map with electronic image superimposition combines the single-image method with an arterial map.[62,64] It is especially helpful for teaching angiography. An electronic angiogram is recorded during the injection of contrast medium into the aorta. This is recorded on track A of the disk recorder and replayed instantly with the rays off to provide a map of the aortic branches. After advancing the catheter, an electronic radiograph that shows the new position of the catheter is superimposed upon the map and can be studied at leisure with the x-rays off (Figs. 5-8 and 5-9). Catheterization of the branch is thus greatly facilitated.

Arterial map with live-image superimposition. The arterial map with live-image superimposition is a procedure in which the live fluoroscopic image of the catheter tip is electronically superimposed on the map.[64] This method offers more flexibility than the superimposition of electronic catheter radiographs but exposes the patient and angiographer to more radiation than either of the first two methods.

In a preliminary clinical trial of electronic selective catheterization of abdominal and cerebral vessels in 20 patients,[62] the three variations described

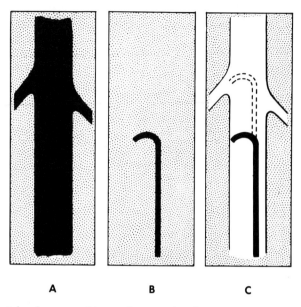

Fig. 5-8. Principle of superposition technique. A, Electronic angiogram is made showing aorta and branch vessels filled with radiopaque contrast medium. B, Electronic radiograph of the noncontrast-filled vessels is made showing catheter. C, Image of catheter is superimposed on reversed electronic angiogram, facilitating rapid selective catheterization.

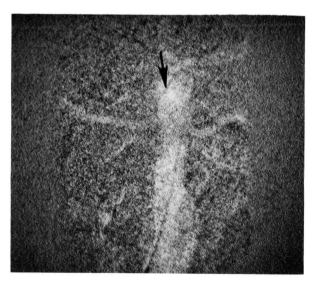

Fig. 5-9. Superposition technique used in 50-year-old man. Electronic radiograph of catheter (arrow) is combined with electronic map and displayed on television monitor screen. Angiogram is electronically reversed to improve visibility of combined images.

were found to simplify the procedure. The single-image method was useful to the experienced angiographer, and the two other variations were most helpful to the novice angiographer. The arterial map methods reduced the search time for specific vessels by positively identifying their location during selective catheterization. In some patients the time required to complete selective catheterization was less than 1 minute, with a total fluoroscopic exposure time of less than 1 second. These methods promise to be an important advance in angiographic training.

By reducing the need for repeated test injections of radiopaque contrast medium, electronic arterial maps greatly decreased the amount of contrast medium injected during catheterization. These reductions amounted to more than 50 ml in some cases.

The limiting resolution of the electronic radiograph was 1.5 lp/mm, a level more than adequate for selective catheterization. Typically, the electronic radiographs required only 1/100 the radiation exposure needed to produce a normal x-ray spot film, and only 1/600 the radiation dose produced by 1 minute of continuous fluoroscopy. Electronic radiography also reduces the time required to perform the examination. Thus the radiation dose is reduced by both factors.

In summary, electronic radiography can be effectively adapted to selective catheterization procedures. By utilizing a series of images stored on a magnetic disk, the electronic technique replaces continuous live fluoroscopy. This requires much less radiation than that needed for conventional fluoroscopy and decreased operating time reduces radiation and risk. The variations possible with this technique simplify the procedure of selective catheterization and serve as a unique training device.

Cardiac catheterization

The stop-action or slide-show capability provided by the magnetic disk has been utilized to obtain radiation dose reduction in cardiac catheterization by Grollman.[27,28]

The system used triggers x-ray pulses at programmed rates from 15/sec down to single pulses, selectable at the control module. A single field of television information, out of the two interlaced fields forming a complete television frame, is recorded in 1/60 second and automatically played back until the next image is to be recorded. A 945-line, 30 frame/sec television system was found to be necessary to deliver acceptable resolution with single field display.

Dosimetry during low pulse–rate fluoroscopy at various rates was undertaken, and it has been demonstrated that the dose is reduced to 35% of the standard mode at a rate of 15 fields/sec and approximately 50% further for each factor of 2 in pulse rate.

The initial application of low pulse–rate fluoroscopy to cardiac catheterization and coronary arteriography employed the 15 pulses/sec mode, which was used for the entire examination. Grollman found both subjectively and objectively that there was no increased difficulty in the performance of these procedures as compared to their performance under standard fluoroscopy. The procedures were performed both from the brachial artery using the more difficult Sones technique[79] and from the femoral artery using the relatively easier Judkins technique.[35] Most important, the duration of the procedure was not prolonged by the use of the 15 pulses/sec mode. The estimated average reduction of dose to patient and paramedical personnel from both fluoroscopy and angiography was approximately 50%.

Subsequently, the 7½ pulses/sec mode was utilized for all routine fluoroscopic monitoring during the physiologic portion of the study and alternated every other case between 7½ and 15 pulses/sec during the actual performance of the coronary arteriographic study. There were 64 patients in each group, and no significant difference was found in the procedural times between both groups of patients. Because those procedures in which the Sones technique was employed are much more difficult and potentially more time consuming, it was decided to compare the patients in each group in which this technique was employed. Again, no difference in overall duration of the procedure was noticed.

During the manipulation of the catheter for coronary arteriography, fluoroscopy at 7½ pulses/sec was generally found to be quite acceptable. All the trainees accepted this rate quite readily, although one of the regular staff members objected on occasion because he felt that he was missing certain movements. In this group in which the 7½ pulses/sec mode was used during the entire procedure there were five instances in which the angiographer requested an increased pulse rate because he felt he was not seeing sufficient detail.

A comparison of the estimated dosage to the patient as well as scatter exposure was carried out. Assuming a total of 3500 cineframes for a case and adding this to the radiation dose accumulated during 40 minutes of fluoroscopy when using low pulse–rate fluoroscopy of 7½/sec, the dose to the patient is reduced to approximately 20% of that of standard fluoroscopy. Even in the group in which 7½ and 15 pulses/sec were both used the radiation dosage was reduced to approximately 30% of the level required in standard fluoroscopy, and corresponding reductions occurred for the scatter dose to the physician, or from 67 to 19 mr at eye level during the typical 40-minute procedure.

Electronic spot imaging for gastrointestinal examinations

Electronic spot imaging (ESI) is a technique whereby the x-ray tube output is momentarily increased during fluoroscopy to produce a single, high-quality television image that is first electronically recorded and then photographed. This technique was developed as a means of improving fluoroscopic spot imaging and thus radiologic studies of the gastrointestinal tract.[61,69] The major advantage of this technique is that high confidence–level decisions are possible during fluoroscopy because of the availability of these recorded images for immediate review. Other benefits of the method include (1) increased diagnostic information by elimination of fluoroscopic "blackouts" during spot recording, (2) faster examination and interpretation as a consequence of reduced film handling, (3) relatively low radiation dose to the patient and fluoroscopic personnel, (4) the elimination of repeat examinations because of film processing malfunctions, and (5) the ability to make unlimited first-quality film copies of recorded images without reexamining the patient.

The installation includes a standard high-resolution 525-line television fluoroscopic unit (Fig. 5-10), which is modified for electronic spot imaging, a 400-track magnetic video disk recorder, and controls providing for record images to be taken at x-ray tube currents of up to 40 mA.

During uninterrupted fluoroscopy, electronic spot images can be recorded either individually or in rapid sequence by completely depressing a two-position fluoroscopic foot pedal. Normally these images are reviewed at the end of each examination, but they may also be replayed at any time during the study. A three-position hand switch at the fluoroscopic table permits the radiologist to select the mode of operation, namely, fluoro-record, reverse, and forward. At the conclusion of each day's fluoroscopy, all electronic spot images

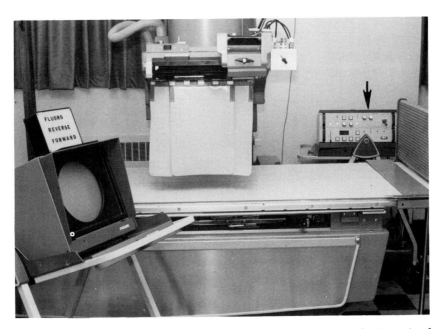

Fig. 5-10. View of installation for electronic spot imaging. Disk recorder (arrow) is located behind fluoroscopic table. Operating mode selected is indicated on panel above monitor.

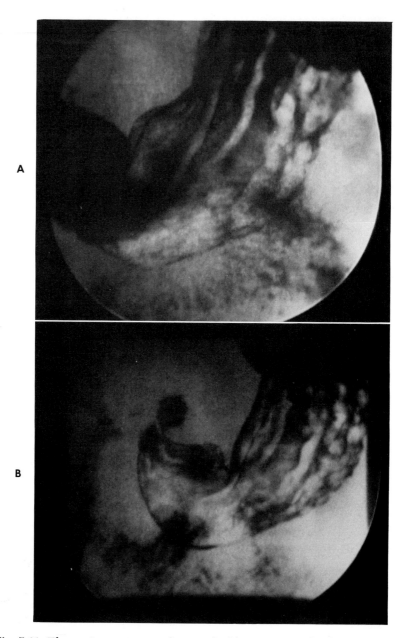

Fig. 5-11. Electronic spot images showing double-contrast study of stomach. **A,** Using 9-inch mode. **B,** Using 6-inch mode. Note that television scan lines have been eliminated by spot-stretching technique.

(Fig. 5-11) are again reviewed in conjunction with the corresponding overhead films before a final diagnosis is rendered. Key electronic images are photographed for a permanent record using an automatic kinescope, thus allowing the disk to be reused the following day.

Preliminary comparison of electronic spot images and modern 105 mm spot films in upper gastrointestinal studies was made by seven radiologists using a double-blind method. The comparison indicated a degree of accuracy for the two methods that was essentially the same, namely, 75.5% and 76.5% for 105 mm spot filming and ESI, respectively.[77] Of the seven radiologists who participated in the evaluation, none with the exception of the original fluoroscopist was experienced in interpretation by either of these techniques, a fact that may have reduced the overall percentage of correct diagnoses in both methods.

Using the technique just described, application of ESI has been made to barium enema examinations.[78] The colon is fluoroscoped during the filling phase and ESI spots are taken of all poorly visualized and noncompressible areas. Once the cecum is filled and the colon is fully distended, ESI spot images are again recorded. These "spots" are quickly reviewed before the patient is allowed to evacuate and possible lesions are noted and further evaluated. Images are made with the 6-inch or magnification mode of the 9-inch image intensifier. Finally, "overhead" radiographs, usually only a postevacuation study, are obtained.

Barium suspensions of 13% weight/volume or less were used because they allowed the best visualization of small colonic filling defects and at the same time fulfilled the need for good visualization of the colonic margins and mucosal patterns. Further refinements in barium preparation are being made.

In an objective evaluation of 25 patients, "phantom" colon polyps made of chewing gum balls 13 mm in diameter were placed in the rectum. In order to avoid confusion with true polyps, a BB shot was inserted into each and electronic spot images as well as standard spot films were obtained for comparison. The chewing gum "polyps" could be seen in all patients examined. However, air bubbles, because of their heightened visibility, were more troublesome but usually identifiable as such.

Electronic tomography

The development of high-resolution electronic imaging systems has opened up the possibility of replacing film in tomographic procedures.

As pointed out by Lasser et al.,[38] the use of film imposes certain restrictions on the utilization of body section roentgenography.

First, a pilot study at the projected depth of interest must be done. Only after inspection of this pilot study and suitable modifications for technique and position have been accomplished can an adequate definitive body section roentgenogram be obtained. This is time consuming, and the dose to the patient is often excessive. If one attempts to overcome this by multiple body plane roentgenograms produced by existing techniques, a certain degree of unsharpness is imposed by virtue of scatter occurring along multiple screen and film interfaces. Furthermore, the definitive plane of interest is often compromised because of patient movement during the interval of time necessary to make additional corrections and to view the resulting roentgenograms.

The use of fluoroscopic presentation overcomes to a very large extent the difficulties outlined by providing the radiologist with the capability of making adjustments in technique and position of the patient rapidly and accurately with a very significantly reduced patient dose. Through the use of a single-scan television system with a video disk recorder as a substitute for the usual film recording it was possible to accomplish recording of true tomograms fluoroscopically.

The method produces a true tomographic image identical to that seen on film. Unlike the method presented by Frimann-Dahl and Kühl,[20] continuous motion and a roentgen-ray input over a period of time sufficient to produce a stationary image are not required. Second, since the monitor is displaying a true tomographic section, it can be photographed and utilized as that portion of the completed study.

The method appears to have the potential for extension to studies of organs having associated motion. The image can be digitized and processed by computer for either quantitative analysis or representation on video after edge enhancement, contrast enhancement, subtraction, etc.

The basic roentgenographic equipment consists of a G.E. Model 73 horizontal table that was modified to accommodate a 6- to 9-inch image intensifier under-table installation that is hydraulically driven in conjunction with the roentgen-ray tube (G.E. B8190, ordography body section attachment).

The most important aspect of the method is the large reduction in patient dose that can be achieved. Exposures 20 cm above the tabletop were 0.43 to 1.4 rad for film planigraphy and 25.5 to 59.5 mr for the electronic recording technique, the image being photographed from the television monitor. Although the initial trials were limited in field size to 3 inches by the curved input phosphor of the intensifier, this curvature permitted section thicknesses of less than 2 mm to be achieved with short travels or less than half of those attained with film.

More recently,[4] a modification of this system was developed by the same group. A series of individual images is recorded at fixed points along the path of tomographic motion and stored in separate channels of the video disk, based on the suggestion of Dümmling[16] and others[41,58] that a finite series of single images can be used to produce an infinite series of planigraphic sections. The individual images are then sequentially transferred to an electronic storage tube and added together with proper displacement so as to create the image for a desired section. As many as 25 individual images have been successfully superimposed to produce the final image.

The principal advantages of this approach are that it can provide sections through portions of the anatomy having pulsating or other forms of motion and that any number of body sections parallel to or partially inclined with respect to the original plane of motion can be obtained with a single set of electronically recorded images.

The greatest improvement in the system would be the substitution of an imaging system with a large, flat input screen in place of the conventional image intensifier. Progress in this direction was recently reported by Baily,[5] who was able to report encouraging results in recording a 14 × 14 inch x-ray fluorescent screen image with a vidicon camera preceded by a three-stage fiber optically coupled image intensifier.

By going to a larger diameter (40 mm) image tube and a larger vidicon, Baily hopes to achieve further improvements in image quality. Already, he has been able to obtain clinically useful images for adult patients at 0.1 ma, indicating that when it is combined with further improvements in the magnetic disk, the technique of large-screen imaging using optically coupled television systems that was initiated by Morgan and Sturm in the early 1950s should solve the problem of field size presented by the use of x-ray image intensifiers, both in tomographic and other applications of electronic radiography.

It should also be possible to eventually apply the technique of multiple electronic image superposition to the technique of transverse axial tomography as developed recently,[17a] thereby achieving a large gain in speed analogous to that realized in nuclear medicine by the development of the gamma camera[2] relative to the mechanical scanner. Clearly, this area of research and development holds considerable promise as a most fruitful application of electronic imaging to the needs of diagnostic radiology.

Remote transmission of electronic images

The development of high-resolution television cameras and recording and display systems within the last few years has also raised the possibility that electronically recorded images can be transmitted to remote locations with sufficient diagnostic quality to finally realize the hopes originally raised but unfortunately not met by the advent of commercial television in the 1950s.[57]

As a first step in the direction of realizing the inherent potential of high-resolution television systems to provide widely acceptable clinical images, such a system was constructed and clinically evaluated as a link from the emergency room to the film reading room of the department of radiology at the University of Pittsburgh.[55] The two areas are some 500 feet apart.

The system was designed to provide a means for a radiologist to diagnose all emergency cases immediately after films are taken and to determine diagnostic accuracy and its change with time as various system parameters are changed and reading experience is gained by the radiologist. The system was specifically designed for maximum resolution, dynamic range, and signal-to-noise ratio obtainable from present components. Furthermore, all important functions at the transmitting end in the emergency room, three floors below and 500 feet distant (Fig. 5-12), were designed to be remotely controlled by the radiologist at the receiving end (Fig. 5-13).

These functions include film position, zoom, amount of light entering the camera, monitoring brightness and contrast, and the size and position of a special blanking feature or circular mask that isolates any desired portion of the image, blanking out the remainder and thereby providing a wider dynamic range than would otherwise be available (Fig. 5-14).

The camera used employed a high-resolution vidicon, giving 1200 television lines limiting resolution with excellent response at low spatial frequencies, using a bandwidth of 30 mHz. Horizontal resolution in the film plane is 1.5 lp/mm for a 14 × 17 inch field of view, and 6 lp/mm for a 3½ × 4½ inch field at maximum zoom.

Seven radiologists viewed a set of 27 preselected film series (45 films total), which were transmitted through the television system; then, 8 weeks later, the radiologists read the same films on a conventional viewbox.[80] The films were selected to represent a typical cross section of emergency room films. Five series were normal, while 22 contained a range of abnormalities that were preclassified as easy, medium, or difficult to diagnose.

The mean accuracy for the 27 film series was 90% for direct viewing and

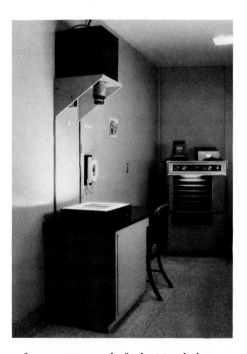

Fig. 5-12. View of transmitting end of television link in emergency room.

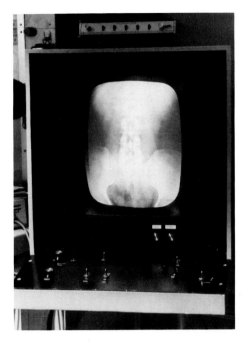

Fig. 5-13. Receiving terminal of television link located in reading room of radiology department.

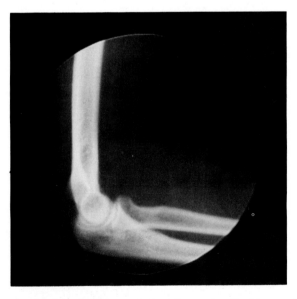

Fig. 5-14. Monitor display of television link with circular blanking applied to vidicon camera to remove bright areas of film.

82% for television viewing (the 95% confidence interval for the true difference between methods is 8 ± 3%). Even though the error rate was slightly higher using the closed-circuit system, radiologist performance was of acceptable accuracy considering the advantages of the system.

The results of the study indicate that the diagnostic accuracy that can be achieved from a televised radiographic image is now approaching the accuracy obtained by conventional reading techniques. It seems reasonable to expect that the incorporation of certain enhancement features and additional television reading experience by radiologists would further improve the diagnostic accuracy of the televised image so that remote diagnosis of electronic images will become a reality.

A logical extension of the present system would be its application to the generally recognized need for transmission of high-quality images between outlying hospitals and major medical centers.[57] It seems highly probable that the combination of a higher interlace ratio and a slightly longer persistence phosphor on the monitor display could reduce the system bandwidth requirement so that a 6 to 12 mHz microwave channel would transmit high-resolution radiographs for a distance of several miles; these radiographs would be of the same diagnostic quality as those now being obtained at Presbyterian-University Hospital.

FUTURE DEVELOPMENTS

The rapid advance of electronic imaging and storage devices that has made all of the aforementioned developments possible is continuing as the electro-optical technology developed for military and space systems in the 1960s is being increasingly applied to the needs of diagnostic radiology.

The following areas of current research and development bear directly on the future of electronic imaging techniques.

1. Coupling to digital computers
   a. Quantitative measurements such as heart volume[85,94] or bone density[11]
   b. Image enhancement, as for the heart,[95] blood vessels,[75] chest,[74] and other body parts
   c. Computer-aided diagnosis such as that presently being developed at the University of Missouri[17]
   d. Transverse axial tomography using silicon storage tubes to increase the speed of imaging,[54] analogous to the scanning system developed by EMI.[17a]
2. Visualization of smaller contrast differences
   a. Utilization of monochromatic radiation by heavy selective filtration of standard tubes for the enhancement of soft tissue contrast, as in mammography,[63] the visualization of soft organs containing naturally occurring high atomic number elements such as the thyroid,[44,45] and the enhancement of contrast media absorption in blood vessels[31,32,69]
   b. Development of new x-ray tubes providing monochromatic radiation in various regions of the spectrum, with intensities adequate for the more efficient electronic technique

    c. Development of analog storage techniques to permit the visualization of small contrast differences down to the limits set by quantum noise ($\leq 0.1\%$), a sensitivity not attainable with film

    d. Development of digital storage techniques to visualize contrast differences set only by the dose or the number of quanta per image element ($\leq 0.1\%$)

3. Visualization of finer detail

    a. Optical imaging of high-resolution, high-efficiency, x-ray fluorescent screens, such as the new family of rare-earth oxide screens recently developed at Lockheed[10] and other screens utilized for electronic mammography at the University of Pittsburgh[63]

    b. Uitilization of x-ray–sensitive vidicons to record fine blood vessels using geometric magnification techniques with ultra-fine focal spots[43,61]

4. Recording of larger fields

    a. Coupling of high-resolution optical image intensifiers to high-resolution camera tubes, as recently begun at San Diego,[4] to record the entire chest

    b. Optical viewing of a large-area, high-efficiency screen by means of low-light level isocon

5. Remote transmission of high-resolution images

    a. Expansion of high-resolution wide-band TV transmission within hospitals to operating rooms and hospital floors

    b. Expansion of remote diagnostic consulting to distant hospitals, using slow-scan techniques to utilize available microwave links

    c. Expansion of remote diagnosis using satellite links[39]

6. Storage, filing, and retrieval of electronic images

    a. Development of low-cost plastic disk for permanent or temporary storage of electronic images

    b. Use of magnetic tape system capable of high-quality storage and recovery of single images[22]

    c. Utilization of 70 to 105 mm film for permanent storage and automated retrieval of electronically recorded images

    d. Electronic beam recording of x-ray images on electron-sensitive tape[3]

SUMMARY

Although application of the technique of electronic radiography in clinical situations has only just begun, it is evident that the development of high-resolution electronic imaging and storage techniques opens up the possibility of earlier detection of neoplasms and other diseases beyond the limitations of ordinary film radiography. Furthermore, the development of entirely new diagnostic and interventional procedures using electronic radiography may make a significant contribution to the future of diagnostic radiology.

References

1. Alksne, J. F.: Stereotactic thrombosis of intracranial aneurysms, N. Engl. J. Med. **284:**171, 1971.
2. Anger, H. O.: Scintillation camera with multichannel collimators, J. Nucl. Med. **5:**515, 1964.
3. Angus, W. M.: Image intensifier fluorography—progress and problems. In Hilal, S. K., editor: Small vessel angiography, St. Louis, 1973, The C. V. Mosby Co.

4. Baily, A., Crepeau, R. L., and Lasser, E. C.: Electronic tomography, Paper presented at the Symposium on electronic imaging techniques in diagnostic radiology, University of Pittsburgh, April, 1973.
5. Baily, N., and Crepeau, R. L.: Performance of a large screen fluoroscopic imaging system, Proc. Soc. Photo-Optic. Instr. Eng. **43**:135, 1973.
6. Banks, G. B.: Television pick-up tubes for x-ray screen intensification, Br. J. Radiol. **31**:619, 1958.
7. Baum, W. A.: The detection and measurement of faint astronomical sources. In Hiltner, A., editor: Astronomical techniques, Chicago, 1960, The University of Chicago Press.
8. Bell, J., Niklas, W. F., Dolon, P. J., and Ter-Pogossian, M. M.: Image intensifying chains for medical scintillation cameras, Adv. Electronics Electron Phys. **22B**:927, 1966.
9. Bertin, E. P.: Intensification of x-ray images by electronic means. In Clark, G. L., editor: Encyclopedia of x-rays and gamma rays, New York, 1963, Reinhold Publishing Co.
10. Buchanan, R. A., Finkelstein, S. I., and Wickersheim, K. A.: X-ray exposure reduction using rare-earth oxysulfide intensifying screens, Radiology **105**:185, 1972.
11. Cameron, J. R., Judy, P. F., Jones, K. M., and Ort, M. G.: Determination of vertebral bone mineral mass by transmission measurements, Paper presented at the Third international conference on medical physics (Conf-72031-1), Göteborg, 1972.
12. Coltman, J. W.: Fluoroscopic image brightening by electronic means, Radiology **51**:359, 1948.
13. Coltman, J. W.: The scintillation limit in fluoroscopy, Radiology **63**:867, 1954.
14. Davis, R. J.: The use of the uvicon-celescope television system for ultra-violet astronomical photometry, Adv. Electronics Electron Phys. **22B**:875, 1966.
15. Dennison, E. W.: An integrating television system for visual enhancement of faint stars, Adv. Electronics Electron Phys. **33B**:795, 1972.
16. Dümmling, K.: A new procedure for multiple layers with the help of a TV picture accumulator, Radiologe **9**:37, 1969.
17. Dwyer, S. J., et al.: Computer analysis of radiographic images, Proc. Soc. Photo-Optic. Instr. Eng. **35**:107, 1972.
17a. EMI-scanner: a new perspective on brain disease, Middlesex, England, 1973, EMI, Ltd.
18. Feist, J. H., Sternglass, E. J., and Sashin, D.: Application of television subtraction techniques to clinical fluoroscopic procedures, Paper presented at the Second international conference on medical physics, Boston, Mass., 1969.
19. Fenner, E., et al.: X-ray image intensifiers: image quality and possibilities for enhancement, Adv. Electronics Electron Phys. **33B**:1049, 1972.
20. Frimann-Dahl, J., and Kuhl, H. B.: Immediate centering and tomographic cut localization by means of roentgen television, Acta Radiol. **10**:236, 1970.
21. Fuchs, H., and Hofman, F. W.: An x-ray image intensifier with improved image quality, Electromedica **3**:94, 1971.
22. Fuchs, H., et al.: Memospot-instant replay television of spot films in internal medicine and pediatrics, Electromedica **5**:156, 1971.
23. Girdany, B.: Symposium on electronic imaging techniques in diagnostic radiology, University of Pittsburgh, April, 1973.
24. Girdany, B., Gaither, E. S., and Darling, D. B.: Large-screen image amplification with closed-circuit television employing television tape recorder, Radiology **77**:286, 1961.

25. Goetze, G. W., and Boerio, A. H.: Secondary electron conduction in low density targets for signal amplification and storage in camera tubes, Proc. IEEE **52:**107, 1964.

26. Graham, S., et al.: Preconception, intrauterine and postnatal irradiation as related to leukemia, Natl. Cancer Inst. Monogr. **19:**347, 1966.

27. Grollman, J. H.: Radiation reduction by means of low pulse-rate fluoroscopy in cardiac catheterization, Paper presented at the Symposium on electronic imaging techniques in diagnostic radiology, University of Pittsburgh, April, 1973.

28. Grollman, J. H., Jr., et al.: Dose reduction in low pulse rate fluoroscopy, Radiology **105:**293, 1971.

29. Hay, G. A., Quantitative aspects of television techniques in diagnostic radiology, Br. J. Radiol. **31:**611, 1958.

30. Hesse, K. R., Improved memory tube, Industrial Products Division Bulletin, Oceanside, Calif., 1972, Hughes Aircraft Co.

31. Huen, A.: Quasi-monochromatic radiation in diagnostic radiology, Sc.D. dissertation, University of Pittsburgh, 1972.

32. Huen, A., and Sternglass, E. J.: Monochromatic radiation in diagnostic radiology, Paper presented at the Third international congress on medical physics, Göteborg, 1972.

33. Jacobson, B.: Dichromography, Acta Radiol. **39:**437, 1953.

34. Jacobson, B., and MacKay, R. S.: Radiological contrast enhancement methods, Adv. Biol. Med. Phys. **6:**201, 1968.

35. Judkins, M. P.: Selective coronary arteriography. I. A percutaneous transfemoral technique, Radiology **89:**815, 1967.

36. Justras, A.: Teleroentgen diagnosis by means of videotape recording, Am. J. Roentgenol. Radium Ther. Nucl. Med. **82:**1099, 1959.

37. Lasser, E. C., Electronic imaging in radiology, Paper presented at the Symposium on electronic imaging techniques in diagnostic radiology, University of Pittsburgh, April, 1973.

38. Lasser, E. C., Baily, N. C., and Crepeau, R. L.: A fluoroplanigraphy system for rapid presentation of single plane body sections, Am. J. Roentgenol. Radium Ther. Nucl. Med. **113:**574, 1971.

39. Lester, R. G., et al.: Transmission of radiologic information by satellite, Radiology **109:**731, 1973.

40. Mackay, R. S.: Radiographic analysis and visualization using x-ray spectral information. In Clark, G. L., editor: Encyclopedia of x-rays and gamma rays, New York, 1963, Reinhold Publishing Co.

41. Miller, E. R., McCurry, E. M., and Hruska, B.: An infinite number of laminagrams from a finite number of radiographs, Radiology **98:**249, 1971.

42. Miller, W. B., Jr., et al.: Design and evaluation of an electronic radiography system, Technical Report DHEW (FDA) 72-8014, Washington, D. C., 1971, U. S. Government Printing Office.

43. Milne, E.: Comments on radiographic magnification and on the design of cathodes for x-ray tubes. In Hilal, S. K., editor: Small vessel angiography, St. Louis, 1973, The C. V. Mosby Co.

44. Mistretta, C. A.: Instrumentation and current results in absorption edge transmission imaging. In Zarnsdorf, W. C., Hendee, W. R., and Carlson, P. C., editors: Proceedings of the conference on applications of optical instruments in medicine, Redondo Beach, Calif., Society of Photo-optical Illumination Engineers. (In press.)

45. Mistretta, C. A., Siedband, M., and Cameron, J.: Absorption edge subtraction imaging, Paper presented at the Symposium on electronic imaging techniques in diagnostic radiology, University of Pittsburgh, April, 1973.
46. Moon, R. J.: Amplification of the fluoroscopic image, Am. J. Roentgenol. Radium Ther. Nucl. Med. **69:**886, 1948.
47. Morgan, R. H., and Sturm, R. E.: The Johns Hopkins fluoroscopic screen intensifier, Radiology **57:**556, 1951.
48. Mouser, D. P.: The image isocon, IEEE Trans. **BC-15:**39, 1969.
49. Mullan, S., et al.: Electrically induced thrombosis in intracranial aneurysms, J. Neurosurg. **22:**539, 1965.
50. Murray, J. P.: Semi-orthometric pelvimetry: an appraisal, Br. J. Radiol. **44:**524, 1971.
51. New, P. F., et al.: Computerized axial tomography with the EMI scanner, Radiology **110:**109, 1974.
52. Oosterkamp, W. J.: Monochromatic x-rays for medical fluoroscopy and radiography, Medica Mundi **7:**68, 1961.
53. Philips Medical Systems, Technical Report No. 142 (Tube No. XG 0200/200), Shelton, Conn.
54. Porti, A., Cho, Z. H., and Sashin, D.: Transverse axial tomography using a scan converter storage tube. In Proceedings of the symposium on transverse axial tomography, Oak Ridge, Tenn., 1974, U. S. Atomic Energy Commission Division of Technical Information.
55. Porti, A., et al.: A high resolution television system for remote viewing of radiographs, Paper presented at the Symposium on electronic imaging techniques in diagnostic radiology, University of Pittsburgh, April, 1973.
56. Princeton Electronic Products: The lithocon. Technical bulletin, Princeton Junction, N. J., Princeton Electronic Products.
57. Report of the task force on x-ray image analysis and systems development, DMRE 69-1, Washington, D. C., 1968, U. S. Department of Health, Education, and Welfare.
58. Richards, A. G.: Variable depth laminagraphy, Biomed. Sci. Instrum. **6:**194, 1969.
59. Robbins, C. D., Enck, R. S., and Sackinger, P.: High performance continuous zoom x-ray intensifiers. In Zarnsdorf, W. C., Hendee, W. R., and Carlson, P. C., editors: Proceedings of the conference on applications of optical instrumentation in medicine, Redondo Beach, Calif., Society of Photo-optical Illumination Engineers. (In press.)
60. Rose, A.: Sensitivity performance of the human eye on an absolute scale, J. Opt. Soc. Am. **38:**196, 1948.
61. Sakuma, S., Ayakawa, Y., Okumura, Y., and Maekoshi, H.: Determination of focal-spot characteristics of microfocus x-ray tubes, Invest. Radiol. **4:**335, 1969.
62. Sashin, D., and Bron, K.: Electronic selective catheterization. (Unpublished data.)
63. Sashin, D., and Morris, C. W.: Electronic mammography in the diagnosis of early breast cancer, Paper presented at Clinical conference on cancer at the M. D. Anderson Hospital and Tumor Clinic, Houston, Texas, November, 1973.
64. Sashin, D., Bron, K., and Sternglass, E. J.: Subtraction technique in fluoroscopy, Paper presented at the Radiological Society of North America annual meeting, Chicago, November, 1970.
65. Sashin, D., Zanetti, P., and Porti, A.: Rapid thrombosis of intracranial aneurysms with electronic radiography, Paper presented at the Third international conference on medical physics, Göteborg, 1972.

66. Sashin, D., Goldman, R. L., Zanetti, P., and Heinz, E. R.: Electronic radiography in stereotaxic thrombosis of intracranial aneurysms and catheter embolization of cerebral arteriovenous malformations, Radiology **105**:359, 1972.

67. Sashin, D., Rocchio, R., Matta, R. K., and Sternglass, E. J.: Resolution, contrast and dose reduction performance of electronic radiography systems, Paper presented at the Second international conference on medical physics, Boston, August, 1969.

68. Sashin, D., Short, W. F., Heinz, E. R., and Sternglass, E. J.: Electronic radiography for spot filming in gastrointestinal fluoroscopy, Radiology **106**:551, 1973.

69. Sashin, D., Sternglass, E. G., Huen, A., and Heinz, E. R.: Dose reduction in diagnostic radiology by electronic imaging techniques. In Proceedings of the symposium in health physics in the healing arts, DHEW Publ. No. (FDA) 73-8029, Washington, D. C., 1972, U. S. Government Printing Office.

70. Sashin, D., et al.: Dose reduction in diagnostic radiology by electronic image storage techniques. In Proceedings of the symposium on reduction of radiation dose in diagnostic x-ray procedures, DHEW Publ. No. (FDA) 73-8009, Washington, D. C., 1972, U. S. Government Printing Office.

71. Sashin, D., et al.: Electronic radiography for pelvimetry and intrauterine transfusions, Paper presented at the American Association of Physics in Medicine, Philadelphia, 1972.

72. Sashin, D., et al.: Pelvimetry with negligible fetal radiation exposure. In Health physics in the healing arts, DHEW Publ. No. (FDA) 73-8029, Washington, D. C., 1973, U. S. Government Printing Office.

73. Schut, T. G., and Oosterkamp, W. J.: The application of electronic memories in radiology, Medica Mundi **5**:85, 1959.

74. Selzer, R.: Improving biomedical image quality with computers, JPL Technical Report 32-1336, October, 1968.

75. Selzer, R.: Computer processing of angiograms. In Hilal, S. K., editor: Small vessel angiography, St. Louis, 1973, The C. V. Mosby Co.

76. Siedband, M. P., and Sternglass, E. J.: Fluoroscopic image differencing by electronic storage means, Paper presented at the Sixth Rochester Cine Conference, Rochester, N. Y., April, 1968.

77. Short, W. F., Sashin, D., Porti, A., and Stanislawczyk, K.: Electronic spot imaging (ESI) for gastrointestinal examinations. (Unpublished paper.)

78. Short, W. F., et al.: Barium enemas utilizing electronic spot imaging. (Unpublished paper.)

79. Sones, F. M., Jr., and Shirey, E. K.: Cine coronary arteriography, Mod. Concepts Cardiovasc. Dis. **31**:735, 1962.

80. Sorby, W. B., Gates, S., Porti, A., and Sashin, D.: An evaluation of a high resolution closed circuit television link. (Unpublished paper.)

81. Sternglass, E. J., and Goetze, G. W.: Field enhanced transmission secondary emission for high speed counting, IRE Trans. Nucl. Sci. **NS-9**:97, 1962.

82. Sternglass, E. J., and Keller, E.: High resolution electronic gamma-ray imaging. In Yen Wang, C. C., editor: Advances in dynamic radioactive scanning, Springfield, Ill., 1968, Charles C Thomas, Publisher.

83. Stewart, A., and Kneale, G. W.: Radiation dose effects in relation to obstetric x-rays and childhood cancers, Lancet **1**:1185, 1970.

84. Sturm, R. E., and Morgan, R. H.: Screen intensification systems and their limitations, Am. J. Roentgenol. Radium Ther. Nucl. Med. **62**:617, 1949.

85. Sturm, R. E., and Wood, E. H.: Roentgen image-intensifier television recording system for dynamic measurements of roentgen density for circulatory studies, In

Heintzen, P., editor: Roentgen-cine and videodensitometry, Stuttgart, 1971, Georg Thieme Verlag.

86. Teves, M. C., and Tol, T.: Electronic intensification of fluoroscopic images, Phillips Tech. Rev. **14:**33, 1952.

87. Ter-Pogossian, M. M.: Monochromatic roentgen rays in contrast media roentgenography, Acta Radiol. **45:**313, 1956.

88. Ter-Pogossian, M. M.: The physical aspects of diagnostic radiology, New York, 1967, Harper & Row, Publishers.

89. Ter-Pogossian, M. M., Kastner, J., and Vest, T. B.: Autofluorography of the thyroid gland by means of image amplification, Radiology **81:**984, 1963.

90. Wallman, H., and Wickbom, I.: Roentgen television equipment for use in surgery, Acta Radiol. **51:**297, 1959.

91. Webster, E. W.: Image intensifier systems and their resolution limitations. In Hilal S. K., editor: Small vessel angiography, St. Louis, 1973, The C. V. Mosby Co.

92. Webster, E. W.: The future of electronic image intensifiers, Paper presented at the Symposium on electronic imaging techniques in diagnostic radiology, University of Pittsburgh, April, 1973.

93. Westinghouse Electric Corp.: Stop-action fluoroscopic storage and display system, Research and development letter, April, 1968.

94. Winter, D. A.: Image enhancement by digital techniques, Paper presented at the Symposium on electronic imaging techniques in diagnostic radiology, University of Pittsburgh, April, 1973.

95. Winter, D. A., et al: Videodensitometry—a clinical approach to the calculation of left ventricular volume. In Zarnsdorf, W. C., Hendee, W. R. and Carlson, P. C., editors: Proceedings of the conference on application of optical instruments in medicine, Redondo Beach, Calif., Society of Photo-optical Illumination Engineers. (In press.)

96. Zucchino, P. M., and Lowrance, J. L.: Recent development of the SEC-vidicon for astronomy, Adv. Electronics Electron Phys. **33B:**801, 1972.

6 Receiver operating characteristic analysis and its significance in interpretation of radiologic images

Lee B. Lusted

The use of receiver operating characteristic or relative operating characteristic (ROC) analysis in the interpretation of radiologic images will be presented as the basis for comments about decision theory, signal detection, and medical diagnosis.

GENERAL CONSIDERATIONS

The problem of detecting signals in noise is really the same as the problem of detecting the presence of unknown systematic influences in celestial mechanics that was described many years ago by Laplace and the same as recent problems of detecting the systematic drift of machine characteristics in industrial quality control. Unfortunately the basic identity of these problems was not widely recognized, and workers in several different fields were forced to rediscover the same ideas over and over again as decision theory penetrated the various disciplines.

More than any other factor, the development of decision theory has led to a revolution in statistical thinking. Except for the introduction of a loss function at the end, there is nothing in decision theory that is not already contained in basic probability theory if we free ourselves from the dogma that "probability statements can be made only about random variables" and use the theory in the full generality given to it by Laplace. As Laplace has said, "Probability theory is nothing but common sense reduced to calculation," and the most important recent advances in statistics have taken us right back to the methods developed by Bayes, Laplace, and Bernoulli in the eighteenth century.

Jaynes[6] has pointed out recently that the present unsettled condition of probability theory has serious implications for problem solving in theoretical physics and engineering, and he proceeds to show that some of the outstanding unsolved problems in both physics and communication theory have their

Supported by U.S.P.H.S. Grant GM-18940.

117

origins in this state of utter confusion that exists in the foundations of probability theory. The issue can be framed as viewpoint A, which denounces any idea that probability theory has anything to do with inductive reasoning and insists that it is, instead, "the exact science of mass phenomena and repetitive events." Viewpoint B holds the opposite opinion and insists that probability theory is exactly what Laplace thought it was, the "calculus of inductive reasoning." Jaynes comes down hard for viewpoint B in science and engineering, and I think we must do so in medicine.

In a series of excellent lectures, Jaynes[6] has shown a great simplification and unification of probability theory and decision theory by the use of a single, very simple set of principles that can be stated in a few lines and that, when applied to specific problems, will be found to give automatically conventional probability theory, the formalism of equilibrium and nonequilibrium statistical mechanics, the results of communication theory, and the newest methods of statistical inference.

The principles just referred to are basic rules of Boolean algebra, probability theory, and decision theory. They have been applied to some specific areas of medical diagnosis with some success and they form the basis for building models of medical diagnosis.[9] The world of medical decision making is too large and too complicated to analyze all at once, so we try to dissect it into several pieces and study these separately. Sometimes we can make a model that represents several features of the pieces; by working with the model we may get new ideas about the pieces, build better models, and so on.

The test of a model is not "Can you prove that it is correct?" but "Is it free of inconsistencies and does it yield predictions in agreement with observable facts?"

In this chapter we are going to look at a rather simple model for studying detection and recognition of a radiologic image. The model uses some of the basic principles referred to previously and represents one of the simplest applications of general decision theory to an aspect of medical diagnosis. The model as presented has limitations, but I think it represents a viewpoint we ought to take in studying medical decision making.

SIGNAL DETECTING AND DECISION THEORY

Suppose that we ask an observer to make the best possible decision about whether a signal is present or not present. The observer is a person looking for a signal in noise. The observer may or may not be a radiologist, and the signal may be anything from the radiographic image of a small gallstonelike object to the image pattern of opacities produced in pneumoconiosis.

From the point of view of the observer, the first thing to do is calculate the probability that the signal is present. If there are only two possibilities for the signal S: either it is present, S_1, or it is not present, S_0. Then after the observer has seen the radiograph, the odds that the signal is present are:

$$\Omega_1(S_1 | I) = \Omega_0(S_1) \frac{P(I|S_1)}{P(I|S_0)} \tag{1}$$

where odds $\Omega(S)$ in favor of signal S are related to the probability $P(S)$ of signal S and the probability $1 - P(S)$ of "no signal" by the condition:

$$\Omega(S) = \frac{P(S)}{1 - P(S)} \tag{2}$$

where:

$\Omega_0(S_1)$ = Prior odds for observer in favor of presence of signal before observer has seen radiograph (It should be emphasized that $\Omega_0(S)$ represents uncertainty of observer's knowledge about S before he has seen radiograph; $\Omega_0(S)$ does not represent "an objective state of the world" unknown to observer.)

I = Any evidence for observer about signal or image S

$P(I|S_1)$ = Probability of evidence I given that image S is present

$P(I|S_0)$ = Probability of evidence I given that image S is not present

$\Omega_1(S_1 | I)$ = Final odds for observer in favor of presence of signal after observer has seen radiograph

Now we tell the observer to make the decision about S that minimizes the expected loss. The observer will use the decision rule[6]:

$$\text{Choose } D_1 \text{ if } \Omega_1(S_1 | I) \equiv \frac{P(S_1 | I)}{P(S_0 | I)} > \frac{L_{FP}}{L_{FN}} \tag{3}$$

where:

D_1 = Observer's decision that S is present

$P(S_1 | I)$ = Probability that image S is present given evidence I

$P(S_0 | I)$ = Probability that image S is not present given evidence I

L_{FP} = Loss or cost of false positive decision (decision that signal is present when signal is not present)

L_{FN} = Loss or cost of false negative decision (decision that signal is not present when signal is present)

To express this in words, the observer decides (S_1) that S is present if, given the evidence, the probability that the signal is present exceeds the probability that it is due to noise alone by a factor greater than the ratio of false positive decision loss to false negative decision loss.

The generality of this decision rule is important. No assumptions are needed about the type of signal or statistical properties of the noise. The left-hand side of expression 3 is a ratio of probabilities and the right-hand side is a ratio of losses. There are different philosophies regarding how you choose the value of probability at which you will change your decision. We are just beginning to explore ideas about this important subject.

Before we proceed to discuss the application of the theory in terms of ROC curves, there are two things to note about the arguments presented. First, on the basis of the Laplace-Bayes "inductive reasoning" form of probability theory and a simple set of principles that form a basic theme for probability theory, communication theory, and statistical inference, we are able to apply ideas about classic matched filters, entropy, information content of a signal, and so on to problems of radiologic image analysis. Second, in the practical situation there may be many different signals to distinguish; this process is called signal recognition. Signal detection may be considered as a special case of signal recognition in which one of the two signals to be discriminated is "no signal," or noise alone. In the recognition situation we may need to decide not only whether a signal is present but also signal size, shape, density, location, and so on. The details of analysis can become complicated. But these extensions, from the Bayesian viewpoint, are straightforward in that they require no new principles beyond those already given.

RELATIVE OPERATING CHARACTERISTIC ANALYSIS AND SIGNAL DETECTION

The use of ROC analysis of observer performance in radiology has a history extending back to the work done in electronic communications in the early 1940s and to psychophysics developments in the early 1950s. In an excellent review, Swets[21] places the relative operating characteristic (ROC) in historical perspective. Swets explains why he prefers the term "relative operating characteristic" to receiver operating characteristic, which is more widely associated with the ROC acronym. It is because the ROC is a comparison of two operating characteristics that Swets describes. We will continue to use ROC to mean receiver operating characteristic and remember that the two terms are synonymous.

Swets emphasizes the ROC in psychology. I wish to discuss the ROC in the context of probability and benefits-costs in order to emphasize a decision theory approach to medical diagnosis.

According to Swet's account,[21] Tanner and Swets were studying sensory psychology at the University of Michigan where Peterson and Birdsall were applying statistical decision theory to radar detection problems and were developing ROC analysis. ROC analysis first appeared in the literature in the transactions of a 1954 symposium on information theory at which both Michigan theorists and Van Meter and Middleton of Harvard University by coincidence discussed decision rules of ROC analysis. Tanner and Swets[22] proposed at that time a new theory of visual detection that presented, from the point of view of psychophysics, a theory of human signal detection based on the physical detection theory proposed by Peterson and Birdsall. It was Peterson and Birdsall[15] who showed how to plot the data to get an ROC curve.

It is interesting to stop here for a moment to look back at the problem of the detection of electromagnetic signals in the presence of noise, which concerned scientists working on radar systems in the early 1940s. In the design of radar receiver input circuits the engineer wished to maximize the signal-to-noise ratio; finding the circuit design to do this led to the classic matched filter. But matched filter theory in engineering and decision theory lead to the same strategy of signal detection; namely, the best statistical analysis you can make of the signal detection problem will always be one in which you calculate the probability that the various signals are present by means of Bayes' theorem.

The central ideas of the Tanner-Swets theory are (1) that noise is present in all discrimination tasks and (2) that the process of detection of a signal is pictured as consisting of two parts, a likelihood ratio (the probability that the signal was present divided by the probability of noise alone) and a straightforward decision procedure based on this likelihood ratio (the observer says "signal present" if the likelihood ratio exceeds a predetermined value). In the initial statements of this theory a general assumption was made that some transformation of the likelihood ratio is Gaussian under both noise and signal-plus-noise hypotheses. Given these ideas, psychophysicists developed detection experiments that involved the simple detection of a sound or a light against a noise background. In these experiments two independent probabilities were developed: a true positive probability (observer says signal when signal plus noise is present) and a false positive probability (observer says signal when there is noise alone).

Peterson et al.[16] plotted the true positive probability on the Y axis and the false positive probability on the X axis. A set of data points was fitted by eye along a single curve called a receiver operating characteristic (ROC) curve because their original work viewed "receiver" in the perspective of communications.

Signal detection theory and ROC curve analysis present a method of separating the decision factors of the observer from the sensory factors that influence his sensitivity as a signal detector. Thus we are able to assess an observer without the necessity of analyzing in exquisite detail all of his decision criteria or of specifying the exact composition of the signal. The separation of decision factors from detection sensitivity permit us to perform some interesting and useful studies of radiologic images. The measures of detection sensitivity and decision criteria will be discussed as we consider some practical applications.

SOME PRACTICAL APPLICATIONS

In 1966 I read books by Swets[20] and Green and Swets[5] on the detection and recognition of auditory and visual signals. I was surprised to find that the false positive–false negative plot of errors that I had demonstrated in the observer error studies of diagnosis of minimal pulmonary tuberculosis by chest radiography[7] was actually a ROC curve (Fig. 6-1). A Laplace-Bayes view of probability underlies signal detection, and I concluded that signal detection theory and ROC curve analysis could be used to study decision-making processes in medicine. Specifically, I wished to study the detection and recognition of radiologic images in terms of observer performance. Some first thoughts along these lines were published in 1967 and 1968.[8,9]

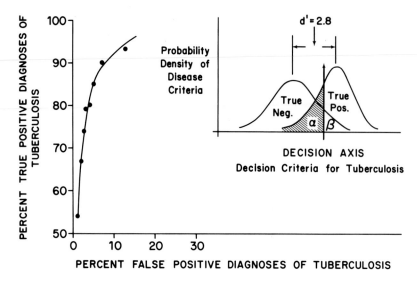

Fig. 6-1. ROC curve for interpretation of chest photofluorograms for presence of pulmonary tuberculosis. Reciprocal relationship is demonstrated between percentage of true positive and percentage of false positive diagnoses. Hypothetical population density curves that generated ROC curve are shown in upper right diagram. The α and β areas represent false negative and false positive diagnoses; d' is index of detectability and is defined as mean separation of two distributions divided by standard deviation of one distribution. This is written:

$$d' = \frac{{}^mTP - {}^mTN}{\sigma}$$

where ${}^mTP$ represents mean of true positive population and ${}^mTN$ represents mean of true negative population. (From Lusted, L. B.: New Engl. J. Med. **284:**416, 1971.)

Now let us look at some selected problems to which signal detection theory and ROC curve analysis have been applied during the past 5 years. We may consider that the analysis has some significance if it provides a viewpoint that seems generally useful in thinking about the problems. I will not present a detailed description of experimental design, decision criteria, and composition of signal and noise for each problem. The reader should consult the cited references.

Problem: to choose an optimum system for a specified task

Suppose that we ask our observer to choose the best screen-film combination to detect low-contrast unsharp images such as the images of certain small gallstones. The observer sets up an experiment with certain specified parameters and obtains a ROC curve for each screen-film combination he is considering (Fig. 6-2).[3,13] As noted earlier, a ROC curve is simply a plot of conditional true positive versus conditional false positive response probabilities observed

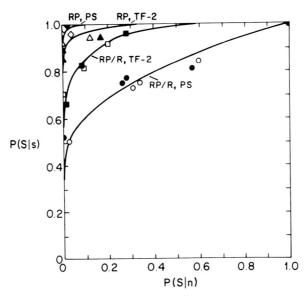

Fig. 6-2. ROC curves generated by single observer. Signal was radiographic image of 2 mm diameter Lucite bead, and noise resulted from radiographic mottle of following screen-film combinations: RP-Kodak RP X-omat medical x-ray film (normal speed); RP/R-Kodak RP Royal X-omat medical x-ray film (fast speed); PS-Dupont Cronex Par Speed Screen (medium speed); and TF-2-Radelin TF-2 Screen (fast speed). Open and solid symbols of a given shape indicate independent trial runs with observer and given screen-film combination. Each independent trial run consists of approximately 100 observations. (From Metz, C. E., Goodenough, D. J., and Rossmann, K.: Radiology **109:**297, 1973.)

in an experiment in which an observer decides whether or not a signal is present. A ROC curve can be generated in several ways. For details see the description by Metz and Goodenough.[12] The ROC curve in the upper left-hand corner of Fig. 6-2 demonstrates the highest true positive rate for a given false positive rate, and the observer concludes that the RP,PS screen-film combination is best for detection of the low-contrast unsharp images used in this experiment.

With the use of the ROC curves in Figs. 6-1 and 6-2 we can illustrate two measures used to assess the observer. One measure defines the observer's sensitivity as a signal detector. An index of detectability, d', has been defined to indicate this measure, and the larger the value of d', the more sensitive the observer. For the RP,PS screen-film combination, d' is larger than 4, whereas for the RP/R,PS screen-film combination, $d' = 1.3 \pm 0.3$. For each point on the ROC defined by the corresponding values of true positive and false positive responses there is a d' value. Swets[20] has provided tables that give d' for a large number of true positive–false positive combinations.

The parameter d' is calculated using the assumption that the signal and signal plus noise can be described by normal probability distributions of equal variance. For many of the problems of interest this seems to be a restrictive assumption that can lead to serious error in ranking observer performance if full ROC curve data are not available[4]; therefore other indices of detectability have been investigated. Metz recently proposed that ROC curve evaluation be considered in terms of information theory, and Metz et al.[13] have shown that the average "information content" of the image can be calculated directly from any point on a ROC curve. In addition, the maximum information content (I_{max}) available on a ROC curve can be determined. Use of this information theoretic approach does not require assumptions concerning physical mechanisms such as normal probability distributions of signal and noise, and observer performance can be determined quantitatively from experimental data in terms of average information obtained per observation.

Use of the information theoretic approach can be applied in two ways: (1) to evaluate maximum information (I_{max}) available on each of two or more ROC curves and (2) to compare the average information content per observation computed for single operating points on one or more ROC curves. This is a great advantage, as we shall see later in a study of pneumoconiosis in which only a percent true positive–percent false positive performance score was obtained for each reader. The average information content (I) does not require knowledge of the entire ROC curve for meaningful application.

For the ROC curves in Fig. 6-2, the d'_e and I_{max} indices of detectability for a single observer are shown below:

	d'_e	I_{max} ± 0.5*
RP,PS	>4	0.95
RP,TF-2	3.0 ± 0.5	0.70
RP|R,TF-2	2.3 ± 0.4	0.50
RP|R,PS	1.3 ± 0.3	0.30

The index of detectability d'_e is defined as the d' value of a ROC curve that would have the same intercept with the negative diagonal (conditional probability of true positive response = $1 -$ conditional probability of false positive response) as the ROC curve under consideration. As an index of detectability, d'_e is somewhat more reliable than d' because d'_e is derived from a ROC curve whereas the d' value is calculated for a single operating point.

A second measure defines the decision factors that lead the observer to choose the odds at which he will change his decision from saying "signal not present" to saying "signal present." This is repeating in words the decision rule of expression 3.

The decision criteria chosen depend upon the goal the observer wishes to achieve. For instance, he might wish to maximize the reduction of uncertainty.

---

*Assume prior signal probability = 0.5.

This is the goal when the I_{max} is calculated for a ROC curve. Other goals the observer could choose include (1) maximizing true positive responses while restricting false positive responses to some specified level, perhaps 10%, (2) maximizing the number of true positive plus true negative decisions, or (3) maximizing the expected value of the decisions.

Although I think that we will wish to use a decision rule that minimizes information loss, it is helpful to think about a loss function of a decision in terms of maximizing the expected value of a decision because we are led to consider the relative benefits and costs of correct and incorrect decisions.

The expected value of a decision strategy in signal detection is the sum of four terms, each of which represents the benefit or cost associated with an outcome weighted by the probability that a particular outcome will occur given the strategy in question.

Maximizing the expected benefit is equivalent to maximizing the expression:

$$L_c = \frac{P(S_0)}{P(S_1)} \cdot \frac{B_{TN} + L_{FP}}{B_{TP} + L_{FN}} \tag{4}$$

where:

L_c = Critical value of decision criteria at which observer changes his decision from "signal not present" to "signal present"

$P(S_1)$ = Prior probability of signal present

$P(S_0)$ = Prior probability of no signal

B_{TN} = Benefit associated with true negative response

L_{FP} = Loss associated with false positive response

B_{TP} = Benefit associated with true positive response

L_{FN} = Loss associated with false negative response

Under the conditions that $B_{TN} = B_{TP} = 0$, equation 4 says the same thing as expression 3, namely, say "signal present" when $\Omega_1(S_1) > L_{FP}/L_{FN}$.

Radiologists have given little thought to relative benefits and costs of decision outcomes, and it will be useful in the future to do so. A ROC curve makes it possible to investigate the values of an observer without asking for an explicit expression of the values. This can be done as follows.

Green and Swets[5] show that the slope of a ROC curve at any point is equal to the likelihood ratio criterion based on the signal-plus-noise response to noise-alone response that generates that point. A point on the ROC curve expresses your attitude about optimal weighting among correct responses and errors coupled with your estimate of the prior probability that a signal is present, so the slope of the curve at this point represents the critical value L_c of your decision criteria.

On the ROC curve shown in Fig. 6-1 my operating point was 80% true positive and 4% false positive diagnoses. At this point the slope is 5. If we assume that this point represents my attitude about the optimal weighting of true positive and false positive diagnoses, then by equation 4 and using data about the prior probabilities of pulmonary tuberculosis[10] we can write:

$$5 = 2000 \cdot \frac{B_{TN} + L_{FP}}{B_{TP} + L_{FN}} \tag{5}$$

With the help of this expression I can explore my preferences for losses in the diagnosis of tuberculosis.

If

$$B_{TN} = B_{TP} = 0 \tag{6}$$

then

$$\frac{1}{400} = \frac{FP}{FN} \tag{7}$$

In words, say (S_1) "tuberculosis present" when the loss of a false negative error is equivalent to 400 times the loss of a false positive error. With this result I can consider the implications of trade-off of one false negative diagnosis for 400 false positive diagnoses. Monetary cost and human costs in terms of such factors as anxiety must be considered. Not much progress has been made in this type of analysis.

The measure of image information content can indicate a point on the ROC curve at which image information loss is minimal, but the observer might choose to operate at a different point on the ROC curve as a result of his assessment of relative benefits and costs for a given diagnosis.

Signal location and signal recognition. If complexity of the detection task is increased to require identification of the location of a signal or to distinguish between two or more different signals, then a somewhat longer analysis is required. Metz and Goodenough[11] have shown an analysis in which the signal location factor is important in the assessment of scan-smoothing processes to improve lesion detectability in clinical scintigraphy.

For a recognition task involving M classes of signals, Metz and Goodenough[12] argue that an analysis can be made in terms of "a generalized ROC hyper-surface" in $M(M + 1)$ dimensional space and that the two distribution-free measures of observer performance, "information content" and "expected value," can be computed for any point in a conditional probability hyper-space. Work on the application of these ideas is in progress.

Problem: to assess observer performance for a specified task

Suppose that you have a program by which you wish to detect pneumoconiosis by chest radiography in a population of miners. You would like to be assured that the maximum number of miners with pneumoconiosis will be detected at a minimum cost. How do you assess the performance of the radiologists who interpret the chest roentgenograms for pneumoconiosis to be sure that they meet a required level of performance as detectors of pneumoconiosis?

Obviously I am going to suggest a procedure based on the decision processes for signal detection and ROC curve analysis that we have just discussed. Morgan et al.[14] recently published an article on decision processes and observer error in the diagnosis of pneumoconiosis by chest roentgenography. Data for the following example come from their work.

The signal to be detected is composed of all of the opacities that are related to the underlying process called pneumoconiosis. There are basically two decisions that the observer may make, namely, "pneumoconiosis is present" or "pneumoconiosis is not present." In the present situation the signal is defined by words that give the diagnostic criteria for the presence of pneumoconiosis. The decision about the presence of pneumoconiosis may be graded as to degree of severity of the disease, but the grades may be divided into two decisions about the presence or absence of disease. A test series of chest roentgenograms, some of which contain the signal, is compiled; for each roentgenogram it is known whether the signal is present or absent. Morgan used a test series of 200 chest roentgenograms, and a panel of five expert radiologists made the decision "pneumoconiosis present" or "pneumoconiosis not present" for each roentgenogram. The use of a test series of proved cases is very important.

The test series is then presented to the observers to be evaluated, and a record of true positive and false positive decisions is kept for each observer. An index of detectability, either d' or information content (I), is calculated for each observer. This index is a measure of the observer's ability to detect pneumoconiosis from the chest roentgenogram.

The performance of seven readers in Morgan's study interpreting a series of 200 test films for pneumoconiosis was as follows*:

Reader	True positive (%)	False positive (%)	Index of detectability (d')
F	84.7	3.1	2.89
B	94.4	14.1	2.66
G	90.2	13.3	2.41
D	93.1	18.0	2.38
A	80.6	9.4	2.25
C	80.6	8.6	2.24
E	57.0	2.3	2.17

Other observers who interpreted the test series showed lower indices of detectability, from 1.33 to 1.84. Morgan hopes to develop quantitative criteria whereby the acceptability of a prospective candidate wishing to engage in the pneumoconiosis program may be determined. If quantitative criteria are interpreted to mean performance criteria, then the previous discussion suggests that the problem might be approached in the following manner.

Metz et al.[13] have shown that, given a specified prior probability of the signal, the average information content per image can be calculated for any

---

*From Morgan, R. H., et al.: Am. J. Roentgenol. Radium Ther. Nucl. Med. **117:**757, 1973.

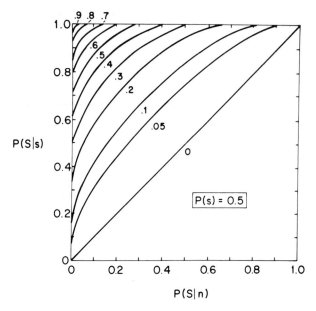

Fig. 6-3. Isoinformation curves. Each curve represents locus of points on ROC graph corresponding to given amount of information (in bits) obtained for observation. $P(S/s)$ = conditional probability of true positive response; $P(S/n)$ = conditional probability of false positive response; $P(s)$ = prior probability of signal = 0.5. (From Metz, C. E., Goodenough, D. J., and Rossmann, K.: Radiology **109**:297, 1973.)

pair of true positive and false positive probabilities. A series of "isoinformation" curves is shown in Fig. 6-3 for 0.5 prior probability of signal. Suppose we decide that minimum acceptable performance must be above isoinformation curve 0.5. The two extremes of the isoinformation curve are true positive = 72%, false positive = 0% at one extreme and true positive = 100%, false positive = 28% at the other. Only observers whose true positive–false positive scores placed above the 0.5 isoinformation curve would be accepted.

I have not said much about how to decide what amounts for benefits and costs to use in the expected benefit relationship (equation 4). This is an important subject that needs a good deal of thought. I hope investigators will publish their ideas about error assessment, possibly expressed as a loss matrix for a specific project.

Problem: to evaluate image transmission or storage by television, Picturephone, or video disk

Revesz and Haas[17] and Revesz and Kundel[18,19] and their colleagues at Temple University have reported on a series of projects to develop and evaluate techniques that would improve the storage and display of radiologic images. Equipment is evaluated in terms of the observer error rate when a series of test radiographs is viewed. These investigators have developed a television display of radiographic images with superimposed simulated lesions that facilitates the testing procedure. The detection measure d′ is calculated and used to evaluate the storage and transmission capability of the system under test.

Nuclear image transmission by Picturephone has been investigated by Anderson et al.[1] at the University of Chicago. A test series of images used single-view scintigram pictures of ^{99m}Tc brain scans recorded on black-and-white Polaroid film. ROC analysis showed that the observer error rate was not increased by Picturephone transmission of the images.

Remote interpretation of chest radiographs can be investigated by ROC analysis. Andrus et al.[2] used a microwave television link between Massachusetts General Hospital and Bedford Veterans Administration Hospital seventeen miles distant to transmit a series of chest radiographs of patients who were normal or had pulmonary tuberculosis or a pulmonary disease that resembles tuberculosis in radiographic appearance. ROC curves were generated to compare the radiologist's ability to recognize tuberculosis on direct view of the films compared with his performance on viewing the transmitted image. The index of detectability for direct viewing was $d'_e = 1.6$ and for television viewing, $d'_e = 1.4$. This study indicates that observer performance was not significantly impaired by television transmission of the radiographic images.

SUMMARY

I have attempted to find a viewpoint from which it is possible to consider the evaluation of radiologic images in the larger context of the reasoning behind medical diagnosis. I think we cannot be far wrong in our methodology if we follow the advice of J. Willard Gibbs, who remarked on the occasion of receiving the Rumford Medal (1881), "One of the principal objects of theoretical research in any department of knowledge is to find the point of view from which the subject appears in its greatest simplicity."

ROC analysis has been presented in terms of decision theory in signal detection because it represents, at present, the viewpoint from which image evaluation appears to me in greatest simplicity. No new mathematics are needed and we can draw on concepts of probability, information theory, and psychophysics.

Future work may provide better viewpoints. That is the challenge.

Acknowledgment

I thank Charles E. Metz, Ph.D., for helpful discussions about ideas presented in this paper.

References

1. Anderson, T. M., et al.: Nuclear image transmission by Picturephone. Evaluation by ROC curve method, Invest. Radiol. **8:**244, 1973.

2. Andrus, W. S., Hunter, C. H., and Bird, K. T.: Remote interpretation of chest roentgenograms. (In press.)
3. Goodenough, D. J.: Radiographic applications of signal detection theory, Ph.D. thesis, The University of Chicago, 1972.
4. Goodenough, D. J., Metz, C. E., and Lusted, L. B.: Caveat on the use of the parameter d' for evaluation of observer performance, Radiology 105:199, 1973.
5. Green, D. M., and Swets, J. A.: Signal detection theory and psychophysics, New York, 1966, John Wiley & Sons, Inc.
6. Jaynes, E. T.: Probability theory—with applications in science and engineering. A series of informal lectures presented at Washington University. (In press.)
7. Lusted, L. B.: Logical analysis in roentgen diagnosis, Radiology 74:178, 1960.
8. Lusted, L. B.: Medical decision making. In Digest of the seventh international conference on medical and biological engineering, Stockholm, Sweden, 1967, Ljunglöfs Litografiska, AB.
9. Lusted, L. B.: Introduction to medical decision making, Springfield, Ill., 1968, Charles C Thomas, Publisher.
10. Lusted, L. B.: Decision-making studies in patient management, N. Engl. J. Med. 284:416, 1971.
11. Metz, C. E., and Goodenough, D. J.: Letter to the editor, J. Nucl. Med. 14:873, 1973.
12. Metz, C. E., and Goodenough, D. J.: Quantitative evaluation of human visual detection performance using empirical receiver operating characteristic curves. In Proceedings of the third international conference on data handling and image processing in scintigraphy, Oak Ridge, Tenn., 1974, USAEC Technical Information Center.
13. Metz, C. E., Goodenough, D. J., and Rossmann, K.: Evaluation of receiver operating characteristic curve data in terms of information theory, with applications in radiography, Radiology 109:297, 1973.
14. Morgan, R. H., et al.: Decision processes and observer error in the diagnosis of pneumoconiosis by chest roentgenography, Am. J. Roentgenol. Radium Ther. Nucl. Med. 117:757, 1973.
15. Peterson, W. W., and Birdsall, T. G.: The theory of signal detectability, Technical Report No. 13, Ann Arbor, 1953, Electronic Defense Group, University of Michigan.
16. Peterson, W. W., Birdsall, T. G., and Fox, W. C.: Trans. IRE Prof. Group Inf. Theory PGIT-4:171, 1954.
17. Revesz, G., and Haas, C.: Television display of radiographic images with superimposed simulated lesions, Radiology 102:197, 1972.
18. Revesz, G., and Kundel, H. L.: Effects of non-linearities on the television display of x-ray images, Invest. Radiol. 6:315, 1971.
19. Revesz, G., and Kundel, H. L.: Videodisc storage of radiographs, Radiology 106:91, 1973.
20. Swets, J. A.: Signal detection and recognition by human observers, New York, 1964, John Wiley & Sons, Inc.
21. Swets, J. A.: The relative operating characteristic in psychology, Science 182:990, 1973.
22. Tanner, W. P., Jr., and Swets, J. A.: Trans. IRE Prof. Group Inf. Theory PGIT-4:213, 1954.

7 Toward optimizing chest x-ray technique

Bob W. Gayler

GENERAL CONSIDERATIONS

Radiographs of the chest are the single most common type of x-ray examination, and in general hospital and office practice they account for 40% to 50% of all radiographic studies. Despite the frequency of this examination, or perhaps because of it, there is no unanimity of opinion on the best way to radiograph the chest. This chapter will review some of the elements of chest radiography. As a preliminary statement, I believe that a good chest radiograph should have good visibility of detail, good soft tissue definition with preservation of some bone detail, and the lowest patient radiation dosage consistent with good detail. A few background observations are pertinent.

For many years, mass survey and screening chest radiographs were taken as 70 mm photofluorograms. This format has a considerable advantage in cost, convenience, and storage ease over the full-size radiograph and still appears to be used on a fairly wide scale. The amount of radiation involved may be several times greater than that required for the full-size radiograph, and use of this modality has been recently discouraged by the Bureau of Radiological Health.[20] However, in the past few years there have been significant technical advances in image intensification tubes, and it is quite possible that there may be a resurgence in the popularity of photofluorography, particularly if a significant silver shortage occurs and if other forms of imaging do not reliably replace silver halide systems. Some stated advantages of the smaller film format, in addition to those listed above, are better penetration in "blind" (retrocardiac and mediastinal) areas of the chest and reduction of observer fatigue.[5] Suffice it to say that chest photofluorograms continue to have an impact on the total subject of chest radiography but will not be discussed further in this section.

The capacity of x-ray generating equipment in the past necessitated that chest radiographs be made at kilovoltages below 90 and milliamperages of from 100 to 300. Some of the timing apparatus was not particularly accurate at times of less than 1/10 second. Routine formats of 10 or 20 milliampere seconds (mAs) with variable kilovoltage of 55 to 70 kilovoltage peak (kVp) for the posterior-anterior projection became very widely used. This produces a visually

131

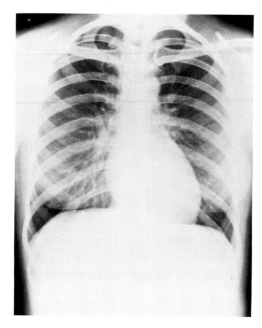

Fig. 7-1. Routine format using 70 kVp, 10 mAs, and no grid for a patient with a 24 cm AP chest diameter. Film taken in 1953 and processed manually.

pleasing radiograph for small- and average-size cooperative patients without requiring the use of a grid (Figs. 7-1 and 7-6, *A*).* Many radiologists received their training observing chest films made with these technical factors and various suggestions for the modification of these techniques have often been less than enthusiastically received. As the kilovoltage and milliampere capacity of x-ray generating equipment has increased, many other combinations of technical factors have been tried and some are in common use. These factors will be considered in more detail later in this chapter.

With x-ray generators of fairly low output, motion-free lateral chest films are frequently difficult to obtain, and for many years the PA view was felt to be a sufficient chest examination in the absence of symptoms. The lateral view, however, with its demonstration of the retrosternal, retrocardiac, and posterior costophrenic angle regions, is now widely accepted as part of the routine chest examination[13,21] and is not held in reserve as a special view.

---

*In the legends for all figures in this chapter, the term "grid" refers to a reciprocating grid (Potter-Bucky diaphragm) except in Fig. 7-19, for which a stationary grid was used. Fig. 7-19 is the only radiograph made with three-phase equipment. Radiographs were processed with a 90-second automatic processor unless otherwise stipulated. All of the photographs exhibit moderate contrast enhancement. The degree of contrast enhancement should be similar for all the radiographs. One can estimate the appearance of the original by looking at Fig. 7-12. The original radiograph for Fig. 7-12, *A*, had approximately the same contrast range as the photographically reduced radiograph in Fig. 7-12, *D*. The original radiograph for Fig. 7-12, *D*, was rather gray, with a wide latitude and low contrast.

FACTORS AFFECTING FILM QUALITY

There are several aspects of chest radiography that affect film quality, and they are individually considered below.

Focal spot to film distance

The most frequently used focal spot to film distance (FFD) is 72 inches. This produces a slight magnification of 10% to 15% of the more distant (with respect to the film) structures, but this does not appear to be of great practical significance. The percent enlargement can be calculated as[9]:

$$\text{Percent enlargement} = \frac{\text{Object to film distance}}{\text{Focal spot to object distance}} \times 100$$

In taking a PA chest film of a patient with a 24 cm AP diameter, the posterior ribs would be about 9 inches from the anterior chest wall and 10 inches from the film surface. Percent enlargement would therefore be $\frac{10}{62} \times 100$, or 16%.

To reduce this to 8%, for example, would require a 140-inch FFD. This rather considerable distance is rarely used, probably because the advantages of reduced magnification do not outweigh the disadvantages of altered room size and layout and increased demands on the x-ray generating equipment at this greater distance. An FFD of greater than 72 inches is used, however, when an air-gap method is employed to reduce scattered radiation. At one time the film produced at 72 inches was called a "teleroentgenogram," but since the 72-inch FFD has become the standard for chest radiographs, no special notation is ordinarily made of this distance.

Equipment

The equipment used for chest radiography in the United States is predominantly single phase, with a 30 to 50 kilowatt capacity and a peak kilovoltage capability of 125. Many x-ray tubes in general use have nominal focal spots of 1 and 2 mm. The actual focal spot size as determined by the pinhole method may be 40% higher than the nominal value and still be acceptable by National Electrical Manufacturers Association (NEMA) standards. This range of tolerance has been very important to manufacturers because there is considerable wastage in tube manufacture within these constraints, and a requirement that tubes have precise adherence to the nominal value would cause rejection rates to be higher than they are with consequent substantial increase in tube prices. This tolerance on the large side of focal spots has, of course, the practical benefit of increasing the safety margin with respect to heat-loading capacity.

Within the last decade, x-ray generators capable of operating at 150 kVp have become available from all manufacturers, and milliamperage in excess of 1000 and kilowattage specifications in excess of 100 are produced by a few. Electronic timing has made possible a wider selection of exposure times than is available if one relies simply on impulse timing devices. Accurate calibration of the available milliamperage settings and precision timing has been a problem, so that federal regulations concerning accuracy of timing and reproducibility have been published in the Federal Register and are in effect as of August 1, 1974.[7]

In response to greatly increased generator output, the x-ray tube manufacturers have made tubes of greater heat-loading capacity with respect to single as well as repeated exposures. For chest radiography, total heat loading is seldom a problem, but it is frequently desirable to use a high milliamperage with a high kilovoltage to get a very short exposure time, and some of these newer tubes are very helpful in this regard, even though the heat unit output may be well under 1000 per exposure. The tube manufacturers have been very interested in making the nominal focal spots smaller so that tubes with focal spots of 0.6 mm and large focal spots of 1 to 1.5 mm are now readily available. These small focal spots frequently have a load capability of 30 kilowatts and are thus suitable for a large percentage of the patients who have chest radiographs. These smaller focal spots with increased heat capacity have been made possible by modifying anode structure as well as decreasing the target angle. A target angle of 12° covers a 17 by 17 inch field at 40 inches. The coverage of an 11° target angle is approximately 14 by 14 inches at an FFD of 40 inches. Targets with these angulations do not impose any restrictions on chest film field coverage at a 72-inch FFD.

Films and intensifying screens

Intensifying screens and x-ray films must be treated together as the recording medium. The standards for comparative comment are the medium-speed screens and medium-speed films. There are numerous manufacturers of screens and films, and the terminology can certainly be confusing. Tables 7-1 and 7-2 give the nomenclature used by several manufacturers for their films and screens. The four major characteristics of film-screen combinations of interest to the radiologist are speed, contrast, latitude, and resolution.

Speed relates film density to exposure values. A high-speed film or screen has a higher density at the same kilovoltage peak and milliampere second values than does a lower speed film or screen. Density may be plotted against

Table 7-1. Manufacturers' film designations and film characteristics

Company	Medium speed	Fast speed	Wide latitude
Dupont	Cronex 4	Cronex 5	Cronex 6
Eastman	RP	RPS, RPR	RPL
Fugi	Rx	RxS	RxL
GAF	HR 1000	HR 2000	HR 3000
Gevaert	RP-1		
Ilford	Red Seal	Rapid-R	

the logarithm of the relative exposure, producing a curve (called the H and D curve, after Hurter and Driffield) that is useful for making comparative evaluations[11] (Fig. 7-2).

Contrast is the difference in the density of a structure by comparison to the density of its surroundings. Film and screen contrast characteristics are important in final image contrast, but image contrast is also affected by the patient's body structures and the quality of radiation.

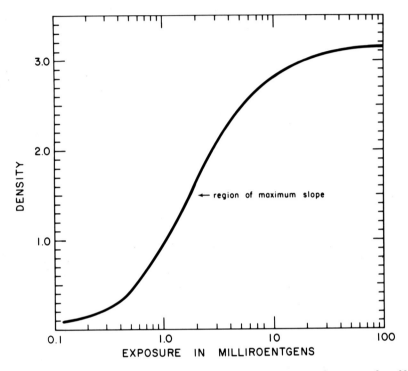

Fig. 7-2. Example of an H and D curve. (Prepared by Dr. Gopalo Rao and Wilfred Sewchand, Physics and Engineering Section, Department of Radiology and Radiological Science, The Johns Hopkins Medical Institutions, Baltimore, Md.)

Table 7-2. Manufacturers' intensifying screen designations

Company	Slow	Medium	Fast
Dupont	Detail, Fast Detail	Par	Hi Plus, Lightning Plus
Eastmen	Fine	Regular	
Fugi	FS	MS	HS
Ilford	Hi-Definition	Standard	Fast
Intensi	Fine	Medium	High-speed
Picker		Medium	High
Rädelin	HD	T-2, TF-2	STF-2
Siemens	Ruby	Sapphire	Diamond

Latitude is a film-screen characteristic related to film and screen contrast and generally used with an opposite connotation. Thus a high-contrast film generally has low latitude and a low-contrast film generally has high (wide) latitude.

Resolution is the ability of the film or screen to record detail and may be expressed in terms of line pairs per millimeter (lp/mm) resolution capability. For further discussion of these four features, refer to textbooks concerned with the physics of diagnostic radiology[18] and to Bates.[4]

There have been numerous articles in the radiologic literature over the last few years giving some of the advantages and disadvantages of various film-screen combinations with respect to these four features. It has been shown that by using fast film and medium-speed screens, one can reduce patient dosage with little loss in resolution.[14,16,17] The exact amount of decrease in patient exposure would, of course, depend specifically upon the film used. One should certainly be able to use this data in radiography of the chest, but there has been a practical problem. High-speed film usable in 90-second processing has not been as uniform in quality as the medium-speed film available for 90-second processing. There have apparently been problems in emulsion stability, and many radiologists have been disappointed in the appearance of the high-speed films available. The practical consequence has been that radiologists wishing to increase the speed of their system and thereby decrease the exposure to the patient have frequently gone to faster screens. Those currently on the market are made with calcium tungstate and are significantly improved over those available only 5 years ago with respect to their resolution capability. Another practical consideration in determining the manner of switching to a high-speed system has been that it is difficult to work routinely with films and screens of different speeds in an x-ray department; however, it is easier to work with cassettes with different screen speeds than it is to work with different speed films loaded into the same cassette. The most significant exception to this general statement, however, occurs in angiography, in which faster films as well as faster screens are very commonly used. Angiographic film is generally easier to keep separate because of the different size involved. Many radiologists would be very hesitant to change to a faster screen-film combination because of concern over the loss of resolution. It will probably be several years before this question is fully resolved.

Film latitude. Most film manufacturers make film with a wider than normal latitude in their medium-speed line. The information about this film emphasizes the changes in the shoulder region of the H and D sensitometric curve, noting that relatively thinner anatomic parts are not overexposed while claiming that contrast in the relatively straight portion of the H and D curve is not affected. This may well be true, but with respect to a chest radiograph or indeed any other common types of radiograph, a wide-latitude film appears to offer significantly less contrast wherever one looks at the film. This is certainly

not necessarily a drawback; many departments have gone entirely to the wide-latitude film, and in any department there may be areas in which having a film of wider latitude is of material benefit. We have used this film routinely for chest examinations made with bedside units, since FFD, patient thickness, and large densities due to disease processes may make an optimal exposure difficult, and the wider latitude of this film means fewer retakes (Fig. 7-3).

Intensifying screens. Appropriate screen care, cleaning routines, and replacement procedures should not be left to unsupervised junior personnel. Screen manufacturers' representatives are generally eager to assist radiology departments with screen care. It should be kept in mind that the abrasion resistance of screens may vary from manufacturer to manufacturer, and indeed from screen type to screen type produced by the same manufacturer. Damage due to abrasion may be manifest by obvious artifacts on the exposed and processed film but may be more subtly expressed in loss of brightness. Minor damage to screens occurs with use, and it will be necessary to replace a few screens because of this damage. For this reason, the screens should be coded in such a manner that when screen-related artifacts are detectable on the film, the responsible cassette can be immediately identified. Intensifying screens should be replaced in pairs, since the minor economy of not doing so will be lost in the increased record keeping necessitated by having screens with different installation dates in the same cassette. If one changes brand or type of

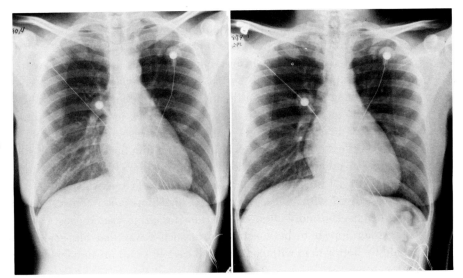

A   **B**

Fig. 7-3. Both films of this average-size woman are made with wide-latitude film. The FFD was approximately the same. There is little difference in appearance of film despite the 10 kVp difference in exposure. **A,** 90 kVp, 4 mAs, and no grid using portable equipment. **B,** 80 kVp, 4 mAs, and no grid using portable equipment.

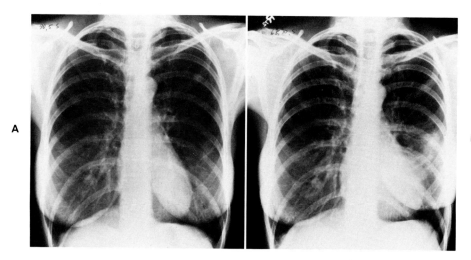

Fig. 7-4. Patient with multiple nodular lesions due to tuberculosis. **A,** 90 kVp, 5 mAs, and no grid. **B,** 65 kVp, 10 mAs, and no grid. The nodules can be seen in both films but are easier to see in **B. A** has poor film-screen contact lateral to cardiac apex.

intensifying screen, it is suggested that the results over the next several years be scrutinized with particular care for evidence of any shortening or lengthening of the normal screen life. Since screens must be replaced on a regular basis, it is well to budget for their replacement at approximately 5-year intervals.

These comments primarily apply to screens and conventional cassettes, since film transport systems involve somewhat different stresses, and the number of films taken may be more important than the age of the intensifying screens in determining appropriate replacement time.

Cassettes. Conventional 14 by 17 inch cassettes are reasonably expensive pieces of equipment and with normal care they should last at least as long as the intensifying screens within them. They are quite easily warped, however, some types much more easily than others, so that areas of poor film-screen contact may develop, causing a marked loss in resolution (Figs. 7-4, *A,* and 7-12, *C*). Unless one is extremely critical about film quality, this loss of resolution may go undetected for a long period of time. It is recommended that screen contact tests be made annually on 14 by 17 inch cassettes. If the cassettes are used with unusual frequency, the film-screen contact should certainly be checked more often. The various magazine-loaded chest changers on the market appear to be constructed in such a way that film-screen contact should be better than with conventional cassettes and presumably will remain better.

Technical factors

Among those persons very interested in chest radiographic technique, one of the ways of starting a spirited discussion is to ask "What kilovoltage do you

like for your chest films?" For most radiologists, however, the kilovoltage peak used is not of great interest, and many do not know how the films made in their section are taken. For this discussion, the question of technical factors will be considered in four groups, according to kilovoltage peak used:

1. Low kVp (55 to 75), no grid
2. Medium kVp (90 to 110), grid or air gap optional
3. High kVp (125 to 150), grid or air gap
4. Very high kVp (250 to 400), grid or air gap

It is obvious that between the low and medium ranges and the medium and high ranges there are significant openings that are probably preferred by many people. Films taken between the major ranges will share characteristics of adjacent types.

The low kilovoltage peak range, as just mentioned, is the one that has been in use the longest, and it produces a visually very attractive film with good definition of bony structures, lung markings, and major outlines (Figs. 7-1, 7-4, *B*, and 7-6, *A*). The major difficulties with this technique arise with larger patients. Even on normal-size patients, however, there may be some difficulty in recording mediastinal patterns and the various borders of the lung zones (Fig. 7-5). Calcifications are normally very easily detected (Fig. 7-6). Patients must be accurately measured since there is not as much latitude as in higher kilovoltage peak ranges, but there is reasonable latitude in the upper aspects of this range. It is common for the lungs of heavier patients to be considerably overexposed. The low intensity of the scattered radiation prevailing with this technique normally does not necessitate the use of a grid for reduction of such radiation. When a grid is used with larger patients, the results may be disappointing due to the high contrast (Figs. 7-7 and 7-8).

The next major step up is the kilovoltage peak range of 90 to 110. The equipment suitable for 55 to 75 kVp exposures is generally suitable for use in this range as well, and with the resultant drop in milliampere second levels to 3.5 to 6.7 without a grid, the small focal spot can be used on many patients. One may effect an appreciable drop in image contrast that is related to a small reduction in tissue absorption and a moderate increase in scattered radiation reaching the film (Figs. 7-4, *A*, 7-9, and 7-10). The significance of this reduced contrast from the standpoint of film interpretation is a point on which there is no general agreement. There are essentially three responses one can make to this: (1) accept it and take advantage of the increased latitude achieved, (2) reject it by taking all chest films with a grid (6:1 or 8:1 in this kilovoltage peak range; Figs. 7-11 and 7-12), or (3) take the smaller- and average-size patients' films without a grid and use a grid for larger patients with a chest diameter of 25 cm AP or greater. The use of a grid negates some of the reduced exposure advantages of the higher kilovoltage peak in that considerably greater milliampere second levels are required for adequate film density, so that the large focal spot or a longer exposure time will have to be used. When one uses a grid and

Text continued on p. 144.

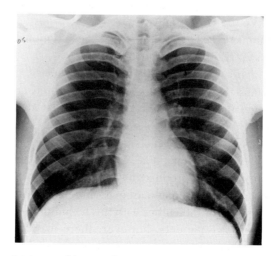

Fig. 7-5. A normal 25-year-old muscular man; 77 kVp, 10 mAs, and no grid. The ribs obscure some lung detail laterally at the crossing areas. Otherwise there is adequate penetration of all areas.

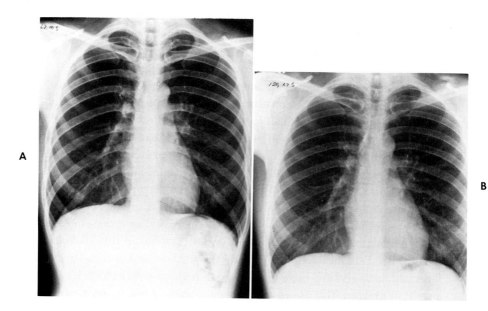

Fig. 7-6. Patient with calcifications. **A,** 62 kVp, 10 mAs, and no grid. **B,** 120 kVp, 1.7 mAs, and no grid. The right hilar node calcification is more easily appreciated in **A.** Both films are a bit dark. Some free air related to recent surgery is evident in **A.**

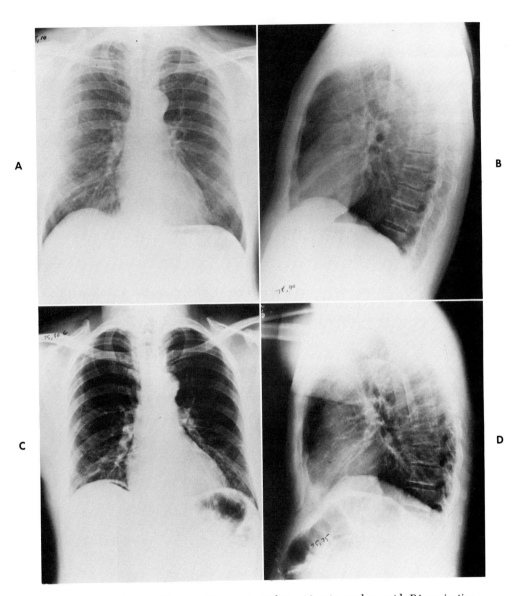

Fig. 7-7. Average-size 57-year-old man. **A,** 78 kVp, 10 mAs, and no grid. PA projection. **B,** 78 kVp, 40 mAs, and no grid. Lateral projection. **C,** 75 kVp, 30 mAs, and grid. PA projection. **D,** 75 kVp, 75 mAs, and grid. Lateral projection. **C** and **D** have high contrast, but mediastinum is insufficiently penetrated in PA projection, and upper lung zones are dark.

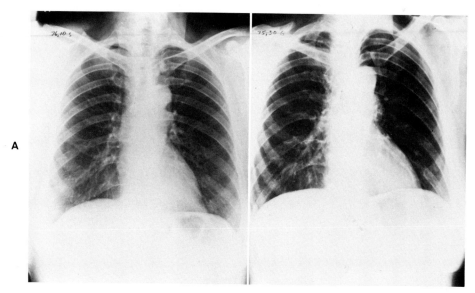

A

B

Fig. 7-8. A 66-year-old woman with a 29 cm AP chest diameter. **A,** 76 kVp, 10 mAs, and no grid. **B,** 75 kVp, 30 mAs, and grid. **B** is somewhat rotated. Lower portion of chest is adequately seen despite large breasts. Lungs are a bit dark.

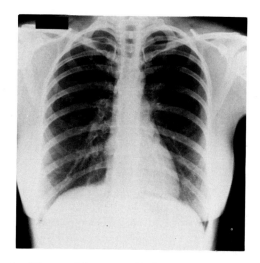

Fig. 7-9. Average-size 39-year-old woman. Technique using 100 kVp, 5 mAs, and no grid. Slow film: 7-minute processing.

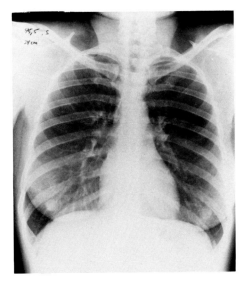

Fig. 7-10. Low-contrast, adequately exposed film using 95 kVp, 5 mAs, and no grid.

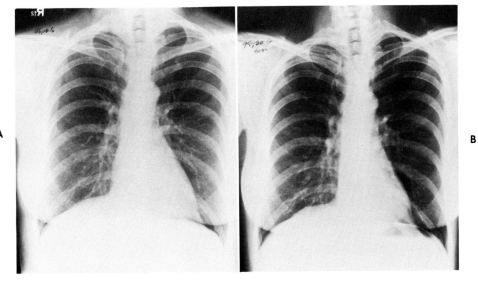

Fig. 7-11. A 51-year-old woman with a 26 cm AP chest diameter. **A,** 95 kVp, 10 mAs, and no grid. **B,** 95 kVp, 20 mAs, and grid. **B** shows poor film-screen contact centrally.

changes only the milliampere seconds, the patient's dosage goes up substantially. The advantage of better mediastinal and behind-the-rib visualization related to higher kilovoltage peak is variably still present (Figs. 7-13 to 7-16).

At this point a brief discussion about some equipment features may be of interest. With the general availability of 125 kVp, 500 mA generators, it is

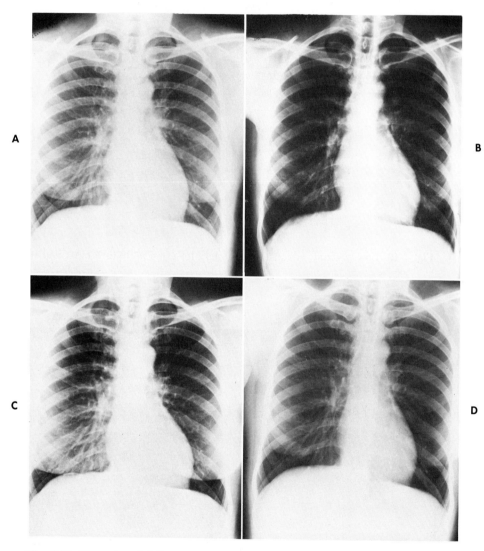

Fig. 7-12. Examples of different contrast with kVp changes and use of grid, also illustrating variability of equipment with respect to kilovoltage peak and milliampere seconds. **A,** 80 kVp, 10 mAs, and no grid. Automatic 7-minute processing. **B,** 110 kVp, 10 mAs, and grid. Automatic 7-minute processing. **C,** 90 kVp, 30 mAs, and grid. Automatic 90-second processing. Note poor film-screen contact over right hilum. **D,** 110 kVp, 5 mAs, and no grid. Automatic 7-minute processing.

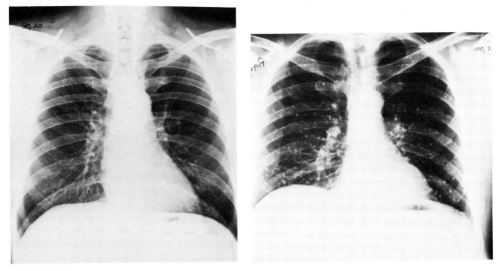

Fig. 7-13   Fig. 7-14

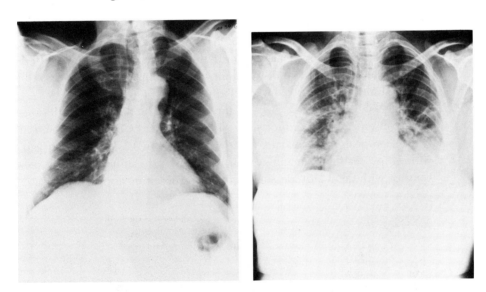

Fig. 7-15   Fig. 7-16

Fig. 7-13. Patient with chest diameter of 24 cm. Mediastinal penetration poor with 90 kVp and 20 mAs.

Fig. 7-14. Good visualization of calcifications due to histoplasmosis using 100 kVp, 20 mAs, and grid. Upper lobes are somewhat dark.

Fig. 7-15. This large patient with scoliosis and mild funneling of thorax presented a radiographic challenge, but a reasonable film was obtained using 100 kVp, 30 mAs, and grid. If patient gains much weight, lower lung tissue will be too light and upper lobes will be too dark.

Fig. 7-16. Relatively high-contrast radiograph of an obese 53-year-old woman with pneumonia using 95 kVp, 30 mAs, and grid. Bases are light; to adequately expose bases would require overexposure of apices with this disease process and body habitus at 95 kVp using a grid.

reasonable to use their kilovoltage peak capacity. There are some serious constraints with some of this equipment. The 500 mA may be only available at 80 kVp or below, and the limitations of single-phase impulse timing make only large changes in milliampere seconds possible if one does use 120 to 125 kVp with less than 5 mAs. As an example, the available times on one such unit are 0.008 second (1 impulse), 0.017 second (2 impulses), 0.025 second (3 impulses), 0.033 second (4 impulses), 0.05 second (6 impulses), and 0.67 second (8 impulses). At 100 mA and 120 kVp this would be the appropriate range available for a PA chest radiograph, and it is obvious that, since the incremental milliampere second steps are large, there is not much potential for changing to accommodate different patient sizes. One can vary kilovoltage peak as well as milliampere seconds, however, and there is moderate latitude with a kilovoltage peak in this range. The advantage of the quite short exposure time, small focal spot, and improved latitude are quite attractive on paper, but the film will be rather low in contrast at 120 to 125 kVp (Figs. 7-17 and 7-18). At 125 kVp, one has the options available for 90 to 110 kVp noted above, but one is much more likely to use a grid or air gap for everyone or start using it at a narrower AP diameter such as 22 cm. In this kilovoltage peak range, a 10:1 grid may be used instead of an 8:1 grid for somewhat more efficiency in reducing scattered radiation with 125 kVp exposures.

High kilovoltage peak films in the range 125 to 150 (Fig. 7-19) are very lucidly discussed in an editorial by Jacobson et al.[10] Chest films taken in this kilovoltage peak range may be made with a 10:1 or 12:1 grid (or air gap) and with either scatter-reducing system the films will exhibit a visually pleasing contrast with good latitude so that minor errors in measuring or disease pro-

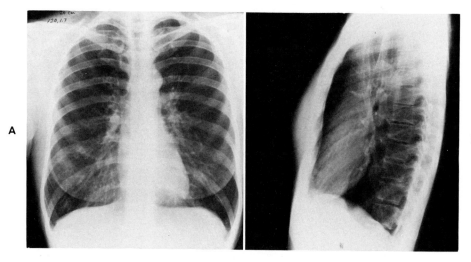

Fig. 7-17. Medium contrast films of a patient with a 22 cm chest diameter. **A,** 120 kVp, 1.7 mAs, and no grid. **B,** 120 kVp, 7.5 mAs, and no grid. Lateral projection.

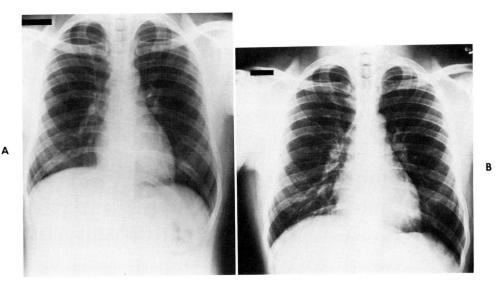

Fig. 7-18. An average-size 27-year-old muscular man. **A,** 120 kVp, 2.5 mAs, and no grid. **B,** 120 kVp, 10 mAs, and grid. **B** has much shorter scale of contrast. Both films have good penetration and good visibility of vascular detail.

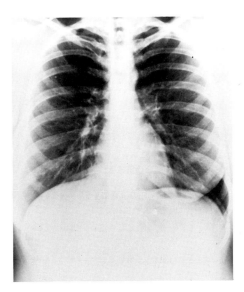

Fig. 7-19. Patient with deformed left breast. Good contrast and good mediastinal penetration obtained with 125 kVp, 6.4 mAs, and 10:1 grid.

cesses that affect total tissue density are well accommodated. It is very desirable to have at least 300 mA available at high kilovoltage peak so that short exposure times may be used. One should keep in mind that it may not be possible to get 300 mA on a small focal spot in this high kilovoltage peak range, but with some of the newer tubes the large focal spot is only 1 or 1.2 mm. It is very likely that the advantages of a short exposure time more than offset going from a 0.6 mm focal spot to a 1.0 or 1.2 mm focal spot. With advances in tube design, a greater capacity 0.6 mm focal spot may soon be available. With regard to the problem patient in chest radiography, the very obese or very muscular person, it is possible to achieve a very reasonable film with good lung detail and soft tissue visualization in most instances, so that the total range of patients appears to be handled better with techniques here than in lower kilovoltage peak ranges (Fig. 7-19).

In July, 1973, the following guidelines were issued for taking chest films of coal miners for pneumoconiosis assessment.

(a) Every chest roentgenogram shall be a posteroanterior projection at full inspiration on a 14- by 17-inch or 14- by 14-inch film.

(b) Miners shall be disrobed from the waist up at the time the roentgenogram is given.

(c) Roentgenograms shall be made only with a diagnostic x-ray machine having a rotating anode tube with a maximum of a 2 mm source (focal spot).

(d) Except as provided in paragraph (e) of this section, roentgenograms shall be made with units having generators which comply with the following: (1) The generators of existing roentgenographic units acquired by the examining facility prior to effective date of the regulations shall have a minimum rating of 200 mA at 100 kVp; (2) Generators of units acquired subsequent to such date shall have a minimum rating of 300 mA at 125 kVp.

NOTE: A generator with a rating of 150 kVp is recommended.

(e) Roentgenograms made with battery-powered mobile or portable equipment shall be made with units having a minimum rating of 100 mA at 110 kVp at 500 Hz, or of 200 mA at 110 kVp at 60 Hz.

(f) Capacitor discharge and field emission units may be used: *Provided,* That the model of such units is approved by ALFORD* for quality, performance, and safety. ALFORD will consider such units for approval when listed by a facility seeking approval under #37.42 of this subpart.

(g) Roentgenograms shall be given only with equipment having a beam-limiting device which does not cause large unexposed boundaries. The use of such a device shall be discernible from an examination of the roentgenogram.

(h) To insure high quality chest roentgenograms:

(1) The maximum exposure time shall not exceed 1/20 of a second except that with single phase units with a rating less than 300 mA at 125 kVp and subjects with chests over 28 cm posteroanterior, the exposure may be increased to not more than 1/10 of a second.

(2) The source of focal spot to film distance shall be at least 6 feet: *Provided,* That where space limitation in mobile units requires a shorter distance, the source of film distance shall not be less than 5 feet. Films made in mobile units with less than 6 feet between the focal spot and film shall be marked with the source to film distance.

(3) Only medium-speed films and medium speed intensifying screens shall be used.

(4) Film-screen contact shall be maintained and verified at 6 month or shorter intervals.

(5) Intensifying screens shall be inspected at least once a month and cleaned when necessary by the method recommended by the manufacturer.

---

*ALFORD is the acronym for Appalachian Laboratory for Occupational Respiratory Diseases, National Institute for Occupational Safety and Health, Box 4258, Morgantown, W. Va. 26505.

(6) All intensifying screens in a cassette shall be of the same type and made by the same manufacturer.

(7) When using over 90 kVp, a suitable grid or other means of reducing scattered radiation shall be used.

(8) The geometry of the radiographic system shall insure that the central axis (ray) of the primary beam is perpendicular to the plane of the film surface and impinges on the center of the film.*

These requirements are rather straightforward, and they are in general agreement with many of the remarks made in this chapter.

The last major kilovoltage peak range is very high. Radiologists trained in radiation therapy as well as diagnostic radiology have known for many years that chest radiographs taken with orthovoltage therapy units or even with vandeGraaff generators have some interesting features. There is excellent visualization of the tracheobronchial tree, good visualization of the vascular structures, and reasonable visualization of lung masses with sufficient latitude so that very little adjustment need be made for different-size patients. The density difference between calcium and soft tissue is lost. Bone detail is very poor, and it is one of the advantages of this technique that the ribs are relatively radiolucent, thus allowing good visualization of the underlying lung tissue. The 300 kVp x-ray generating equipment specifically for chest radiographs that is now available may have a very important place in chest radiology. The current feeling is that 300 kVp film will supplement rather than supplant the more widely used low, medium, and high kilovoltage peak techniques mentioned.[8]

Films made with mobile x-ray units

The so-called portable film is a significant part of hospital chest radiology and to consider it appropriately would require a fairly lengthy section. A few brief comments will be made. With the vagaries of hospital power supplies available on patient floors, it is well to consider a battery-powered or condenser-discharge type of unit in order to achieve reasonably short exposure time. For reasonable latitude, we feel that it is very helpful to be able to use 90 kVp or more and fairly low milliampere seconds. Most of the work should be done without a grid, since centering the beam to the grid is quite difficult when a patient is confined to bed. This is a good place to use wide-latitude film for the reasons mentioned, and if there is a problem with patient motion, fast screens may be employed to advantage.

Radiation dosage

Table 7-3 gives some comparative dosage values for specified conditions. Comparative numbers are somewhat more meaningful than the absolute numbers, since there will be some minor differences because of current equipment variation.

---

*Federal Register **38**(144):20079, July 27, 1973.

Table 7-3. Approximate skin dosage for 25 cm thick patient, medium-speed screens, medium-speed film, 72-inch FFD, full-wave rectification, 2.5 mm aluminum total filtration*

kVp	mAs	Grid		Skin dosage (mrad)
70	30.0	None		24 + 20%, BSF = 29
100	5.0	None		18 + 20%, BSF = 22
100	20.0	8:1,	80 lines/inch	73 + 20%, BSF = 88
125	1.5	None		8.5 + 20%, BSF = 10
125	6.7	8:1,	80 lines/inch	36 + 20%, BSF = 43
125	6.7	10:1,	133 lines/inch	36 + 20%, BSF = 43
125	9.0	12:1,	80 lines/inch	51 + 20%, BSF = 61
145	3.3	10:1,	133 lines/inch	24 + 20%, BSF = 29
145	5.0	12:1,	80 lines/inch	36 + 20%, BSF = 43

*Dosage values supplied by Dr. Gopala Rao, based on published values and measurements used in the Department of Radiology, The Johns Hopkins Medical Institutions. kVp and mAs values selected for similar densities, based on Dupont bit system and Rao Radiographic Technic Calculator. Values are not absolute but provide a basis for comparison. BSF = back scatter factor.

Processing

Automatic processors for x-ray film became available in the 1950s. A 7-minute dry-to-dry processing cycle was the standard until the mid-1960s, when 3½-minute processors and appropriate film became available. In the late 1960s, 90-second processors and film capable of passing through them became available, and these processors have taken over the major share of the market (Fig. 7-11). It should be noted that the first films used for 90-second processors were not very good in comparison to their immediate 7-minute predecessors, but there have been steady improvements, so that the 90-second film available today is quite good. The early films had a low contrast and rather muddy appearance in some instances, and a very high contrast, very mottled appearance with other types. The appearance of the film has improved considerably, but there is still a distinct sparkle or crispness to a 7-minute or 3½-minute processed film that is absent from the general 90-second films made by the same manufacturer. The high temperature and short time in the development cycle of the 90-second processor are felt to be factors in this difference. To many radiologists this sparkle is a positive feature, although quite a few others will not notice the difference. The esthetic qualities of a 7-minute processed film may be surpassed by manually processed film, but the difficulties with space, quality control, and rapid interpretation make it difficult to recommend manual processing except in very special circumstances. The most practical processing arrangement with current technology is an automatic processor with either a 3½-minute or 90-second cycle. The 3½-minute cycle gives a greater safety margin with regard to technical factors and processor variables. The 90-second cycle certainly does speed up examination time in those instances in which subsequent filming may be determined by earlier films in the examination. This is not true for chest examinations, of course, nor is it true for most other radiographic examinations.

Reduction of unwanted radiation by air gap or grid

Scattered and secondary radiation may be reduced by either intercepting the radiation with a stationary or moving grid or by using the air-gap method. With the air-gap method, the patient is separated from the film by from 5 to 9 inches so that some dispersion of the scattered radiation can occur. Ardran[2] indicates that some 25% of the radiation dose leaving the patient does not reach the film if a 6-inch air gap is used. To avoid the effects of magnification with this system, it is necessary to increase the FFD. Distances of from 9 to 12 feet have been advocated.[12] The air gap has much the same function as a grid but does not require as great a patient dose as does an 8:1 grid at the conventional 72-inch FFD because no primary radiation is absorbed by the air gap and a considerable amount of primary radiation is absorbed by a grid.[1,15] Use of the air gap requires a specific place for chest radiography or some time for setup of equipment. There are many staunch advocates of the system, while others have felt that use of a grid results in better definition and films of a more uniformly high quality. From a practical standpoint it may be noted that the various manufacturers of x-ray equipment have not been as interested in air-gap equipment as they have in grid equipment, so that it may be somewhat awkward to set up an effective air-gap system for trial. The potential advantages in the reduction of patient dosage appear to indicate the validity of their continued consideration and further development of appropriate equipment.

Grids. When a grid is used, the question of which ratio to use arises. Although grid ratio and grid lines per inch are the generally used indicators of effectiveness in reducing scattered radiation, the efficiency of the grid in reducing this radiation is primarily related to the lead content of the grid. A high grid ratio and many lines per inch normally mean a high amount of lead per unit area, however, so there is little reason to change the current terminology. For research and comparative evaluation it would be of interest to know the total lead content.

For abdominal work, a grid ratio of 10:1 or above is ordinarily used for kilovoltage peaks in excess of 100, but the scatter associated with chest radiography is not the same as that produced for abdominal work. Trout and Kelley indicate that the contrast of a chest film taken at 70 kVp without a grid is similar to that of a film taken at 100 kVp with a 6:1 grid, to a film taken at 115 kVp with an 8:1 grid, or to a film taken at 130 kVp with a 10:1 grid using single-phase equipment.[19] A 10:1 grid for films at 125 to 145 kVp[10] has been independently recommended; since there is only slight difference between a 10:1 and 12:1 grid, either would produce similar results. A high-quality fine-line grid of 100 to 110 lines/inch generally has lines that are so slender that they are not objec-

Table 7-4. Data from Table 7-3 rearranged in separate no-grid and grid groupings*

kVp	mAs	Grid	Skin dosage (mrads, including BSF)
70	30.0	None	29
100	5.0	None	22
125	1.5	None	10
100	20.0	8:1	88
125	6.6	8:1	43
125	9.0	12:1	61
145	3.3	10:1	29

*It should be noted that not all of these values will produce a film with acceptable characteristics.

tionable. This use of a stationary grid avoids the problems occasionally associated with high-speed grid movement for short exposure times (Table 7-4).

Film size and patient positioning

The film size in most common use for the adult PA chest film is 14 inches wide by 17 inches high. Some departments have used a 14 by 14 inch size, however, which is about 15% less costly. One of the advantages of the 14 by 17 inch size (it should be noted that the nomenclature used in the United States gives the short side first, while the Canadian and British usage gives the long side first) is that it may be turned so that the long dimension is horizontal to accommodate the wide patient. This horizontal orientation seldom causes exclusion of any lung tissue from the film, since the transverse dimension is generally greater than the vertical lung dimension in wide patients.

Audsley et al.[3] in 1970 evaluated two different groups of male laborers in the United Kingdom with respect to appropriate film size. The details of their findings are quite interesting. In one group of 714 men, only 66% fit conveniently on a 14-inch wide film (35.5 cm), whereas 99.9% fit on a 15.7-inch (40 cm) wide film. Regarding the vertical dimensions, 83% of patients easily fit a 14-inch high film, while 99.9% fit a 40 cm high film. Their conclusions were that a 40 by 40 cm film would not exclude any of the lung tissue from the film in 99.9% of male manual laborers. The surface area of a 40 by 40 cm film is 340 cm² larger than a 35.5 by 35.5 cm (14 by 14 inch) film, but only 66 cm² (4%) larger than a 35.5 by 43.2 cm (14 by 17 inch) film.[3]

With this in mind, the chest sizes (as approximated from a chest radiograph) of 300 coal miners in the eastern United States were evaluated, and the results are shown in Table 7-5. Measurements included the outer rib margin on each side of the widest portion of the chest. Three categories were made. Persons 34 cm wide or less would have a total of 1.5 cm or more leeway for positioning. Patients between 34 and 35.5 cm were considered borderline, since it takes meticulous positioning to avoid excluding a small area of the lung or adjacent rib from the film in these persons. The third category included those who

Table 7-5. Evaluation of chest sizes of 300 coal miners

Less than or equal to 34 cm	210 (70%)
Borderline, 34 to 35.5 cm	47 (15.7%)
Greater than 35.5 cm (14 inches)	43 (14.3%)
Taken on 14-inch wide film	212 (70.7%)
Taken on 17-inch wide film	88 (29.3%)

would not be adequately radiographed with a 14-inch wide film regardless of the positioning.

Of this group of 300 men, 40 (13.3%) had an estimated 1 cm or more of lung tissue excluded from the film. Obviously some 17-inch films were taken of patients who would have fit on a 14-inch wide film, and some films should have been taken on 17-inch rather than 14-inch wide film. In this entire group only films of two persons, or less than 1%, excluded the top of the apex, and films of five persons excluded a costophrenic recess. Our impression is that about 30% of this male population either will not have their entire lung shadow and adjacent rib projected on the film 14 inches wide or will require very careful positioning to avoid having a portion of lung or adjacent rib excluded. The question then raised is whether the conventional 14 by 17 inch format is appropriate. If one considers the total population, the percentages of persons difficult or impossible to position on a 14-inch film would be diminished by about half, since it is very uncommon for women not to be adequately positioned on a 14-inch film (less than 1% in our informal experience), and the population studied included larger men in general than if a total adult male population were surveyed. There would be major problems in attempting to change the current chest film format to a 40 by 40 cm size in the United States, since viewboxes, film envelopes, and filing shelves are designed with the 14 by 17 inch film as the maximum film size. The various high-volume chest changers make it rather inconvenient to use other than a 14-inch format. The 14-inch film will no doubt continue to be the predominant size, but we believe manufacturers should be encouraged to make it easier to accommodate larger persons who are such a significant portion of the population.

The possibility of using a smaller film size for the lateral position frequently arises, and many radiologists use an 11 by 14 inch film size with a consequent savings of money and ultimately of natural resources. This does necessitate an extra decision by the technologist and slows down the examination slightly, but it is worth considering in a practice with a significant number of patients who can easily have their chest projected into an 11 by 14 inch area in the lateral position.

VIEWING RADIOGRAPHS

After considerable care and expense go into producing a radiograph of good quality, it is only reasonable to view it under very good circumstances. The radiographic viewbox should have the diffusing plate cleaned both front and back on a regular schedule. The fluorescent lights should be of uniform color and should be changed as soon as they begin to deteriorate. The plastic or glass diffusing material may color with age and therefore should be replaced when necessary. The on-off switches should be convenient to the hand of the radiologist so that it is not awkward to switch off viewboxes not being used. The instant-on feature for the fluorescent illumination is extremely important since the radiologist will tend not to switch off lights if they do not come back on instantly. The presence of extraneous light from unused viewboxes is very distracting since extraneous light dispersed within the eye reduces contrast. There should be a regular viewbox maintenance program just as there is a maintenance program for other equipment; in this program the light output of the viewbox is checked, the light switches are checked, and the viewing boxes are cleaned. Use of a photographic light meter is simple and provides objective readings of the light getting past the diffusing glass. It makes no economic sense to use a poor viewbox at a saving of $10 or $15 per viewing space if this is going to cause any irritation and therefore distraction of the radiologist. A magnifying lens and a minifying lens should be at hand. The reading area should be comfortable and free of visual and acoustic distractions. Every radiologist with any experience can remember many instances in which films initially interpreted one way under distracting circumstances were subsequently read differently when conditions of environmental tranquility prevailed.

SUMMARY AND RECOMMENDATIONS

Several aspects of chest radiography have been considered. Suggestions and comments are summarized here.

Photofluorography is currently not recommended for mass screening chest radiography. The standard focal spot to film distance is 72 inches, except where an air gap is used, and the FFD should then be 9 to 12 feet. X-ray generating equipment capable of exposure times of 1/20 second or less at selected kilovoltage peaks and milliampere second values should be used. X-ray tubes with focal spots of 0.6 mm (small) and 1.0 to 1.2 mm (large) are suitable for all chest radiography except for magnification radiography. This is a dynamic field, and tubes with smaller focal spots may be suitable in the future.

Although medium-speed screens and film have been the standard in use, it may be possible to use a faster system without diagnostically significant loss of information. Improvements in intensifying screens and x-ray film necessitate that periodic appraisal of new products be part of the radiologist's standard operating procedure, either directly or through the literature. Cassette and screen maintenance programs should be carefully set up and implemented.

For new installations, use of 125 to 150 kVp with grid or air gap is recommended as the best technique with regard to patient exposure, film quality, and a low repeat rate. When using older equipment, low kilovoltage peak and no grid are recommended for average and smaller patients and an intermediate kilovoltage peak and grid or air gap are recommended for larger patients. If the equipment permits, the increase in "technique" necessitated by a grid should be made by increasing the kilovoltage peak, not by increasing milliampere seconds. Increasing the milliampere seconds alone considerably increases patient dosage. With 80 kVp or less, one can produce overall good films with no grid up to a patient size of about 26 cm. Low kilovoltage peak-grid films of the chest suffer from excessive contrast and, frequently there are problems with patient motion. In the medium kilovoltage peak range of 90 to 110, one can produce good films without using a grid of patients of a size of about 24 cm. There are problems of excessive contrast with use of a grid for thicker patients here as well as at the lower kilovoltage peak. It is quite possible that a grid ratio lower than 8:1 would be preferable for larger patients in the low kVp settings. For higher kilovoltage peaks, a grid or air gap should be used. Detection of calcium in the 130 kVp range does not appear to be a major problem if a grid or air gap is used. The 14 by 17 inch film size routinely used for chest work is not perfect, but practical considerations make it difficult to change.

Thus far, nothing has been said about collimation. Collimation to the field of interest is very important in reducing patient exposure but also greatly improves film quality. This has been fully discussed in several other presentations, however.[6]

Radiographs should be viewed under favorable visual and acoustical circumstances.

Acknowledgments

I would like to express my appreciation to Dr. Russell Morgan for his review of the manuscript, to Dr. Gopalo Rao and Dr. Lloyd Bates for consultation, to Miss Patricia Bailey for typing the manuscript, and to Henri Hessels and Willie Ragsdale for their photographic expertise.

References

1. Ardran, G. M.: New techniques in diagnostic radiology, Br. J. Radiol. **46:**149, 1973.
2. Ardran, G. M., and Crooks, H. E.: The reduction of scatter fog in chest radiography, Br. J. Radiol. **37:**477, 1964.
3. Audsley, W. P., Latham, S. M., and Rossiter, C. E.: Film sizes for radiography of the chest, Radiography **36:**70, 1970.
4. Bates, L. M.: Some physical factors affecting radiographic image quality: their theoretical basis and measurement, Publication No. 999-RH-38, Washington, D. C., 1969, United States Public Health Service.
5. Deasy, J. B.: Mass radiography, Br. Med. J. **3:**48, 1970.
6. Epp, E. R., Weiss, H., and Laughlin, J. S.: Measurement of bone marrow and gonadal dose from the chest x-ray examination as a function of field size, field alignment, tube kilovoltage and added filtration, Br. J. Radiol. **34:**85, 1961.
7. Federal Register **37**(158):16461, Aug. 15, 1972.
8. Field Emission Corporation: Technical Bulletin No. 26, 1972.
9. Goodwin, P. N., Quimby, E. H., and Morgan, R. H.: Physical foundations of radiology, ed. 4, New York, 1970, Harper & Row, Publishers.

10. Jacobson, G.,Bohlig, H., and Kiviluoto, R.: Essentials of chest radiography, Radiology **95**:445, 1970.
11. Mees, C. E. K.: The theory of the photographic process, New York, 1948, Macmillan Publishing Co., Inc.
12. O'Donnell, E. B.: Concerning high voltage technique and accessories, X-Ray Tech. **36**:71, 1964.
13. Pfister, R. C., Oh, K. S., and Feracci, J. T.: Retrosternal density, Radiology **96**: 317, 1970.
14. Rao, G. U. V.: Do high detail screens always yield better resolution than high speed screens? Am. J. Roentgenol. Radium Ther. Nucl. Med. **112**:812, 1971.
15. Rao, G. U. V., Clark, R. L., and Gayler, B. W.: Radiologic magnification: critical, theoretical and practical analysis, Applied Radiol. **2**(1):37, 1973; **2**(2):25, 1973.
16. Rossman, K., and Wiley, B. E.: The central problem in the study of radiographic image quality, Radiology **96**:113, 1970.
17. Rossman, K., Hans, A. G., and Dobben, G. D.: Improvement in the image quality of cerebral angiograms, Radiology **96**:361, 1970.
18. Ter-Pogossian, M. M.: The physical aspects of diagnostic radiology, New York, 1967, Harper & Row, Publishers.
19. Trout, E. D., and Kelley, J. P.: A phantom for the evaluation of techniques and equipment used for roentgenography of the chest, Am. J. Roentgenol. Radium Ther. Nucl. Med. **117**:771, 1973.
20. United States Department of Health, Education, and Welfare: The chest x-ray as a screening procedure for cardiopulmonary disease, Publication No. (FDA) 73-8036, Washington, D. C., 1973, U. S. Government Printing Office.
21. Vix, V. A., and Klatte, E. C.: The lateral chest radiograph in the diagnosis of hilar and mediastinal masses, Radiology **96**:307, 1970.

Suggested readings

Christensen, E. E., Curry, T. S., III, and Nunnally, J.: An introduction to the physics of diagnostic radiology, Philadelphia, 1972, Lea & Febiger.
Lynch, P. A.: A different approach to chest roentgenography: TRIAD technique (high kilovoltage, grid, wedge filter), Am. J. Roentgenol. Radium Ther. Nucl. Med. **93**:965, 1965.
United States Department of Health, Education, and Welfare: Volume of x-ray visits, Publication No. (HSM) 73-1507, Vital and Health Statistics Series 10, No. 81, Washington, D. C., 1973, U. S. Government Printing Office.

8 Special procedures in pulmonary radiology

John V. Forrest and Stuart S. Sagel

GENERAL CONSIDERATIONS

Although plain films of the chest are the most common study in radiology, the use of adjuvant radiologic procedures in chest diagnosis has received relatively little recent attention. Which technique to use, when, and why in chest disease is the subject of this chapter.

Radiologists, chest physicians, and surgeons have individual approaches to the evaluation of a chest abnormality. Available time, equipment, and personal experience modify almost any situation. Bronchial brushing or aspiration needle biopsy require an experienced cytologist for completion of the study. Similar limitations apply to all the procedures described in this chapter, and the individual physician must decide which procedure meets his needs in any given situation.

There is a definite need to abandon unproductive radiologic examinations and establish criteria for use as definitively as possible. Laminagraphy and bronchography, which have specific, limited uses in chest diagnosis, are techniques overutilized in many institutions. Bronchial brushing and needle biopsy are more time consuming, costly, and potentially dangerous, and they require expertise. However, in certain instances they provide the final and often only significant information about a lung lesion.

Other chest special procedures that are less frequently used will not be discussed in this chapter. Vascular studies fill a specific, limited role in certain types of lung disease. Diagnostic pneumothorax, pneumomediastinum, and pneumoperitoneum all can be used in certain situations but are not in common usage and have limited application. Other techniques are still in an experimental stage. Nordenström and his colleagues at the Karolinska Institute have been pioneers in chest special procedures, helping to popularize high-kilovoltage plain-film techniques, bronchial brushing and related studies, and various needle biopsy techniques, some of which have now received wide usage and acclaim.[15]

157

FLUOROSCOPY AND SPOT FILMS

Fluoroscopy with spot filming is a technique available in almost all radiology departments. It is easily and quickly done at low cost to the patient.

Pulmonary nodules

Confirmation of the presence of a small nodular density seen on the plain film is usually easily obtained. Occasionally a nodule or mass is only seen on the frontal or lateral film, and localization to a particular lobe or segment can usually be done with ease fluoroscopically. Fluoroscopy and spot films often can readily distinguish nonpulmonary lesions that may mimic pulmonary disease (for example, a healed rib fracture). The pleural or extrapleural location of a density is often only appreciated on fluoroscopy with spot films taken at the proper degree of obliquity (Fig. 8-1).

Certain abnormal densities often have characteristic shapes or configurations that fluoroscopy and spot films with the proper degree of obliquity can bring out. Enlarged bronchi due to bronchiectasis, bronchocele, or mucoid impaction may be demonstrated. Enlarged or abnormal blood vessels also may be laid out in this manner. During fluoroscopy, characteristic pulsation or response to the Valsalva or Mueller maneuver may confirm the presence of a vascular lesion (Fig. 8-2).

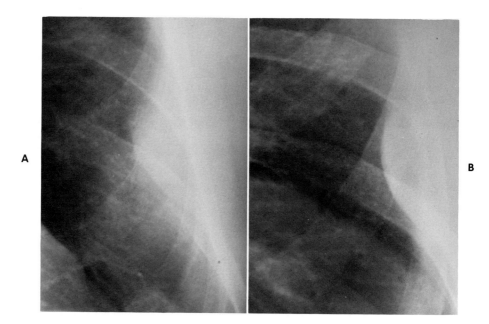

Fig. 8-1. A, Poorly defined soft tissue density is seen at left base. **B,** Spot film of density with proper degree of obliquity reveals characteristic extrapleural configuration. This was pleural lipoma.

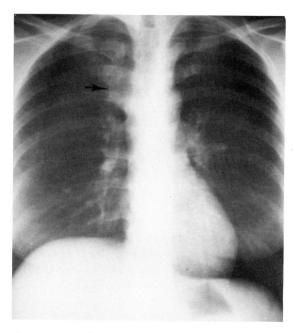

Fig. 8-3. Slight elevation of right hemidiaphragm with phrenic nerve paralysis due to bronchogenic carcinoma invading mediastinum (arrow).

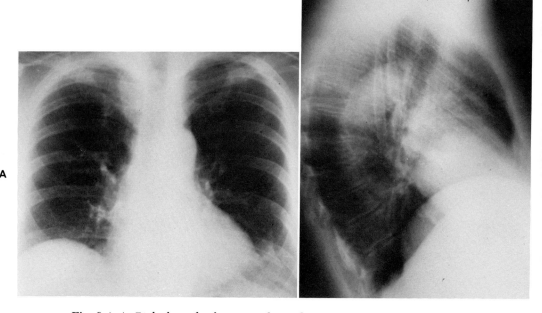

Fig. 8-4. A, Right hemidiaphragm is elevated, giving an appearance similar to that in Fig. 8-3. **B,** Lateral view of same patient shows elevation is anterior. Posterior right hemidiaphragm is at its normal level. Fluoroscopy confirmed normal movement of posterior right hemidiaphragm while anterior portion moved paradoxically. This is characteristic appearance of eventration.

Good quality plain films usually reveal the presence of calcification in a pulmonary nodule, but occasionally spot films in different obliquities are more definite.

Diaphragmatic abnormalities

An elevated hemidiaphragm may be due to an intra-abdominal mass, adjacent acute inflammatory disease, paralysis, eventration, subpulmonic effusion, lung volume loss, or postinflammatory adhesions. Fluoroscopy is often the best means of differentiating among these possibilities.

With paralysis, the diaphragm either does not move at all or it moves paradoxically; that is, it moves upward on inspiration. Sniffing may accentuate paradoxical movement. Probably the commonest cause is mediastinal neoplasm of any sort but especially carcinoma of the lung (Fig. 8-3). There are many other causes of diaphragmatic paralysis, but in many instances no particular etiology is found. Diaphragmatic paralysis is rarely if ever due to an occult mediastinal neoplasm. Radiographic evidence of a mediastinal mass has always been present in our experience.

Eventration or weakness and thinning of the diaphragm is a common entity that frequently mimics diaphragmatic paralysis. Its characteristic location is anteromedially on the right. Plain-film findings are frequently characteristic

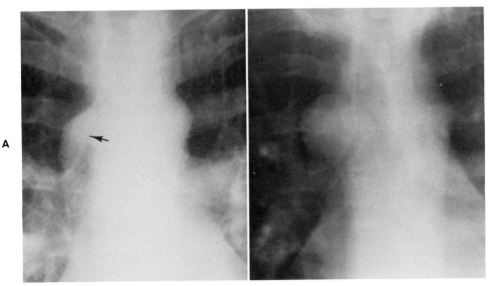

Fig. 8-2. A, Soft tissue mass in inferior right paratracheal area (arrow). **B,** Supine position and use of Valsalva maneuver greatly increase size of shadow, indicating its vascular nature. This is typical appearance of enlarged azygous vein. Patient had congenital azygous continuation of inferior vena cava.

enough to be diagnostic when eventration occurs in this area (Fig. 8-4). Fluoro-scopically, the eventrated area moves poorly, if at all, and may move para-doxically. Differentiation from a paralyzed diaphragm is made by rotating the patient to permit observation of the most posterior portion of the diaphragm, which almost always has intact functioning muscle that moves normally. A paralyzed diaphragm will not exhibit this normal posterior motility.

Adjacent inflammatory disease, particularly subphrenic abscess, also may cause an elevated diaphragm. Fluoroscopic movement is weak or absent, but paradoxical movement does not occur. Associated atelectasis and pleural ef-fusion help in the radiographic differential diagnosis (Fig. 8-5). Clinical find-ings usually allow an easy distinction between adjacent inflammatory disease and paralysis or eventration.

Postinflammatory adhesions often result in tacking of the lateral portion of the dome of the diaphragm to the lateral pleura. There is decreased or absent motion of an elevated diaphragm at the site of the adhesions. The rest of the diaphragm moves normally.

A subpulmonic effusion can usually be best evaluated by the appropriate lateral decubitus film (Fig. 8-6). The pseudohemidiaphragm moves with a somewhat decreased amplitude. Often the moving, breathing patient causes some change in the configuration of the fluid while the fluoroscopy is in prog-ress, and the cause of the apparent diaphragmatic elevation is apparent.

Patients with intra-abdominal masses or volume loss in a hemithorax will

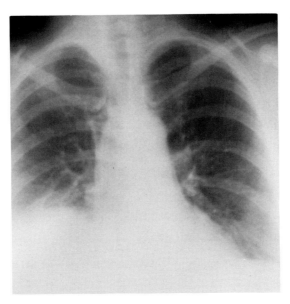

Fig. 8-5. Elevation of right hemidiaphragm with associated basilar pleural and paren-chymal disease in patient with right subphrenic abscess.

usually have normal diaphragmatic movement, although sometimes decreased amplitude of excursion is seen. Associated radiographic and clinical findings usually make the cause of the diaphragmatic elevation clear.

Vascular structures

Certain vascular structures are seen on chest films and usually are readily distinguished by their characteristic location and shape. Fluoroscopy with

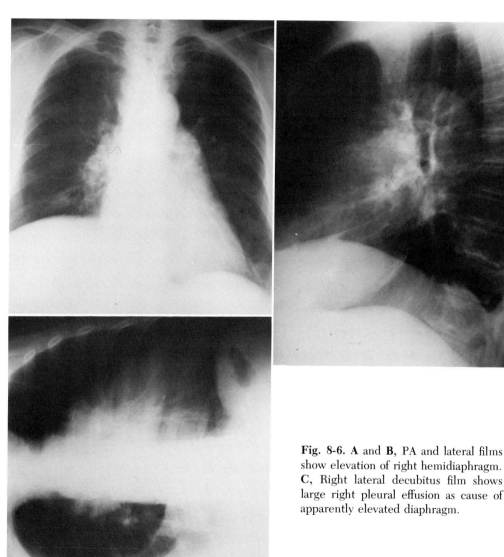

Fig. 8-6. **A** and **B**, PA and lateral films show elevation of right hemidiaphragm. **C**, Right lateral decubitus film shows large right pleural effusion as cause of apparently elevated diaphragm.

spot films may confirm or identify their vascular nature. Arteries usually pulsate. Venous structures will often change significantly in size with the Valsalva or Mueller maneuver and on movement from a supine to an erect position. The azygous vein is readily evaluated and almost always can be distinguished from an enlarged azygous lymph node with this technique (Fig. 8-2).

Fluoroscopy may allow differentiation between a vascular and a solid mass, as between an enlarged pulmonary artery and an enlarged lymph node or between a tortuous or aneurysmal aorta and a mediastinal mass. This can be done by following contours and changes in shape on rotation and not relying completely on pulsations.

Masses, particularly if they are cystic, may pulsate if adjacent to a major artery or to the heart. Distinguishing this transmitted pulsation from intrinsic pulsation is usually impossible (Fig. 8-7). Also, aneurysms often contain clot and do not pulsate.

A thorough discussion of cardiac fluoroscopy is beyond the scope of this paper. Intracardiac calcifications are best evaluated fluoroscopically since they are almost constantly in movement. The kinetics of cardiac aneurysms and damaged areas of cardiac muscle can often be appraised with the fluoroscope. Pericardial effusions dampen cardiac pulsations but are not different in this regard from a myocardiopathy or other severe form of heart disease. If separa-

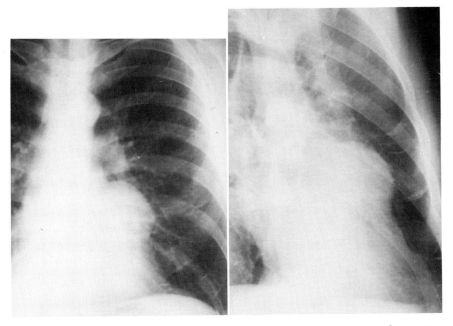

Fig. 8-7. Abnormal soft tissue density is seen adjacent to area of pulmonary outflow tract. Fluoroscopy showed pulsation indistinguishable from that of adjacent cardiovascular structures. At surgery this proved to be cystic teratoma.

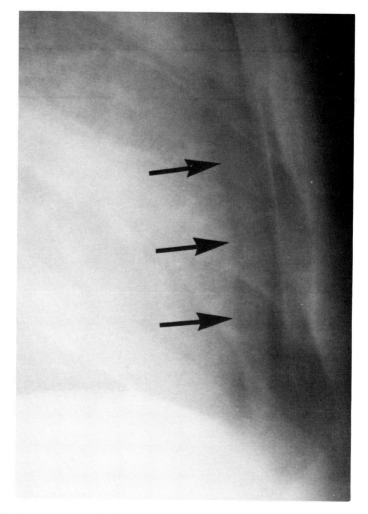

Fig. 8-8. Large pericardial effusion is separated from heart by prominent epicardial fat pad (arrows). Fluoroscopy confirmed this finding. In many cases this sign of pericardial effusion is seen only fluoroscopically.

tion of the epicardial fat pad from the edge of the cardiac shadow is seen, a pericardial effusion can be definitely diagnosed. This is usually best done in the lateral projection (Fig. 8-8).

LAMINAGRAPHY

Laminagraphy, or body section radiography, is performed in most radiology departments. It has the advantage of being a procedure performed almost entirely by a technician. Unlike some of the other special procedures described in this chapter, the demand upon the radiologist's time is small.

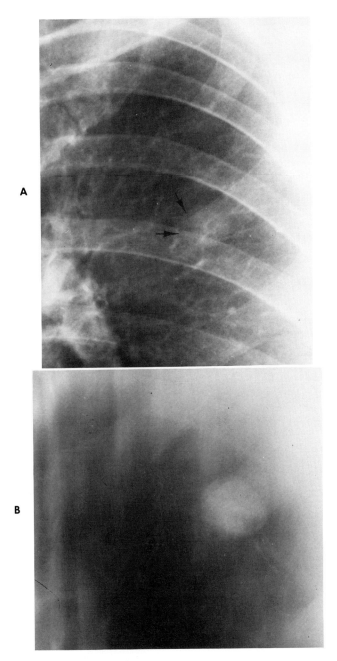

Fig. 8-9. A, Small nodule is seen in left midlung field (arrows). **B,** Tomography confirms far anterior location of nodule, contiguous with anterior rib. Tomogram also shows apparent soft tissue density to be irregularly calcified. Characteristic appearance of healed rib fracture mimicking pulmonary nodule.

However, to do laminagraphy correctly and well, it is essential that the radiologist carefully monitor the procedure. Large numbers of films covering the entire chest or uninvolved areas add greatly to patient x-ray exposure, the cost of the examination, and technician and room time. The films necessary in each instance should be decided upon by the radiologist, and the study should be monitored as it proceeds to decide upon necessary additions or deletions. Full-chest laminagrams taken routinely or the use of laminagraphy to evaluate all lung lesions is unjustifiable.

Laminagrams may define the exact location of an abnormal density, the shape or margins of the lesion, calcification in a nodule or mass, cavitation, the cause of hilar enlargement, or the presence of hidden lung nodules. The

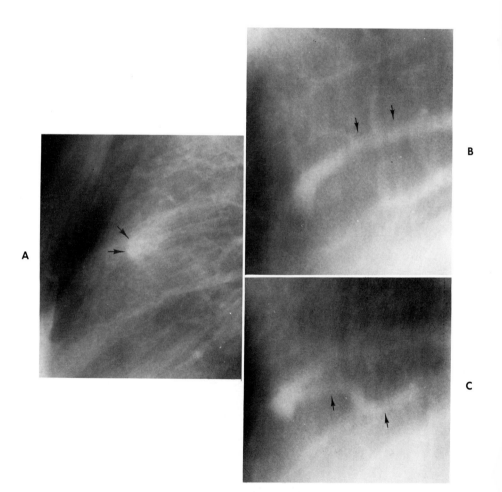

Fig. 8-10. A, Poorly defined soft tissue nodule overlies root of aorta in lateral projection (arrows). **B** and **C,** Feeding artery (arrows in **B**) and draining vein (arrows in **C**) reveal that nodule is arteriovenous malformation.

use of high-kilovoltage technique in plain films of the chest has greatly reduced the number of laminagrams necessary to evaluate "hidden" lesions.

Rarely the exact location of a pulmonary density of nodule cannot be determined from the PA and lateral films. Either fluoroscopy with spot films or a few selected laminagrams will usually resolve this problem (Fig. 8-9).

The characteristic configuration of some densities may be shown by laminagraphy. This includes extrapleural masses, arteriovenous malformations (Fig. 8-10) and other pulmonary vascular lesions (Fig. 8-11), and dilated bronchi as might be seen with allergic aspergillosis, a bronchocele (Fig. 8-12), bronchiectasis, or mucus plugs.

In problem cases the question of whether calcification (Fig. 8-13) is present in a nodule or cavitation (Fig. 8-14) in a pulmonary lesion can be resolved laminagraphically.

Enlargement of the hila may be due to engorged pulmonary arteries, lymphadenopathy, or other mass lesions. Differentiation among these possibilities may be impossible without laminagrams (Fig. 8-15).

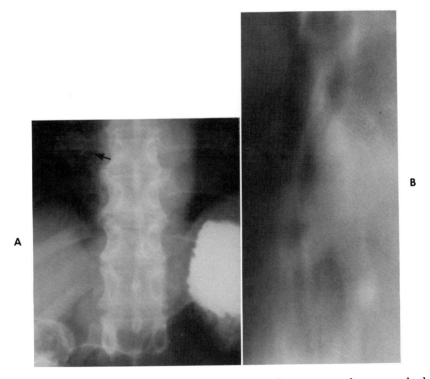

Fig. 8-11. A, Films taken during upper gastrointestinal tract series show a poorly defined nodule at right lung base (arrow). **B,** Tomography of this nodule shows multiple vessels entering it. This is typical appearance of prominent confluence of pulmonaary veins.

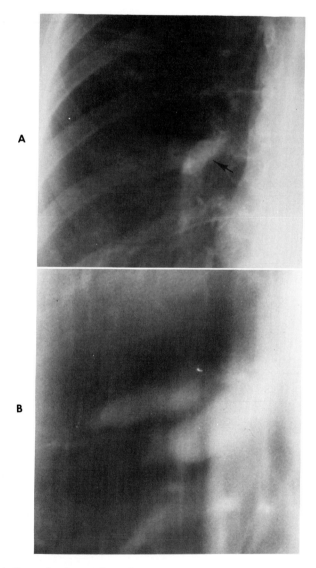

Fig. 8-12. A, Irregular density lies adjacent to and over right hilum (arrows). **B,** Laminagram reveals branching tubular nature of these shadows in patient with bronchocele.

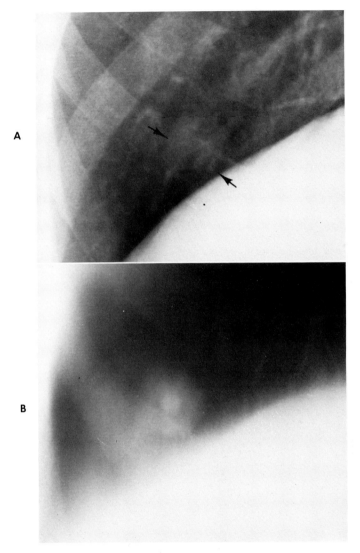

Fig. 8-13. A, Poorly defined nodule is seen at right lung base (arrows). **B,** Laminagram reveals central calcification, indicating that this is a benign lesion.

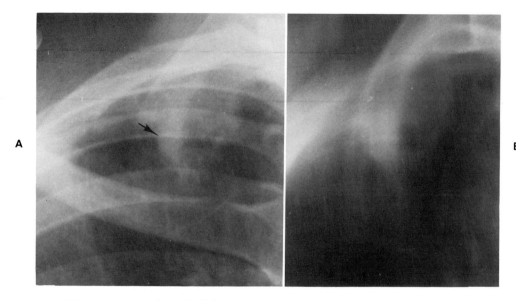

Fig. 8-14. A, Poorly defined density at right apex (arrow) is partially obscured by overlying ribs. **B,** Laminagraphic cut reveals definite central cavitation in this patient with pulmonary tuberculosis.

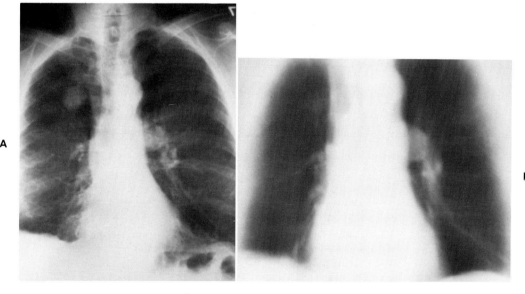

Fig. 8-15. A, Patient with emphysema and right upper lobe bronchogenic carcinoma has very prominent left hilum. **B,** Laminagraphic cut shows characteristic configuration of enlarged left main pulmonary artery.

Laminagraphy can be used to discover other lung nodules or to locate a nodule or nodules in a patient with suspected metastatic disease. Our experience has been that full-chest laminagrams at 1 cm intervals will occasionally reveal a nodule in patients, particularly if obese, not seen on routine frontal or lateral projections. This is of value when radical surgery may be contemplated. Repeated laminagrams after a suitable interval (4 to 6 weeks) often allows distinction of small metastases (growth) from healed granulomas.

BRONCHOGRAPHY
Technique

Contrast material may be placed into the tracheobronchial tree by many methods. The contrast medium can be placed at the base of the tongue and aspirated by the patient, metallic powders may be inhaled, or bronchi may be catheterized through the nose, mouth, or cricothyroid membrane. The use of a catheter under fluoroscopic control permits local studies to be performed,

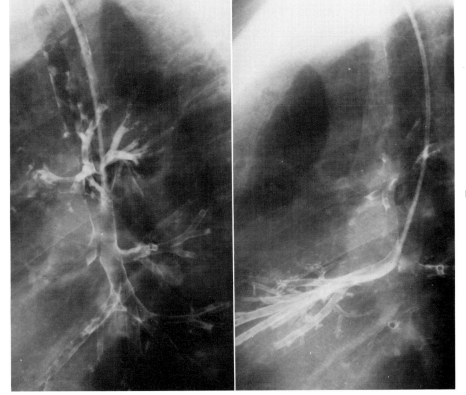

A   **B**

Fig. 8-16. A, Right middle lobe bronchi are not filled, suggesting possibility of broncho-occlusive disease. **B,** Selective catheterization of right middle lobe bronchus allows filling and excludes bronchial occlusion.

better control of filling, and selective refilling of poorly visualized areas (Fig. 8-16). We personally favor the use of the cricothyroid membrane approach for greater patient comfort, reduction in the amount of local anesthetic needed, and better control of the catheter for selective studies. The procedure is often combined with bronchial brushing when specimens are needed for cytologic or bacteriologic examination.

Oily Dionosil, a solution of organically bound iodine in peanut oil, is the only contrast medium material currently approved by the Food and Drug Administration for bronchography in the United States. The merits and problems of the various contrast agents in bronchography is beyond the scope of this chapter, and because other media are not approved for general use, such a discussion will not be of practical interest for the average practitioner.

Preparation of the patient for the bronchogram must include obtaining an informed consent. Most important to the success of the procedure, the patient must be well informed and relaxed, since an uncooperative or anxious patient greatly increases the difficulty of the examination. Fasting before the examination reduces the possibility of aspiration of gastric contents during the procedure, but with a cooperative, healthy patient this is not a problem. Premedication consists of the administration of 0.4 to 1.2 mg atropine sublingually to decrease secretions, the intramuscular injection of 50 to 100 mg of codeine to dull the cough reflex, and the intramuscular injection of 5 to 10 mg diazepam (Valium) as a sedative. The value of these drugs has not been satisfactorily examined in controlled studies, and when one or several are eliminated, the examination usually does not suffer. Rapid performance of the examination and patient understanding and cooperation are much more important than any of these medications. The materials on p. 173 are keyed in the text by their corresponding designations in the list.

Following premedication, the patient is placed supine upon the fluoroscopic table, and the anterior neck is cleansed and draped. The skin and soft tissues over the cricothyroid membrane are anesthetized.[a] The membrane is punctured and 2 ml of anesthetic is placed in the larynx and upper trachea. Then a small incision with a scalpel blade[b] is made in the skin, and a curved needle[c] is inserted through the membrane with the tip pointing distally. An additional 3 ml of local anesthetic is injected during inspiration. A guide wire[d] is next inserted through the needle, which is then withdrawn. A preshaped catheter[e] is subsequently placed over the guide wire and inserted into the lower trachea. Under fluoroscopic control the catheter is advanced to the area to be studied. The contrast medium is instilled after the patient is moved into the lateral position with the side to be studied down. If both sides are to be studied, the right side is usually done first for better visualization of the middle lobe orifice in the lateral projection. When sufficient coating is obtained, spot films are obtained in various projections. Lateral and steep oblique films usually show the major bronchial orifices better than frontal films (Fig. 8-

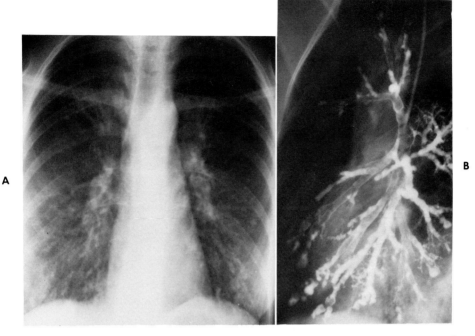

Fig. 8-17. A, Patient with chronic productive cough has diffuse increase in interstitial lung markings. **B,** Tubular and varicose bronchiectasis involves all segments of right lung as demonstrated on this bronchogram. Notice how well oblique projection shows orifices of many segmental bronchi.

17). Depending upon the quality of the spot films, appropriate overhead films may be obtained. A postcough film has been advocated to evaluate more peripheral airways, particularly to see bronchiectasis involving only smaller bronchi. This film is of questionable value since it produces a very low yield of pertinent information.

Special materials required for bronchography, bronchial brushing, and needle biopsy

a. 1% lidocaine (Xylocaine) in 10 ml syringe fitted with 25-gauge needle
b. No. 11 scalpel blade (Bard-Parker)
c. 16-gauge, thin-walled cricothyroid needle (Cook BN-16-150)
d. 60 cm long 0.035 safety spring guide wire (Cook TSF-35-60)
e. Green-Kifa catheter (USCI-4608)
f. Controllable bronchial brush (USCI-2701)
g. Catheter deflector (Cook TDH-100)
h. Polysal balanced electrolyte solution (Cutter) or ether alcohol
i. Multi-slide holder filled with 95% alcohol
j. 18-gauge aspirating biopsy needle (Cook TBN-18-600)
k. Disposable Vim needle (Travenol)
l. 9-inch straight sponge forceps (Storz Instrument Co. N7175)
m. 20 ml Luer-Lok glass syringe (Becton-Dickinson 2313)

Indications

There is a wide discrepancy in opinion regarding the uses of bronchography. Some authorities rarely use the study,[12] whereas others use it frequently to evaluate many sorts of chest disease.[22] It is the definitive method of evaluating the severity and extent of bronchiectasis (Fig. 8-18). Clinical and plain-film findings are unreliable in determining the anatomic distribution of bronchiectasis, and surgical correction for bronchiectasis is only feasible when the disease is localized.

We have also found bronchography helpful in searching for broncho-occlusive disease, particularly broncholithiasis (Fig. 8-19), the right middle lobe syndrome, and its variants (Fig. 8-20). The use of bronchography to evaluate neoplastic disease (Fig. 8-21), particularly to distinguish lung cancer from benign forms of broncho-occlusive disease, has been unproductive in our hands (Figs. 8-33 and 8-34). It is useful as a map in bronchial brushing for decisions as to which areas to brush and for delineating the anatomy to reveal the course the brush must take to reach a more peripheral lesion.

Bronchography is widely used to evaluate hemoptysis of unknown etiology.[6] We feel it is of little help in this group of patients, particularly if the plain film is normal. In our recent series of 146 patients with hemoptysis who were studied by bronchography, the examination was of significant clinical help in only six cases.

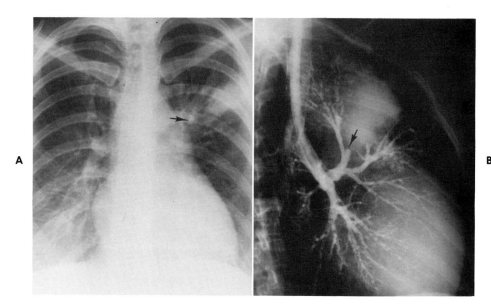

A
B

Fig. 8-18. A, Area of consolidation is seen in left upper lobe. Small calcification is evident centrally (arrow). **B,** Bronchogram reveals complete obstruction of anterior segment of left upper lobe due to broncholith (arrow).

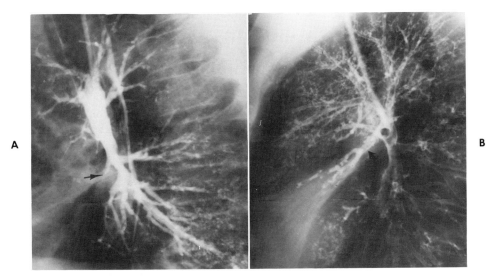

Fig. 8-19. A, Right middle lobe syndrome with chronic pneumonia and atelectasis. Right middle lobe bronchus is occluded on bronchogram (arrow). **B,** Another example of right middle lobe syndrome with chronic atelectasis and consolidation. In this instance, right middle lobe bronchus is patent (arrow).

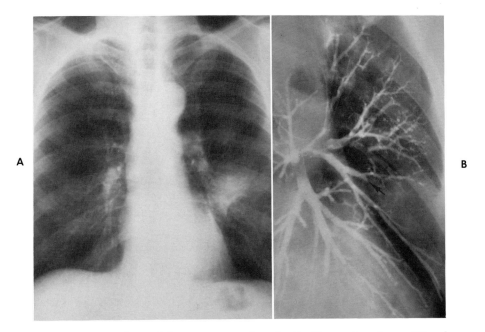

Fig. 8-20. A, Area of consolidation is seen in lingula. **B,** Obstruction of one of lingular subsegments due to bronchogenic carcinoma (arrow) is seen on bronchogram. This is often impossible to distinguish from benign causes of broncho-occlusive disease.

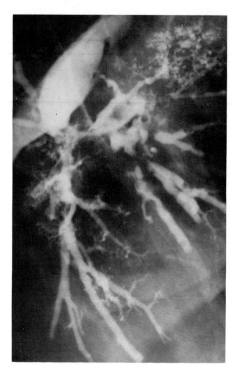

Fig. 8-21. Bronchogram of patient with severe chronic bronchitis shows slight dilatation and irregularity with incomplete filling and lucent defects due to spasm and increased secretion.

Certain bronchographic findings have been associated with chronic bronchitis and emphysema. These include irregularity of bronchial walls, slight dilatation, spasm, increased secretions (Fig. 8-22), filling of mucous glands (Fig. 8-23), and bronchiolectasis (Fig. 8-24). The use of bronchography to evaluate these disease processes is unrewarding, since clinical and laboratory studies are more reliable. Most middle-aged or elderly patients in the urban population have radiographic findings of chronic bronchitis on bronchography, and the severity of these findings is not well correlated with clinical status.

Contraindications

True allergy to the contrast material is rare, but when present it certainly is a contraindication to the examination. An alternative contrast material with different chemical properties such as tantalum powder might be indicated in this situation. Allergy to a local anesthetic agent is more common, and if a study is necessary in such a person, a general anesthetic must be used.

A patient with a very labile medical condition, particularly a cardiac arrhythmia, would not be a candidate for bronchography. Severe respiratory insufficiency is also an absolute contraindication, since the bronchographic con-

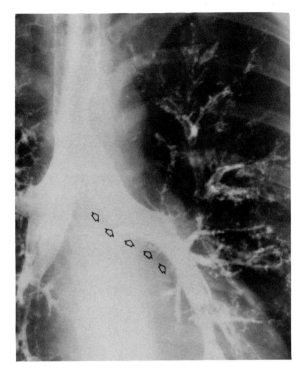

Fig. 8-22. Bronchogram of another patient with chronic bronchitis shows filling of many dilated mucous glands (arrows).

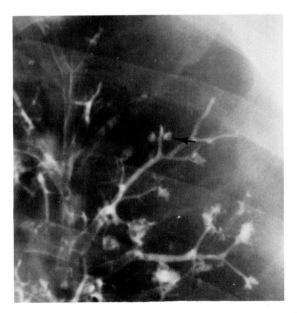

Fig. 8-23. Bronchogram of patient with emphysema shows sparse peripheral filling of bronchi ("pruned-tree" appearance) and bronchiolectasis (arrows).

trast will occlude or partially occlude some airways during the course of the examination.

The tolerance of asthmatics to bronchography is difficult to predict. Severe bronchospasm will occasionally occur locally where the contrast is instilled, but other patients with severe asthma tolerate the procedure well. The study should not be performed during an acute attack.

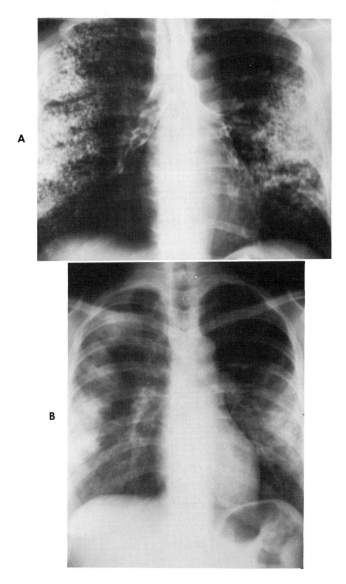

Fig. 8-24. A, Film at end of bronchogram shows diffuse alveolarization. **B,** Four days later there is extensive peripheral consolidation; patient was febrile with symptoms of pneumonia. Chemical and superimposed bacterial pneumonia have been caused by "alveolarized" oily Dionosil.

Complications

The most common serious complication is due to the local anesthetic. Allergic reactions and an overdose of the local anesthetic are potentially fatal. Respiratory embarrassment from spasm or occlusion of the bronchi is almost exclusively seen in those with serious respiratory insufficiency or asthma.

If a large amount of oily Dionosil is coughed or aspirated into the most peripheral airways, the characteristic appearance of "alveolarization" is seen (Fig. 8-25). This contrast may cause no effect on the patient, or a secondary chemical or superimposed bacterial pneumonia may ensue. Coughing during the procedure or overfilling with contrast increases the risk of this complication. Decanting half the oil from the unmixed bottle of oily Dionosil will increase the viscosity of the contrast agent and decrease alveolarization.

Laryngeal spasm and edema may occur occasionally. The transcricothyroid membrane approach can result in a neck infection that may spread to the mediastinum. Contrast material left in the soft tissues of the neck after such a study may cause a small sterile abscess. Subcutaneous emphysema due to air leakage at the wound site is a frequent complication of this approach but is usually of no significance. Occasionally large amounts of air will collect subcutaneously and dissect into the mediastinum (Fig. 8-26); air rarely perforates into the pleural space, where it causes pneumothorax. Massaging the neck

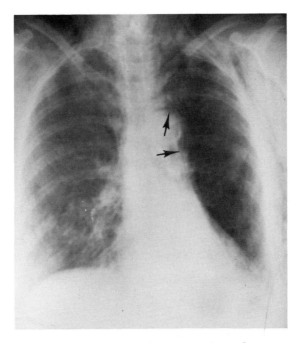

Fig. 8-25. Twenty-four hours after bronchogram performed using transcricothyroid membrane technique. Extensive subcutaneous emphysema and mediastinal emphysema (arrows) are obvious.

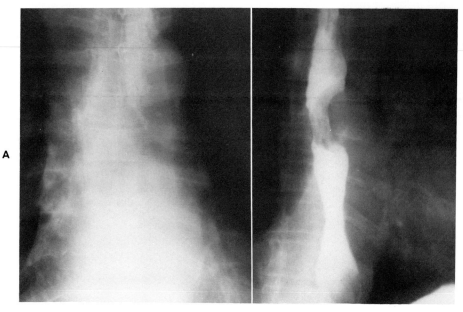

Fig. 8-26. A, Close-up PA view of mediastinum shows diffuse widening but no specific abnormality. **B,** Esophagogram shows large subcarinal mass in this patient with bronchogenic carcinoma metastatic to mediastinum.

wound for 5 minutes after the procedure and instructing the patient to cover the wound with a finger for the next day whenever he has to cough will reduce the incidence of air leakage into the surrounding tissues.

ESOPHAGRAPHY

Since the esophagus passes through the middle of the mediastinum, abnormalities in this area may be reflected by an esophagram. Patients with esophageal symptoms will almost invariably have undergone a barium swallow examination. However, this study should not be overlooked in patients with questionable mediastinal abnormalities (Fig. 8-27), mediastinal masses, severe chronic cough, or recurrent pneumonias of unknown etiology (Fig. 8-28). Because of its safety and simplicity this study should be used early in the evaluation of mediastinal disease.

RADIOLOGIC-ASSISTED LUNG BIOPSY TECHNIQUES

The determination of the etiology of an infiltrate or mass lesion seen in the lung on a chest radiograph is a common clinical problem. Usually the chest roentgenogram contributes only a tentative diagnosis. In some instances the disease process cannot be diagnosed by the usual clinical workup—sputum examination and culture, serologic studies, bronchoscopy, or bone marrow examination. The establishment of the true nature of the lesion then depends

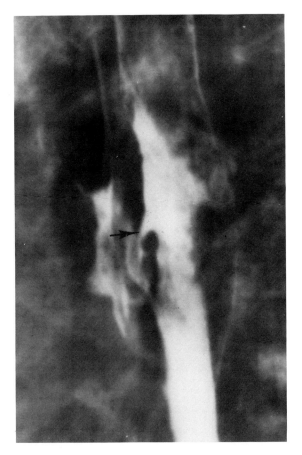

Fig. 8-27. Barium swallow on this patient with chronic cough shows fistulous tract between esophagus and distal trachea (arrow). At surgery caseous lymph nodes and fibrosis were found adjacent to fistula.

upon examination of tissue from the radiographically demonstrated pulmonary density.

The ideal diagnostic test, with no risk and a 100% yield, unfortunately does not exist. In the past, pulmonary tissue usually was obtained via a diagnostic thoracotomy, which is still unquestionably the most reliable method of diagnosis. However, it is also the most expensive, painful, and dangerous. A fundamental logic in medicine dictates that attempts to establish a diagnosis should be made in order of increasing risk and expense to the patient; the procedure less likely to injure should be used first before progressing to the more dangerous, discomforting, and expensive techniques. Using this philosophy, the two nonoperative fluoroscopically assisted lung biopsy techniques—transcatheter bronchial brushing and percutaneous needle biopsy—have proved to be highly accurate diagnostic modalities while maintaining low morbidity and

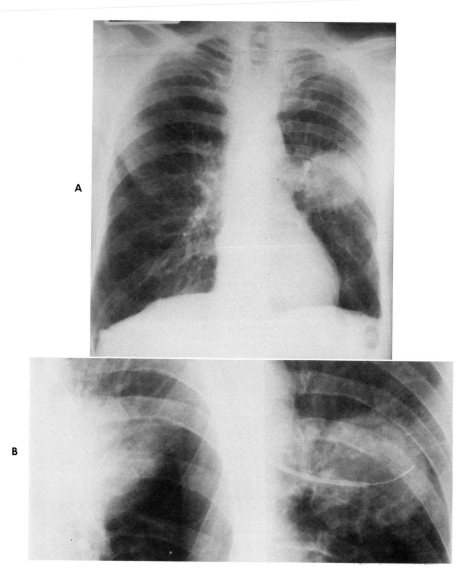

Fig. 8-28. A 60-year-old man with confusion and gait disturbance. Brain scan revealed multiple areas of abnormal uptake. **A,** Chest roentgenogram demonstrates left lung mass. Results of sputum examination and bronchoscopy were negative. **B,** Spot films in steep oblique and frontal projections demonstrate correct position of brush tip within mass. Cytologic specimens were positive for oat cell carcinoma and chemotherapy was instituted.

low financial cost. The availability of image-intensification fluoroscopy has made it possible to guide a brush or needle to pulmonary lesions situated in virtually any portion of the lung with a minimum of difficulty. Either of these techniques is capable of providing tissue for cytologic or microbiologic study, and either can usually provide the basis for the definitive diagnosis of a pulmonary lesion when thoracotomy is not desirable.

Indications

The patients that benefit most from these procedures include those who are clinically inoperable with suspected lung neoplasm, those with suspected pneumonic infiltration, and those with an indeterminate solitary pulmonary lesion.

Suspected lung neoplasm in clinically inoperable patients. Patients with pulmonary mass(es) are unlikely to benefit from surgery, either because of known metastatic disease or severe cardiopulmonary disorders. An accurate tissue diagnosis is required before radiotherapy or chemotherapy can be instituted (Figs. 8-28 and 8-29).

Suspected pneumonic infiltration. A specific etiologic diagnosis is extremely important for the immunologically deficient patient (whether the deficiency is due to immunosuppressive drugs, as after transplantation surgery or for leukemia therapy, or to an underlying disease such as hypogammaglobulinemia) because of the large variety of opportunistic infectious agents that might be responsible (Fig. 8-30). The differentiation of opportunistic infection from neoplastic pulmonary infiltration is often possible through the use of bronchial brushing or needle biopsy (Fig. 8-31). This becomes important because many organisms responsible for opportunistic infection and metastatic neoplastic cells are difficult to recover from routine sputum samples or bronchoscopic washings. The same techniques are also useful in diagnosing the problem of a patient whose condition deteriorates while he is receiving antibiotic therapy (Fig. 8-32).

Indeterminate solitary pulmonary lesion. Thoracotomy may become justified in a patient with severe medical problems who is a poor surgical candidate if a definite diagnosis of lung carcinoma can be established through a radiologically assisted lung biopsy technique. Such a technique is also indicated for patients from whom an infectious organism has not yet been recovered and when the diagnosis of a neoplastic process has not been excluded with certainty (Fig. 8-33 and 8-34). Neither bronchial brushing nor needle biopsy is indicated for a patient in good clinical condition with a solitary lung lesion when a thoracotomy is planned regardless of the results of the diagnostic procedure.

TRANSCATHETER BRONCHIAL BRUSHING

Many techniques for transcatheter bronchial brushing have been described,[9,35,38,39] and all are relatively simple and readily learned. Our preferred

Text continued on p. 190.

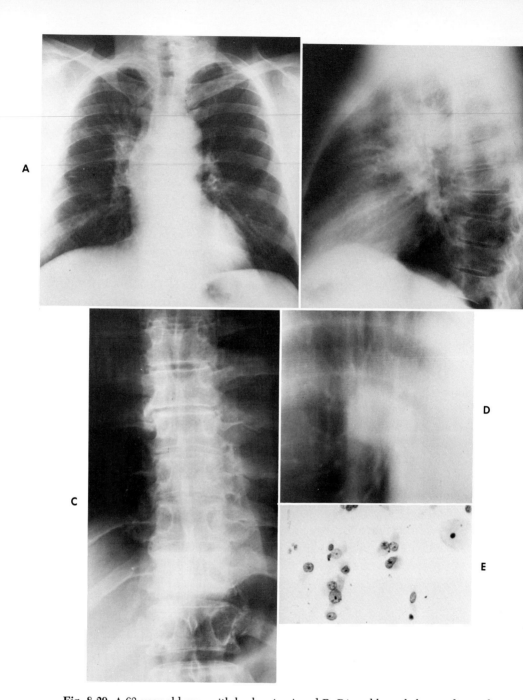

Fig. 8-29. A 63-year-old man with back pain. **A** and **B**, PA and lateral chest radiographs demonstrate mass lesion in superior segment of right lower lobe and right hilar lymph node enlargment. Sclerosis of T-10 vertebral body is noted on lateral projection. **C**, Cone-down view of lower thoracic spine shows blastic lesion of T-10 vertebral body and left paraspinal mass. **D**, Tomogram demonstrating mass in right lower lobe. Sputum examination and bronchoscopy were negative. **E**, Cytologic specimen of material obtained from aspiration needle biopsy of right lower lobe mass shows adenocarcinoma cells.

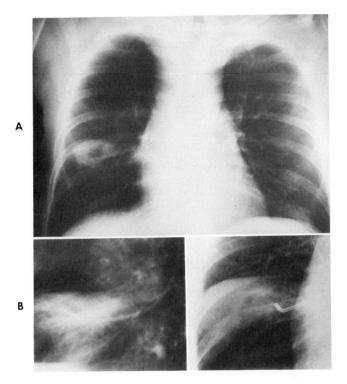

Fig. 8-30. A 37-year-old man on long-term, high-dose corticosteroid therapy who has cough and low-grade fever. **A,** AP chest roentgenogram demonstrates cavitary infiltrate within lateral segment of middle lobe. Mediastinal widening due to fat deposition incidently noted. Sputum examination and transtracheal aspiration were negative. **B,** Spot films in lateral and frontal projections confirming correct position of catheter tip within middle lobe infiltrate before bronchial brushing. Culture of brush specimens revealed *Cryptococcus neoformans*.

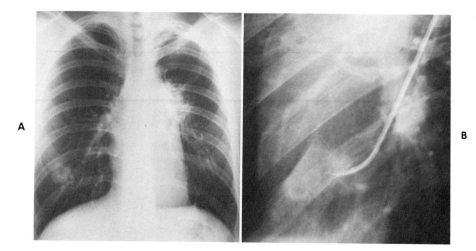

Fig. 8-31. A 26-year-old asymptomatic man treated with radiation therapy 1 year previously for mediastinal Hodgkin's disease. **A,** PA chest radiograph demonstrates radiation fibrosis in left upper lung field and cavitary nodular infiltrate in anterior basal segment of right lower lobe. **B,** Oblique spot film confirming tip of brush within cavitary infiltrate. Culture of brush specimens was negative, but cytologic preparation showed abnormal cells compatible with Hodgkin's disease.

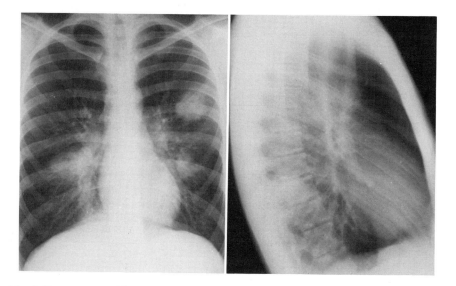

Fig. 8-32. A 19-year-old man with cough and fever. PA and lateral chest roentgenograms demonstrate bilateral pneumonic infiltrates more extensive than on radiographs obtained 5 days previously despite interim treatment with tetracycline. Sputum examination was negative. Smears from percutaneous aspiration needle biopsy of right lower lobe infiltrate showed multiple cocci in clumps. Subsequent treatment with methicillin resulted in complete resolution of patient's symptoms and abnormal chest radiograph.

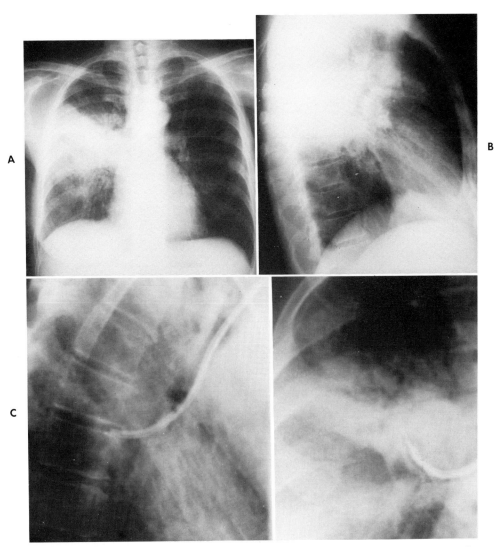

Continued.

Fig. 8-33. A 56-year-old woman with cough and fever. Patient had had a left radical mastectomy 6 years previously. **A**, and **B**, PA and lateral chest roentgenograms demonstrate consolidation in right upper and lower lobes. **C**, Spot films in lateral and frontal projection demonstrate proper positioning of brush and catheter within lesion. **D**, Postbrush bronchogram shows complete obstruction of superior segment bronchus of right lower lobe. **E**, Gram stain of material obtained from bronchial brushing reveals coccobacillary organisms with long mycelial filaments, later confirmed to be *Nocardia asteroides*.

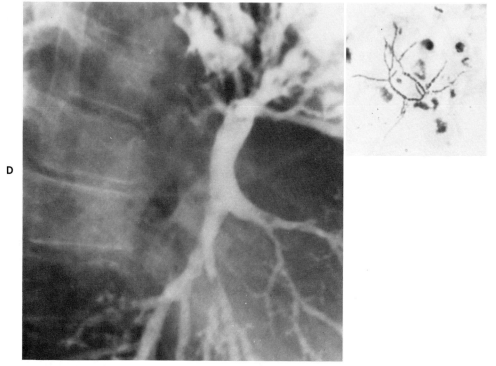

Fig. 8-33, cont'd. For legend see p. 187.

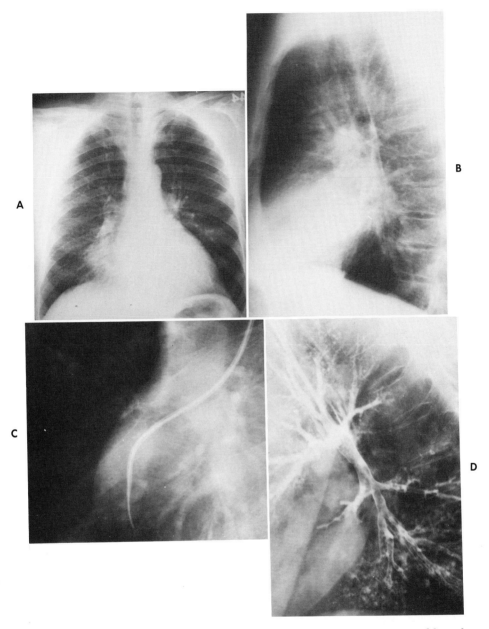

Fig. 8-34. A 57-year-old male alcoholic with cough and fever. **A** and **B,** PA and lateral chest roentgenograms demonstrate middle lobe consolidation unchanged from radiograph taken 1 week previously despite interim antibiotic therapy. Sputum examination negative. **C,** Spot film confirming brush in proper location within middle lobe infiltrate. **D,** Post-brush bronchogram demonstrating poor peripheral filling of middle lobe bronchi. Bronchial brush specimens were positive for large cell undifferentiated carcinoma.

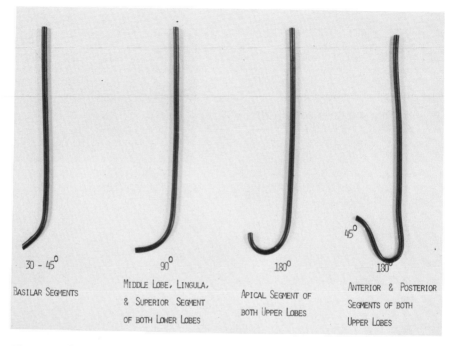

30 – 45°

BASILAR SEGMENTS

90°

MIDDLE LOBE, LINGULA,
& SUPERIOR SEGMENT
OF BOTH LOWER LOBES

180°

APICAL SEGMENT OF
BOTH UPPER LOBES

45°

180°

ANTERIOR & POSTERIOR
SEGMENTS OF BOTH
UPPER LOBES

Fig. 8-35. Shape of tip of catheter usually required for selective catheterization of orifices of segmental bronchi.

method is to introduce preshaped arterial catheters (specific curves are put in the distal tip of the catheter for selective placement in the desired bronchial segment (Fig. 8-35) through the transcricothyroid membrane using the Seldinger technique. This approach is quick and easy and permits optimal control of the catheter for positioning.

Premedication and entry into the tracheobronchial tree are the same as described in the section on bronchography. Under image-intensification fluoroscopic control, the tip of the catheter can usually be easily advanced into the segmental or subsegmental bronchus in which the lesion is situated. Peripheral bronchi can be probed with the flexible end of the guide wire or a controllable brush[f] as the catheter is manipulated until the bronchus leading to the lesion is entered. A special catheter tip deflector[g] may be used when the lesion is not readily reachable. The catheter is generally sufficiently small to enter even a partially occluded bronchus. The catheter is advanced until it is as close to the lesion as possible. In dealing with cavitary lesions, the stiff end of the guide wire may be used in an endeavor to puncture the cavity wall if there is difficulty in entering the cavity.[11] Correct positioning of the catheter should be verified by spot films (Figs. 8-28, 8-30, and 8-33) in at least two projections. (One should not despair if after several attempts the lesion cannot be

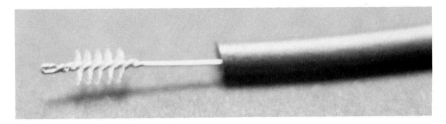

Fig. 8-36. Close-up view of nylon-bristled brush protruding through tip of catheter.

reached with the catheter, as brushings and washings from a nearby position may be positive.)

When optimal positioning of the catheter is achieved, a small, disposable, flexible, nylon-bristled brush[g] (Fig. 8-36) is passed through the positioned catheter and advanced toward and, if possible, into the substance of the lesion. The region is vigorously scrubbed by forward and backward movements of the brush in an attempt to tear off and catch pieces of tissue on the bristles. The brush may be removed and replaced as many times as necessary to obtain material for study. Generally, following a slight repositioning of the catheter, brushings from a number of other small bronchi closely associated with the lesion are obtained.

Brush scrapings are manually agitated in test tubes containing sterile saline solution to remove pieces of tissue. Depending upon the clinical situation, smears and cultures are subsequently prepared for routine bacteriologic studies, mycobacterium, fungus, and so on. If anaerobic infection is suspected, the brush scrapings are inoculated into a special "nitrogen-gas" tube. For cytologic study, the brushings are agitated in a special preservative solution, which is then centrifuged; the sediment is placed on both a frosted slide and a Millipore filter and subsequently stained by the Papanicolaou technique. Some brush scrapings are placed directly on frosted glass slides, which are fixed immediately prior to staining. If *Pneumocystis carinii* is suspected, slides are fixed in 10% formalin.

The catheter is then pulled back proximally from the wedged position within the small bronchus, and 5 ml of sterile saline solution is injected and vigorously aspirated. This material is divided for the appropriate diagnostic studies mentioned previously.

In patients with a solitary indeterminate lung lesion a localized selective bronchogram is usually done, especially in patients who are poor surgical candidates. This permits examination of the bronchial tree adjacent to the lesion. The finding of patent bronchi extending through an area of infiltration or localized bronchiectasis proximal to or within the lesion (Fig. 8-37) is an ancillary indication that the lesion is not neoplastic if the cytologic examinations of the brush scrapings are negative.[8,21] The extent of broncho-occlusive

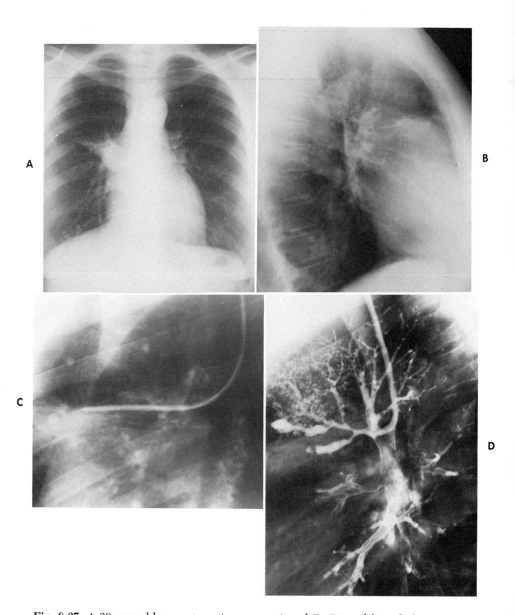

Fig. 8-37. A 39-year-old asymptomatic woman. **A** and **B**, PA and lateral chest roent-genograms demonstrate mass density in anterior segment of right upper lobe and old healed calcified granulomatous disease. **C**, Spot film confirming proper location of brush and catheter within right upper lobe density. Culture and cytologic preparations of brush specimens were subsequently negative. **D**, Post-brush bronchogram demon-strates localized bronchiectasis in anterior segment of right upper lobe. Lesion was thought to be postinflamatory in view of negative brushings and bronchographic find-ings; diagnostic thoracotomy was not performed.

disease can also be determined and the possible need for pneumonectomy can be predicted should the cytology be positive. Bronchography should be performed after the brushings have been obtained, since contaminating Dionosil makes cytologic diagnosis more difficult.

The patient is then returned to his room, where he is allowed nothing by mouth for an additional 3 hours. He is instructed to hold his thumb over the cricothyroid membrane puncture site whenever he coughs to prevent air from leaking into surrounding tissues. Sputum is collected for the 24-hour period following brushing. Occasionally, when the brush biopsy results have been negative, the sputum collected after the brushing has revealed positive results. Probably the trauma caused by the brush and the coughing that occurs when the local anesthetic wears off accounts for this result.

Fluoroscopically controlled transcatheter bronchial brushing produces specimens that yield a positive cytologic diagnosis in approximately 80% of patients with a peripherally located bronchogenic carcinoma.[9,26] This is a considerable improvement over the accuracy obtained from sputum samples or rigid bronchoscopic washings in peripheral carcinomas. Brushings obtained through the fiber optic bronchoscope may be slightly more accurate in the case of central or midzone lesions when the brush can be applied directly to a visualized bronchial mass.[39] In our experience with distal lesions, fiber optic bronchoscopic brushings produce results as accurate as transcatheter brushings if the bronchoscopy is also done under fluoroscopic control. Fluoroscopy aids immeasurably in documenting the relationship of the instrument tip and a lesion beyond the segmental bronchus (Fig. 8-38). Previous reports[30,39] also emphasize that fluoroscopy is critical in ensuring that the proper peripheral area is brushed.

Bronchial brushing is much less accurate in the diagnosis of metastatic lesions, which are frequently extrabronchial and thus are not brushed. Needle biopsy is the preferred diagnostic procedure when metastatic disease is suspected.

Positive results from smears and cultures (about 70% overall accuracy) have been obtained from brushing in a myriad of infectious conditions[9] (Figs. 8-39 to 8-42), including mycobacteriosis, nocardiosis (Fig. 8-33), aspergillosis,[13] and *Pneumocystis carinii* pneumonitis,[25] when sputum specimens were consistently negative. Our accuracy has now increased to about 80%, after an initial report[11] following brushing of undiagnosed cavitary lesions (Figs. 8-43 and 8-44). Catheterization of a large fluid-filled abscess may have therapeutic as well as diagnostic value.[14] Purulent material can be aspirated because widening of the bronchial communication via the catheter facilitates drainage. Antibiotics may be instilled directly into the cavitary lesion if desired.

In our own experience with more than 600 bronchial brushings this procedure has proved to be virtually free of significant complications. A pneumothorax has occurred in four patients. Two of these cases occurred because in-

Text continued on p. 201.

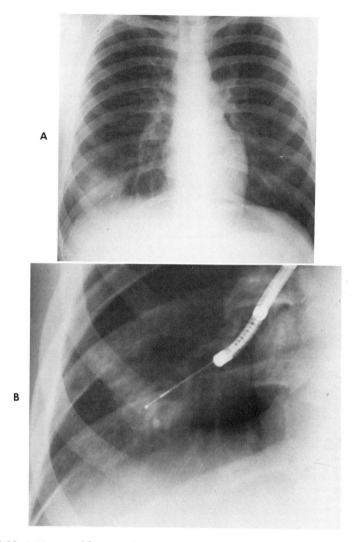

Fig. 8-38. A 19-year-old man with cough and fever. **A,** PA chest roentgenogram demonstrates infiltrate within anterior basal segment of right lower lobe. **B,** Spot film obtained following insertion of brush through fiber optic bronchoscope, confirming tip of brush within lesion. Subsequent culture of brush scrapings revealed anaerobic streptococci.

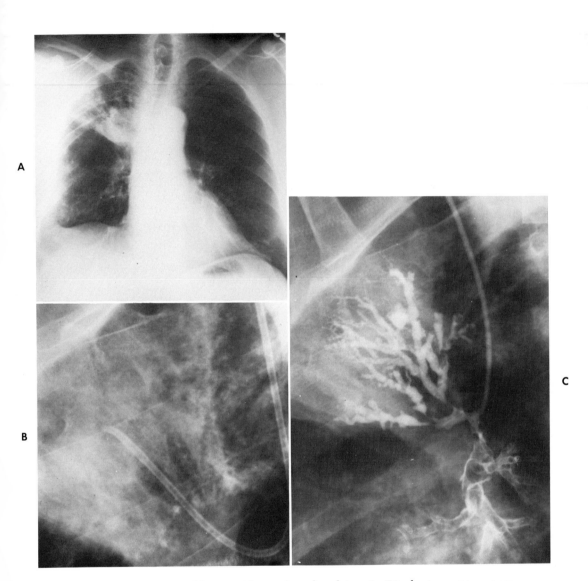

Fig. 8-39. A 72-year-old man with cough and malaise. **A,** PA chest roentgenogram demonstrates some infiltrate and volume loss within right upper lobe. Sputum examination and bronchoscopy negative. **B,** Spot film showing bronchial brush catheter within right upper lobe infiltrate. Brush scrapings revealed acid-fast bacilli on smear, which subsequent culture confirmed as *Mycobacterium* tuberculosis. **C,** Post-brush bronchogram demonstrates stenosis of right upper lobe segmental bronchi with dilatation of subsegmental branches.

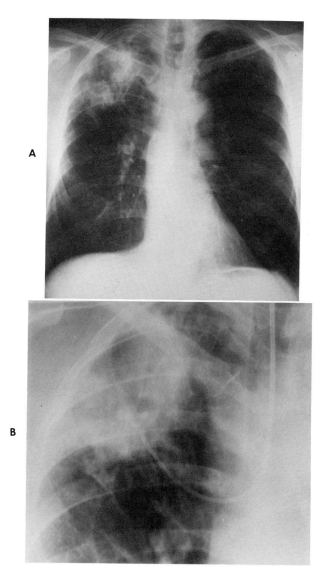

Fig. 8-40. A 57-year-old man with cough, weight loss, and dyspnea. **A,** PA chest radiograph demonstrates evidence of chronic obstructive pulmonary disease and right upper lobe infiltrate. Sputum examination and culture were negative. **B,** Spot film showing tip of bronchial catheter within right upper lobe infiltrate. Brush scrapings revealed acid-fast bacilli on smear, which subsequent culture confirmed as *Mycobacterium kansasii.*

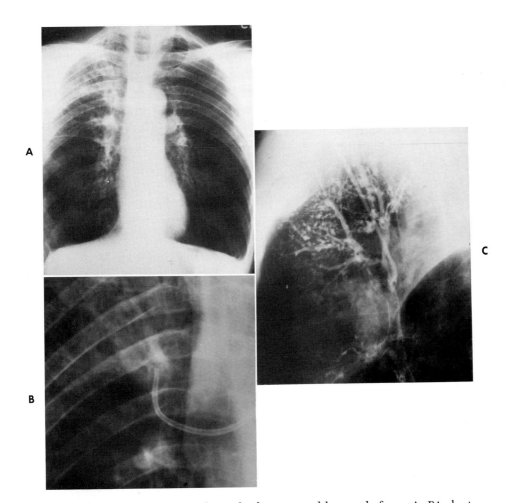

Fig. 8-41. A 68-year-old man with cough, dyspnea, and low-grade fever. **A,** PA chest roentgenogram demonstrates evidence of chronic obstructive pulmonary disease and some infiltrate and volume loss within right upper lobe. (Note similarity of plain chest radiograph to those in Figs. 8-39 and 8-40.) **B,** Spot film showing tip of catheter in place within right upper lobe infiltrate. Cytologic material of brush scrapings revealed squamous cell carcinoma cells; no acid-fast bacilli were obtained on smear or culture. **C,** Lateral projection of post-brush bronchogram reveals occlusion of posterior segmental bronchus of right upper lobe.

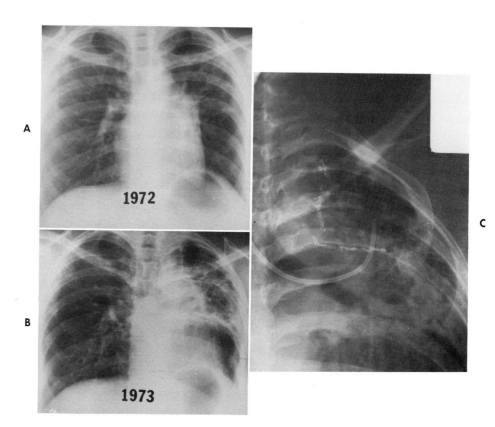

Fig. 8-42. A 30-year-old woman. **A,** PA chest radiograph reveals left upper lobe infiltrate and left hilar lymph node enlargement. Open-lung biopsy demonstrated noncaseating granulomas. Patient placed on corticosteroids and isoniazid. **B,** PA chest radiograph shows progressive infiltrate with cavitation and volume loss in left upper lobe. Sputum examination negative. **C,** Spot film showing catheter tip within left upper lobe. Culture of brush scrapings revealed *Blastomyces dermatitidis.*

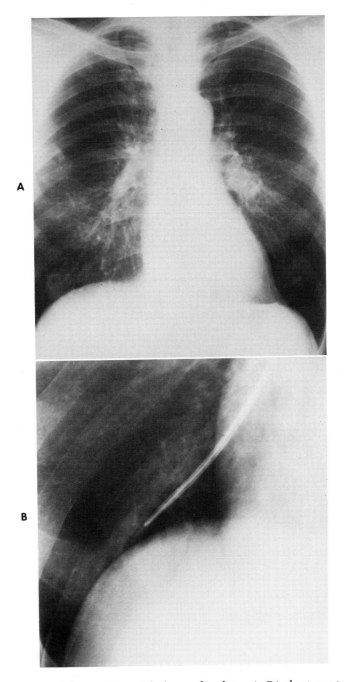

Fig. 8-43. A 60-year-old man with weight loss and malaise. **A,** PA chest roentgenogram shows several nodular densities throughout both lung fields with cavitation within nodular mass in anterior basal segment of right lower lobe. Sputum examination and bronchoscopy were negative. **B,** Spot film demonstrating brush in optimal position within right lower lobe cavitary nodule. Brush scrapings revealed adenocarcinoma cells. Barium enema showed constricting carcinoma of rectosigmoid area.

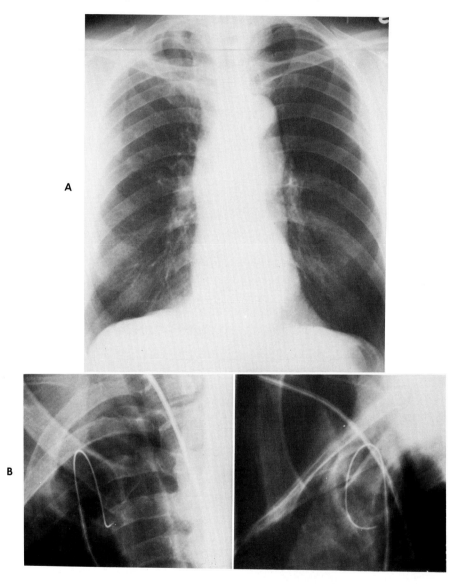

Fig. 8-44. A 70-year-old male alcoholic admitted for delirium tremens. No chest symptoms. **A,** PA chest roentgenogram demonstrates a thin-walled cavitary lesion containing small amount of fluid within apical segment of right upper lobe. Lesion was considered to be probably an infected bulla. Sputum examination and bronchoscopy were negative. **B,** Spot films showing bronchial brush within proper location coiled within cavity. Cytologic preparation of brush scrapings revealed squamous cell carcinoma cells. Surgical resection confirmed a primary cavitating lung carcinoma, which had presented with an atypical radiographic appearance.

experienced residents brushed a peripheral lesion so vigorously that they perforated into the pleural space with the brush. The other two were the result of mediastinal air that dissected into the pleural space, complicating the transcricothyroid membrane puncture. These few pneumothoraces were easily managed by thoracostomy tube drainage.

Minor transient blood streaking of the sputum not uncommonly occurs; this is usually an indication that the brush was in the proper spot in the abnormal tissues. While it has not occurred in our experience, significant and even fatal intrapulmonary hemorrhage has been reported in four patients who suffered from thrombocytopenia or hemoptysis prior to the brushing.[10]

PERCUTANEOUS NEEDLE BIOPSY

Percutaneous needle biopsy is certainly not a new technique, as it was described more than a century ago before radiologic assistance was even available. The introduction of sensitive image-intensification fluoroscopy, permitting the direction of small needles to even very small pulmonary lesions with acceptable risk, and the development of highly reliable cytologic techniques have resulted in a revived interest in this diagnostic modality.[7,17,18,26,31]

Basically, two different methods of percutaneous needle biopsy of the lung may be employed; these are aspiration with a spinal-type needle and true biopsy with a cutting-type needle.

Aspiration biopsy with a spinal-type needle

Aspiration biopsy with a spinal-type needle is a simple, relatively painless method of diagnosis through which lesions situated in virtually any portion of the lung or even in the mediastinum may be aspirated. When it is suspected that the pulmonary lesion is neoplastic, an 18-gauge spinal-type needle whose inner cannula is sharp,[j] making it possible to cut off some cellular material, is used (Fig. 8-29).[32] If the lesion is thought to be infectious, a 20-gauge simple spinal needle is used (Fig. 8-32).

True biopsy with a cutting-type needle

The advantage of the cutting needle is that it provides a tissue specimen for histologic rather than cytologic study. A Vim biopsy needle[k] is occasionally used if the simple aspiration biopsy of a lesion has been negative (Fig. 8-45), and it is used primarily when metastatic neoplasm or granulomatous angiitis is suspected and a definitive histologic diagnosis is necessary (Fig. 8-46). The use of the cutting biopsy needle[33] is restricted to solid lung lesions greater than 2 cm in diameter abutting upon or invading the chest wall.[37] We no longer employ percutaneous cutting needle biopsy in patients with diffuse pulmonary infiltrates such as chronic interstitial disease.[19] In this type of lesion the complication rate increases significantly, and we believe that an open limited thoracotomy is the preferable diagnostic procedure for diffuse lung lesions,

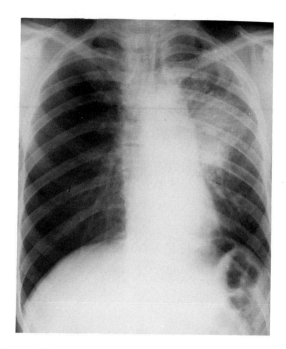

Fig. 8-45. A 28-year-old asymptomatic man who had received mediastinal radiation therapy 1 year previously for Hodgkin's disease. PA chest roentgenogram demonstrates consolidation and some volume loss in left upper lobe. Sputum examination, fiber optic bronchoscopy with brushing, and aspiration needle biopsy were negative. Histologic preparation of tissue specimens obtained from cutting Vim needle biopsy of left upper lobe revealed parenchymal Hodgkin's disease.

since the complications are no greater and a more satisfactory histologic specimen is obtained. (Alternative methods to open thoracotomy, with which we have had no experience, are the suction excision biopsy[23] and the trephine drill needle biopsy.[5])

Technique

No complex materials are needed for percutaneous needle biopsy of the lung. In order to assuage apprehension and reduce the minimal pain, 75 mg of meperidine (Demerol) is usually administered intramuscularly as a premedication, but this may be omitted in the severely ill patient.

Prior to performing the percutaneous pulmonary needle biopsy, the patient is placed in a horizontal position on the fluoroscopic table with the affected area closest to the radiologist. Thus the patient would assume a supine position for an anteriorly situated lesion and a prone position if the lesion is posterior. A posterior approach is always used for apical lesions to avoid injury to brachial vessels and nerves. In the patient with multiple pulmonary lesions the most peripheral accessible lesion is biopsied.

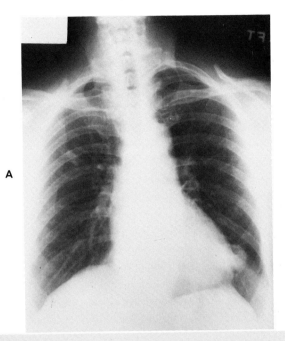

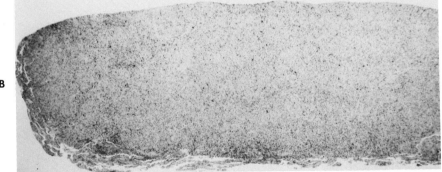

Fig. 8-46. A 70-year-old asymptomatic woman. One year previously she had undergone resection of fibrosarcoma of right axilla, at which time her chest roentgenogram was normal. **A,** PA chest roentgenogram showing large cavitating nodular density in left lower lobe (noted to be adjacent to posterior chest wall on lateral projection) and smaller nodule in right upper lobe. Physical examination was negative; a tuberculin skin test was positive. Sputum examination and bronchoscopy were negative. **B,** Histologic preparation of tissue specimen (original size 2 by 6 mm) obtained from cutting needle biopsy of left lower lobe mass reveals metastatic fibrosarcoma. (Cutting needle was used because of poor likelihood of diagnosing fibrosarcoma cytologically.)

After optimal fluoroscopic positioning, the skin over the lesion is marked in midexpiration. The site chosen should be such that the needle will pass over the rib in its approach to the lesion, thus avoiding injury to intercostal vessels or nerves. The skin in the area is cleansed with disinfectant and draped, and then the skin and soft tissues of the chest wall over the lesion are anesthetized[a] down to the level of the pleura. A small incision is made in the skin with a scalpel blade.[b]

The biopsy needle is now inserted into the skin, advanced over the superior aspect of the rib, and then quickly thrust through the pleura while the patient is holding his breath in midexpiration. The needle tip is guided to the periphery of the lesion by intermittent image-intensification fluoroscopy (a television monitor is greatly preferable to mirror optics). Proper position and direction of the needle are confirmed while the needle is held by a long forceps with a jaw,[1] thus avoiding irradiation to the hand. If necessary, the patient may breathe shallowly after penetration of the lung by the needle.

Determination of the depth of the lesion almost always can be accomplished using single-plane fluoroscopy, which is much less cumbersome and certainly much more readily available than biplane fluoroscopy. A fairly accurate estimate of the depth of the lesion can be calculated by study and measurement of the patient's PA and lateral chest radiographs. Occasionally, if it is necessary for better localization, oblique views or laminagrams can be obtained; these are helpful in providing a more detailed assessment of the size and depth of the lesion. Precise determination of the depth of the lesion prior to needle insertion is not necessary. Verification that the needle is in the periphery of the lesion is often achieved by a feeling of increased resistance when the lesion is penetrated. This sensation almost always occurs with solid neoplastic lesions. If there is concern about the position of the needle tip relative to the lesion, fluoroscopy can demonstrate whether movement of the tip of the needle and the lesion is synchronous during quiet respirations; if this is the case, penetration of the needle tip to the proper depth is confirmed. As a further check, if doubt still remains, the patient can be rotated slightly to an oblique position, and the tip of the needle with respect to the lesion can be checked fluoroscopically in this new projection.

If the mass to be biopsied is large, the specimen should be obtained from the periphery rather than the center of the lesion, since large neoplasms are often necrotic in the center. Cavitary lesions should be aspirated from both their inner and outer margins. If the lesion is neoplastic, the biopsy from the interior will often contain only necrotic material, while tissue obtained from the outer margin may establish the diagnosis. The converse is true when inflammatory cavities are biopsied.

With the needle tip placed optimally within the periphery of the lesion, fluoroscopy is discontinued and the patient is instructed to stop breathing.

When the aspiration-type needle is used, the stylet is removed, and a syringe[m] filled with 2 ml of sterile saline solution is attached to the needle hub. (When the stylet is removed and before attaching the syringe, the radiologist should place his thumb over the hub of the needle to prevent the possibility of air embolism[34] if the patient should inadvertently breathe). Constant suction is now applied to the syringe, and the needle is rotated clockwise and counterclockwise while it is moved slightly forward and backward within the lesion. With solid lesions this permits the sharp bevel of the needle to cut off very small fragments of tissue. With suction still applied, the needle is withdrawn from the thorax. The contents of the syringe and needle are then expressed into test tubes containing a special preservative[h] or sterile saline solution, depending upon whether cytologic or bacteriologic studies or both are indicated. The syringe is then disconnected from the needle and filled with about 3 ml of sterile saline solution. The needle is then reconnected to the syringe and flushed through with the saline solution into the test tubes. If a small core of tissue is obtained, it is placed in a jar of formalin and sent for histologic study (Fig. 8-47). This biopsy procedure may be repeated two to three times until good specimens for all required studies are obtained. The solutions in the test tubes are subsequently processed, as are the specimens obtained from bronchial brushing.

When the Vim cutting needle is used, the needle is inserted during suspended midexpiration, the usual biopsy maneuver is performed, and the needle is quickly withdrawn from the thorax. The specimen is teased from the cutting blades with a needle and placed on a clean microscopic slide (a "touch preparation" is thus prepared if desired). A portion of tissue is cut off with a scalpel blade and placed in sterile saline solution for subsequent smear and culture. The remainder of the specimen is immersed in formalin prior to histopathologic study. The biopsy maneuver should not be repeated if a satisfactory tissue specimen was obtained on the first attempt.

A PA chest radiograph taken in expiration is routinely obtained following the completion of the lung needle biopsy, and the patient is observed closely for about 4 hours following the biopsy procedure. If a complication occurs, it will almost always be apparent in the radiology suite or shortly after the patient returns to his room.

Complications

The possible complications of pulmonary needle biopsy are pneumothorax, pulmonary hemorrhage, empyema, and implantation of tumor cells into the needle tract.

In our series of more than 300 percutaneous needle biopsies, pneumothorax has been by far the most common complication. The incidence is quite variable, depending upon the location, type, and size of the lesion biopsied. A pneumothorax developed in approximately 20% of the patients after an aspiration biopsy and in about 30% after a cutting needle biopsy (of large, solid

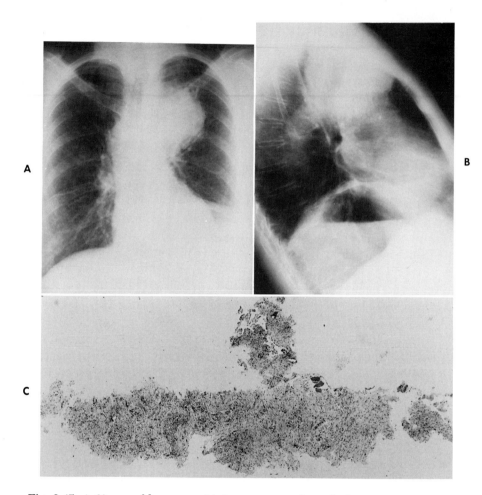

Fig. 8-47. A 63-year-old woman with hemoptysis and weight loss. **A** and **B,** PA and lateral chest radiographs demonstrate large left upper lobe mass extending into mediastinum. Right paratracheal lymph node enlargement is noted. Elevated left hemidiaphragm was confirmed as due to phrenic nerve palsy by fluoroscopy. Sputum examination, bronchoscopy, and bronchial brushing were negative. **C,** Histologic preparation of small tissue fragment (original size 0.8 by 3 mm) obtained by percutaneous aspiration needle biopsy demonstrates poorly differentiated squamous cell carcinoma. Cytologic preparation revealed same findings.

peripheral lesions) had been performed. As in other reported series,[7,16,31] in most instances the pneumothorax was small and resolved spontaneously. When it was large or dyspnea occurred, as happened with each of the eight patients requiring positive-pressure ventilation prior to needle biopsy, closed intercostal drainage was quickly instituted and maintained for about 24 hours. If desired, chest tube drainage can be easily performed by the radiologist using either a 14-gauge Intracath or inserting a No. 8 Teflon catheter with side holes via the Seldinger technique into the second anterior intercostal space on the side of the needle biopsy.[29] Attachment of a Heimlich valve,[4] which permits only unidirectional air flow, usually suffices; underwater sealed drainage is rarely necessary. The possible complication of a large pneumothorax is insufficient justification for preferring diagnostic thoracotomy over needle biopsy, since the insertion of a chest tube into the pleural space is no more difficult after needle biopsy than when it is inserted into 100% of patients after surgery. A recently described technique,[20] which we are now evaluating, may well avoid or diminish greatly the threat of a pneumothorax after aspiration needle biopsies.

Hemoptysis is unusual and invariably mild when an aspiration needle biopsy of the lung has been done.[7,31] Sometimes when a cutting needle is used, however, intrapulmonary hemorrhage may be fairly massive. This is particularly true if diffuse pulmonary disease is biopsied, but it is extremely rare when biopsies of large, solid peripheral lesions are performed. Death due to intrapulmonary hemorrhage from cutting needle biopsy of the lung has been reported; almost all these patients had clinically detectable pulmonary hypertension before the biopsy.

The risk of spread of infection to the pleural space is small and more theoretical than actual.[18] The incidence of empyema appears to be no greater than in comparable cases managed without needle biopsy[28] and to be of no great significance since the introduction of antibiotics.[7]

Implantation of tumor cells into the needle tract, resulting in intrapulmonary, pleural, or subcutaneous dissemination, is extremely rare.[3,18,24,36] This complication usually is seen only in advanced malignant neoplasms, when the risk is of little clinical importance compared to the establishment of a diagnosis. We generally do not perform percutaneous pulmonary needle biopsy in a potentially operable patient with a solitary pulmonary lesion. The exception is the rare patient with a solitary indeterminate lesion whose tolerance for surgery is uncertain. The small inherent risk of tumor dissemination is accepted because a positive diagnosis might justify the need for surgical intervention or radiation therapy. Another exception is the use of percutaneous needle biopsy in patients with suspected superior sulcus tumor. Here needle biopsy is used to establish a histologic diagnosis if bronchial brushing has been negative before the administration of preoperative irradiation therapy (Fig. 8-48).

Contraindications

The contraindications to pulmonary needle biopsy are listed below. Most are relative, rather than absolute.

1. Uncooperative patient
2. Uncontrollable cough
3. Suspected echinococcal lesion

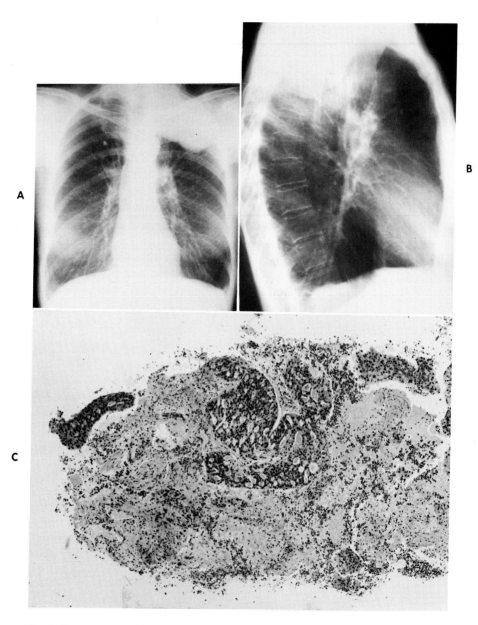

Fig. 8-48. A 59-year-old man with left shoulder pain. **A** and **B**, PA and lateral chest roentgenograms demonstrate large mass lesion in apical posterior segment of left upper lobe. Sputum examination, bronchoscopy, and bronchial brushing were negative. **C**, Histologic preparation of percutaneous cutting needle biopsy reveals poorly differentiated adenocarcinoma.

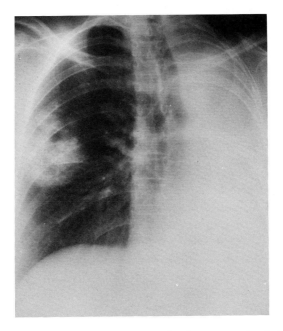

Fig. 8-49. A 58-year-old asymptomatic woman who 2 years previously had a left pneumonectomy for alveolar cell carcinoma. PA chest radiograph demonstrates fluffy infiltrate with some cavitation in right midlung field. Sputum examination, bronchoscopy, and bronchial brushing were negative. Cytologic preparation of material obtained from percutaneous aspiration needle biopsy showed alveolar cell carcinoma cells.

    4. Systemic bleeding diathesis
    5. Severe emphysema with pulmonary insufficiency
    6. Pneumonectomy on contralateral side
    7. Clinically suspected pulmonary hypertension

    If an echinococcal etiology of a pulmonary lesion is suspected, or if the patient is uncooperative or has an uncontrollable cough, needle biopsy is contraindicated. Cutting needle biopsy is absolutely contraindicated in the presence of a systemic bleeding diathesis, clinically suspected pulmonary hypertension, severe emphysema with pulmonary insufficiency, pneumonectomy on the contralateral side, or suspected vascular etiology of a pulmonary lesion. These latter categories are only relative contraindications to aspiration needle biopsy, which can be performed following platelet transfusions and when apparatus to immediately treat a pneumothorax are readily available (Fig. 8-49).

    The fear of puncturing vascular structures with an aspirating needle is generally unfounded. Aspirating needles have been inadvertently placed in the thoracic aorta, right atrium, superior vena cava, and pulmonary artery and veins, all without ill effects.[40] All that is necessary is that the needle be withdrawn and appropriately redirected. The injection of contrast media through the aspirating needle has even been advocated if blood is aspirated from the needle to confirm an intrapulmonary vascular anomaly.[40]

Results

The accuracy of pulmonary needle biopsy is greatly dependent upon the size, type, and location of the lung lesion. A success rate of close to 100% has been achieved in large, solid peripheral lesions, while smaller central lesions produce far less satisfactory results. An overall accuracy of about 80% using the aspiration needle is accepted in the literature,[2,27,31] and these data correlate closely with our own experience.

Recent reports[24,41] emphasize a 95% accuracy in diagnosing neoplastic lesions with the aspiration-type needle and emphasize the ability of this procedure to exclude malignancy with a very high degree of reliability. Because of this high accuracy, aspiration needle biopsy is advocated in all cases of indeterminate lung lesions, including solitary lesions, if routine sputum samples and bronchoscopic washings are negative. If a diagnosis of granulomatous disease or oat cell carcinoma is made, surgery is contraindicated. It is recommended that solitary pulmonary nodules be followed roentgenographically if aspiration biopsy is negative since the chance of malignancy is less than 5%.

Summary

Transcatheter bronchial brushing and percutaneous needle biopsy should be considered complementary procedures, each technique having advantages and disadvantages. Generally, bronchial brushing is the first procedure chosen because it is safer. This is especially true with central or midlung pulmonary lesions. Suspected metastatic pulmonary neoplasm usually is best approached initially by needle biopsy. While the likelihood of significant complications occurring with bronchial brushing is virtually nil, it occasionally is extremely time consuming (sometimes requiring 90 minutes). For this reason needle biopsy, which rarely requires longer than 10 minutes of a busy radiologist's or sick patient's time, may become the procedure of choice.

These diagnostic modalities, which are inexpensive, relatively safe, simple, and highly accurate, should be part of the armamentarium of every radiologist involved with the diagnosis of pulmonary disease. They are efficacious not only in providing a definitive diagnosis in patients with suspected lung neoplasm but can also usually provide the definitive etiology of a pneumonic infiltrate in the immunologically compromised patient when the routine methods (examination and culture of sputum samples or transtracheal aspirates) fail. Direct and often immediate evidence of the pathologic agent can be provided, uncontaminated by the upper respiratory tract flora. All radiologists should be familiar with and competent to perform lung biopsy using either method.

References

1. Adamson, J. S., Jr., and Bates, J. H.: Percutaneous needle biopsy of the lung, Arch. Intern. Med. **119:**164, 1967.
2. Bandt, P. D., Blank, N., and Castellino, R. A.: Needle diagnosis of pneumonitis: value in high risk patients, J.A.M.A. **220:**1578, 1972.
3. Berger, R. L., Dargan, E. L., and Huang, B. L.: Dissemination of cancer cells by needle biopsy of the lung, J. Thorac. Cardiovasc. Surg. **63:**430, 1972.
4. Bernstein, A., Wagaruddin, M., and Shah, M.: Management of spontaneous pneumothorax using a Heimlich flutter valve, Thorax **28:**386, 1973.
5. Boylen, C. T., Johnson, N. R., Richters, V., and Balchum, O. J.: High speed trephine lung biopsy: methods and results, Chest **63:**59, 1973.
6. Bronchography: a report of the committee on bronchoesophagraphy, Dis. Chest **51:**663, 1967.
7. Dahlgren, S., and Nordenström, B.: Transthoracic needle biopsy, Chicago, 1966, Year Book Medical Publishers, Inc.
8. Felson, B.: Fundamentals of chest roentgenology, Philadelphia, 1960, W. B. Saunders Co.
9. Fennessy, J. J.: Bronchial brushing and transbronchial forceps biopsy in the diagnosis of pulmonary lesions, Dis. Chest **53:**377, 1968.
10. Fennessy, J. J., et al.: Transcatheter biopsy in the diagnosis of diseases of the respiratory tract, Radiology **110:**555, 1974.
11. Forrest, J. V.: Bronchial brush biopsy in lung cavities, Radiology **106:**69, 1973.
12. Fraser, R.: Bronchography 1972, J. Can. Assoc. Radiol. **23:**236, 1972.
13. Genoe, G. A., Morello, J. A., and Fennessy, J. J.: The diagnosis of pulmonary aspergillosis by the bronchial brushing technique, Radiology **102:**51, 1972.
14. Groff, D. B., and Marquis, J.: Treatment of lung abscess by transbronchial catheter drainage, Radiology **107:**61, 1973.
15. Jereb, M., and Sinner, W.: The use of some special radiological procedures in chest disease, Radiol. Clin. North Am. **11:**109, 1973.
16. Klein, J. O.: Diagnostic lung puncture in the pneumonias of infants and children, Pediatrics **44:**486, 1969.
17. Lalli, A. F.: The direct fluoroscopically guided approach to renal, thoracic, and skeletal lesions, Curr. Probl. Radiol. **2:**30, 1972.
18. Lauby, V. W., Burnett, W. E., Rosemond, G. P., and Tyson, R. R.: Value and risk of biopsy of pulmonary lesions by needle aspiration: twenty-one years' experience, J. Thorac. Cardiovasc. Surg. **49:**159, 1965.
19. Manfredi, F., and Krumholz, R.: Percutaneous needle biopsy of lung in evaluation of pulmonary disorders, J.A.M.A. **198:**1198, 1966.
20. McCartney, R., Tait, D., Stilson, M., and Seidel, G. F.: A Technique for the prevention of pneumothorax in pulmonary aspiration biopsy, Am. J. Roentgenol. **120:**872, 1974.
21. Mintzer, R. S., et al.: The significance of localized bronchiectasis adjacent to pulmonary coin lesions, Chest **64:**155, 1973.
22. Nelson, S. W., and Christoforidis, A. J.: Bronchography in diseases of the adult chest, Radiol. Clin. North Am. **11:**125, 1973.
23. Newhouse, M. T.: Suction excision biopsy for diffuse pulmonary disease, Chest **63:**707, 1973.
24. Nordenström, B.: Needle biopsy, Paper presented at the Fleischner Society meeting on diseases of the chest, London, England, May 1974.
25. Repsher, L. H., Schröter, G., and Hammond, W. S.: Diagnosis of Pneumocystis

carinii pneumonitis by means of endobronchial brush biopsy, N. Engl. J. Med. **287**:340, 1972.

26. Sagel, S. S.: Current practices in chest roentgenography, Adv. Surg. **5**:51, 1971.
27. Sanders, D. E., Thompson, D. W., and Pudden, B. J. E.: Percutaneous aspiration lung biopsy, Can. Med. Assoc. J. **104**:139, 1971.
28. Sappington, S. W., and Favorite, G. O.: Lung puncture in lobar pneumonia, Am. J. Med. Sci. **191**:225, 1936.
29. Sargent, E. N., and Turner, A. F.: Emergency treatment of pneumothorax: a simple catheter technique for use in the radiology department, Am. J. Roentgenol. **109**:531, 1970.
30. Schoenbaum, S. W., et al.: Fiberoptic bronchoscopy: complete evaluation of the tracheobronchial tree in the radiology department, Radiology **109**:571, 1973.
31. Stevens, G. M., Weigen, J. F., and Lillington, G. A.: Needle aspiration biopsy of localized pulmonary lesions with amplified fluoroscopic guidance, Am. J. Roentgenol. **103**:561, 1968.
32. Turner, A. F., and Sargent, E. N.: Percutaneous pulmonary needle biopsy: an improved needle for a simple direct method of diagnosis, Am. J. Roentgenol. **104**:846, 1968.
33. Vitums, V. C.: Percutaneous needle biopsy of the lung with a new disposable needle, Chest **62**:717, 1972.
34. Westcott, J. L.: Air embolism complicating percutaneous needle biopsy of the lung, Chest **63**:108, 1973.
35. Willson, J. K. V., and Eskridge, M.: Bronchial brush biopsy with a controllable brush, Am. J. Roentgenol. **109**:471, 1970.
36. Wolinsky, H., and Lischner, M. W.: Needle track implantation of tumor after percutaneous lung biopsy, Ann. Intern. Med. **71**:359, 1969.
37. Zavala, D. C., and Bedell, G. N.: Percutaneous lung biopsy with a cutting needle, Am. Rev. Respir. Dis. **106**:186, 1972.
38. Zavala, D. C., Rossi, N. P., and Bedell, G. N.: Bronchial brush biopsy, Ann. Thorac. Surg. **13**:519, 1972.
39. Zavala, D. C., et al.: Use of bronchofiberscope for bronchial brush biopsy, Chest **63**:889, 1973.
40. Zelch, J. V., and Lalli, A. F.: Diagnostic percutaneous opacification of benign pulmonary lesions, Radiology **108**:559, 1973.
41. Zelch, J. V., Lalli, A. F., McCormack, L. J., and Belovich, D. M.: Aspiration biopsy in diagnosis of pulmonary nodule, Chest **63**:149, 1973.

9 The role of radiology in asbestos-related disease

Heber MacMahon and John V. Forrest

Physicians have long been aware of the occurrence of asbestos-related disease in certain occupational groups. More recently, asbestos exposure has been shown to be widespread among the general urban population secondary to atmospheric pollution.[23] This should be cause for concern, especially in light of a documented increased incidence of neoplasia in asbestos workers.[2,11]

Asbestos-related disease is of particular relevance to the radiologist, in that the radiographic manifestations are frequently more striking, and indeed more diagnostic, than the clinical findings. In this paper we hope to underline the importance of this subject and to demonstrate the potential role of the radiologist in the diagnosis and management of asbestos-related diseases. The radiographic manifestations of asbestos exposure may be outlined as follows:

Asbestosis
    Pleural plaques
    Parenchymal fibrosis
    Cor pulmonale
Associated neoplasms
    Malignant mesothelioma (pleural or peritoneal)
    Bronchogenic carcinoma
    Gastrointestinal carcinoma (?)

It has been repeatedly pointed out in the medical literature that a great number of the diagnostic "misses" in this area are due to unfamiliarity on the part of the clinician or radiologist regarding the multiple uses of asbestos and the resultant potential exposure to asbestos in a given occupational group.[18] For this reason we feel it will be useful to describe briefly the nature of asbestos, the method of its production, and the situations in which it is likely to be used. The relationship of asbestos exposure to various forms of malignant disease is of particular radiologic interest; in this respect we shall discuss malignant mesothelioma, bronchogenic carcinoma, and gastrointestinal carcinoma.

NATURE OF ASBESTOS

Asbestos is a fibrous mineral silicate characterized by a tendency to break into fibers when crushed, secondary to strong molecular linkages in one

213

Table 9-1. Commercially useful types of asbestos

Varieties of asbestos	Major producer
Chrysotile	Canada
	Soviet Union
Crocidolite	South Africa
	Australia
Amosite	South Africa
Anthophyllite	Finland
Tremolite	
Actinolite	

direction.[9] The commercially useful types of asbestos are listed in Table 9-1. Chrysotile is the most important of these and accounts for approximately 90% of total world asbestos production. It is a hydrated magnesium silicate characterized by high heat resistance, long fibers, and low acid resistance. It is produced largely in Canada and the Soviet Union. Crocidolite is a sodium ferrous silicate. The bulk of asbestos produced in South Africa is crocidolite, and much of the earlier medical literature relating asbestos to malignancy came from that country.[42] This stimulated interest in the possible variable carcinogenicity of the different types of asbestos, although such differences have not as yet been reliably documented. Amosite is a ferrous magnesium silicate produced largely in South Africa. Anthophyllite, tremolite, and actinolite are of lesser importance in that they are produced in smaller quantitites, although in areas of Finland and other European countries they are the predominant form. The majority of commercially used asbestos in the United States is imported, although chrysotile is mined in Vermont, Arizona, and California.[14]

The various forms of asbestos occur naturally in rock formations, and the initial stage of production is therefore a mining operation. The asbestos is then transported to a milling plant, where it is separated from the rock.

EXPOSURE

Miners and transport personnel are subject to asbestos exposure. The milling operation is particularly dusty, and this is the point at which some of the heaviest exposure to both workers and local residents has occurred in the past. "Open mining" can also lead to heavy environmental contamination.[21] Following the milling operation, further potential personnel exposure and environmental contamination occur as the product is distributed to the numerous industries in which it is used. The extent of the uses of asbestos in modern technology is not widely appreciated. Selikoff, one of the foremost medical authorities on this subject, has stated that no less than 3000 different commercial products now contain asbestos.[36] Some of the principal occupational groups likely to be exposed to asbestos are the following:

Heavy exposure
    Workers directly involved in asbestos mining, milling, and processing
Variable exposure
    Shipyard workers
    Building material manufacturers
    Construction workers
    Insulation workers
    Automobile manufacturers
    Garage attendants
    Electrical appliance manufacturers
    Carpenters
    Masons
    Filter material manufacturers

Asbestosis or related malignant disease has been described in virtually all of these occupations. In the United States 15,000 people are employed in the production and manufacture of asbestos, and there are more than 100 companies involved in the manufacture of asbestos products. Overall, approximately 50,000 to 100,000 people incur occupational exposure to asbestos in this country.[18]

Investigators have been aware of the possibility of significant asbestos inhalation among the general urban population for some time, but reliable documentation of the exact extent of such exposure was lacking until quite recently. In 1957 Kiviluoto drew attention to this in a survey of the general population in an area of Finland immediately adjacent to several open asbestos mines. He found extensive pleural calcification among several hundred people who had never worked with asbestos and who were largely asymptomatic.[21] Pleural calcification is one of the most reliable radiographic indicators of exposure to asbestos.[17]

At approximately the same time, Thomson[40] and others in South Africa had noted several cases of mesothelioma with associated pleural calcification and asbestos bodies in the general population. Whereas the series in Finland had involved a selected population, Thomson attempted to determine the exposure among the urban population in the average city. The cities chosen for the survey were Capetown, South Africa, and Miami, Florida. The criterion for asbestos exposure was the presence of asbestos bodies in the lung. The survey was based on material obtained from 500 consecutive autopsies in each of the cities. Smears were made from cut sections of lung bases and examined for asbestos bodies by light microscopy. In Capetown, asbestos bodies were found in the lungs of 30% of the men and 20% of the women at autopsy. The relatively low yield below 20 years of age was felt to be purely a reflection of the shorter length of time that these subjects had been breathing city air. The results obtained in Miami were strikingly similar. The increased positive rate in men was felt to be due to increased occupational exposure. Among all of these cases there were five with overt asbestosis, although only one of these had documented occupational exposure.

Thomson therefore concluded that these results were probably representative for other cities and indicated contamination of urban air by asbestos fibers. The immediate sources for this contamination would include car brake and clutch linings and various building materials. The validity of Thomson's findings was borne out by Elmes and Wade,[7] who examined specimens from random autopsies on 200 men 50 to 69 years of age in Belfast. Asbestos bodies were present in approximately 25% of those from 60 to 69 years of age.[26]

Asbestos bodies have been shown to be associated with the inhalation of asbestos.[23] A proportion of inhaled fibers, depending upon their length, become coated with a gelatinous material that stains positive for ferritin (Fig. 9-1). Although large asbestos fibers can be seen by light microscopy, generally asbestos bodies can be identified much more easily. The presence of asbestos bodies has therefore been used widely as a criterion for measuring asbestos exposure. In view of the startling implications of Thomson's survey, the question as to whether asbestos bodies might be caused by foreign materials other than asbestos has been raised.

In 1969 Gross et al.[10] reported on city dwellers who had asbestos bodies in their lungs at surgery. He preferred to call them ferruginous bodies because in his study, which was specifically directed toward determining the nature of

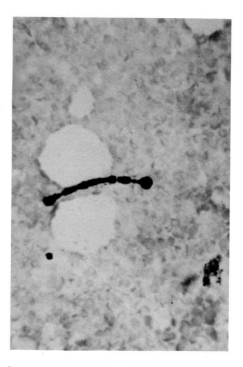

Fig. 9-1. Asbestos body demonstrated with iron staining technique.

the core of these bodies, no chrysotile was demonstrated. Gross et al. therefore concluded that asbestos bodies in city dwellers were not necessarily related to asbestos. More recently, electron microscopic studies have confirmed that the majority of asbestos bodies do indeed contain some part of an asbestos fiber. In 1971 Langer et al.[23] published the results of investigations they had conducted on this subject in New York City. Using electron microscopy, they had demonstrated that, following inhalation, chrysotile asbestos largely breaks into fine fibrils of less than 0.5 micron in diameter (that is, beyond the limits of resolution of the light microscope). Using light microscopy alone, 45% of the lung specimens from 3000 consecutive autopsies were found to contain asbestos bodies. Twenty-eight random specimens were then examined by electron microscopy. Sixteen had asbestos bodies, the core content of which contained material thought to represent chrysotile, which was partially degraded by enzymatic action. More significantly, actual chrysotile fibrils were clearly demonstrated in 24 of the 28 cases. Langer et al.[23] cite the work of Pooley, who used similar methods and found chrysotile fibrils in 80% of a sample of the London population. These findings would seem to indicate conclusively that the vast majority of city dwellers are exposed to asbestos.

INDUSTRIAL BACKGROUND

How serious are the affects of exposure to asbestos in its various forms? It is interesting to review the historical evidence. As with other industrial diseases, there was an initial period of ignorance of the harmful effects of the product that was followed by denial of responsibility by the industry long after the dangers were manifest. There is a parallel here with the osteosarcoma developed by radium watch dial painters, berylliosis in fluorescent lamp workers, and chemical workers who developed bladder carcinoma secondary to benzidine exposure.[5]

Asbestos was first mined in Canada in 1878. In 1890 the first asbestos spinning and weaving factory was established there. No special ventilation was provided in the working area, and no less than 50 workers died in the first 5 years of the factory's operation.[1] However, in 1912 the United States Department of Labor investigation sponsored by the asbestos industry produced no evidence of occupational damage among 600 miners.[5] In 1916 the United States Bureau of Labor Statistics had a record of only 13 deaths among asbestos workers during the preceding 17 years.[15] Interestingly enough, although the industry and insurance carriers were relieved of financial responsibility by these findings, the asbestos workers were denied life insurance due to the "assumed health injurious conditions of the industry."[15]

Asbestosis per se was first described by Murray[30] in London in 1900. A second case was reported by Cooke[4] in 1924. Autopsy findings showed extensive pulmonary and pleural fibrosis and multiple asbestos fibers in the lung. However, it was not until 1931, when Merewether and Price[28] showed pulmonary fibrosis to be present in 25% of 363 asbestos workers, that asbestosis became a compensable disease.

ASBESTOS-INDUCED DISEASE
Pulmonary fibrosis

It has been shown by experimental work in animals that a small percentage of inhaled fibers reach the respiratory bronchioles. Fibers 50 to 200 microns long are deposited in the wall of the respiratory bronchioles and alveoli. The initial reaction is one of peribronchiolar edema, which is followed eventually by interstitial fibrosis (Fig. 9-2). Shorter fibers may be converted to asbestos bodies. Bronchiolar and alveolar fibrosis can eventually lead to an alveolar-capillary block with inadequate gas exchange, and this is the primary physiologic abnormality in asbestosis.[8]

These pathologic findings are associated with a clinical picture of progressive dyspnea, basilar rales, and finger clubbing. Pulmonary interstitial fibrosis can lead to cor pulmonale. In the preantibiotic era, bronchopneumonia and tuberculosis were common complications.[11] Indeed, these terminal infections were probably named on the death certificates of the early asbestos workers as the cause of death: hence the apparent underreporting of the primary disease.

Pleural plaques

Calcified pleural plaques are the most characteristic radiographic feature. The reason for the occurrence of these plaques is not certain, although

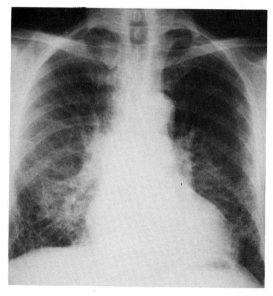

Fig. 9-2. Predominantly basilar pulmonary fibrosis in asbestosis.

Kiviluoto[21] postulated that asbestos fibers penetrate the visceral pleura and, by virtue of differential movement between the pleural surfaces, produce microhemorrhages that subsequently calcify. Interestingly, the early descriptions of the disease make no mention of calcified plaques. In fact, as late as 1955, pathologic and even radiologic studies of asbestos workers failed to mention this entity, although it was described in talc workers in 1952.[39] Selikoff's work regarding the relationship of duration of exposure to the development of calcified pleural plaques (Table 9-2) provides a possible explanation of the previous apparent rarity of this finding.[35] His data show pleural calcification is rare with less than 10 years' exposure but occurs in the majority of those with more than 40 years' exposure. Although it might appear that the total amount of exposure is the only significant factor, this is not the case. The total time elapsed since the first exposure is also important. Hence pleural calcification may be seen in people who worked briefly with asbestos 30 to 40 years earlier and have not had subsequent occupational exposure (Fig. 9-3). This is because once the fibers have been inhaled, progressive pulmonary fibrosis and pleural calcification may ensue, regardless of removal from the contaminated environment.[3]

The pleural calcification almost always affects the parietal pleura. This may be appreciated at fluoroscopy or more clearly in the presence of a pneumothorax. Often the plaques are bilateral and preferentially affect the diaphragmatic pleura. Asbestosis has long superseded tuberculosis as the most common cause of bilateral pleural calcification.

Other causes of pleural calcification must be distinguished from asbestos exposure. A previous empyema, either pyogenic or tuberculous, is a common cause of pleural calcification. However, this type of calcification is generally unilateral and tends to have a distribution that roughly corresponds to the distribution of the previous pleural fluid. Intrapleural hemorrhage, secondary either to trauma or thoracotomy, also leads to calcification. Again this tends to be unilateral, and the presence of healed rib fractures or a regenerating rib are helpful in making the diagnosis. These entities usually cause calcification of

Table 9-2. Roentgenographic evidence of pleural abnormality among 1117 asbestos insulation workers*

Years from onset of exposure	Number examined	Normal pleura	Abnormal pleura	
			Fibrosis	Calcification
40+	121	28	65	70
30-39	194	96	62	67
20-29	77	47	25	8
10-19	379	340	36	5
0-9	346	342	4	0

*From Selikoff, I. J.: Ann. N. Y. Acad. Sci. **132:**351, 1965.

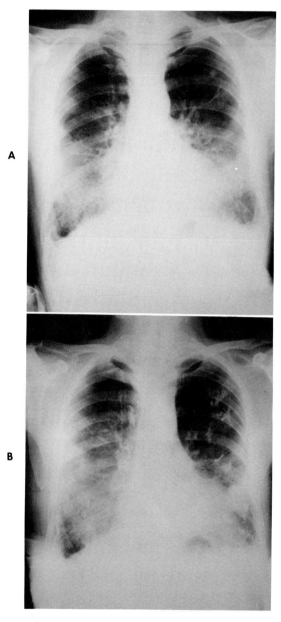

Fig. 9-3. Progressive pleural calcification secondary to previous asbestos exposure. Patient had worked with asbestos for only 6 months 20 years prior to initial radiograph. No further industrial exposure occurred. He died in 1972 of bronchogenic carcinoma. **A,** Chest radiograph taken in 1956 shows basilar fibrosis and several areas of pleural calcification. **B,** Examination 10 years later shows progression of calcification.

the visceral pleura, in contradistinction to asbestosis, which, as mentioned, affects the parietal layer. Neither old empyema nor hemothorax produces the characteristic localized calcified pleural plaques of asbestosis. Since talc contains tremolite, talc exposure can cause pleural disease indistinguishable from that due to asbestos.[35]

Ultrasonic examination has been shown to be more sensitive than the chest radiograph in detecting pleural plaques. Viikeri[41] correlated ultrasonic, radiographic, and pathologic findings in 10 cadavers. Plaques less than 2 to 3 mm in thickness were missed by x-ray examination but were detected successfully by ultrasound.

Malignant mesothelioma

The relationship of asbestosis to malignant mesothelioma is well established.[2,6,16] Mesothelioma is a primary neoplasm of serosal membranes and may be benign or malignant. Various pathologic subclassifications are used; it can occur in solitary fibrous form that is usually benign or in a diffuse invasive form that is malignant. Asbestosis is associated only with the latter. The tumor may arise from visceral or parietal pleura, peritoneum, or pericardium. It tends to spread by direct extension and by serosal seeding. Table 9-3 summarizes the evidence for an association between asbestosis and malignant mesothelioma. The overall incidence of malignant mesothelioma in asbestos workers is approximately 4%, as compared to 0.07% in 60,000 autopsies in the general population. Indeed, one might question the role of asbestos in that 0.07% of the general population, in view of the high incidence of asbestos in the lungs of urban dwellers.[23] The average latent period for the development of malignant mesothelioma after asbestos exposure appears to be about 32 years.[19]

Table 9-3. Association of mesotheliomas with asbestosis*

Hochberg (1951, Germany)	60,000 autopsies		43 mesotheliomas (0.07%)
Study	**Deaths in asbestos workers**	**Pleural mesothelioma**	**Peritoneal mesothelioma**
Konig (1960, Germany)	36	4	3
Elwood and Cochrane (1964, England)	144	1	0
Elmes and Wade (1965, Ireland)	30	2	3
Vigliani et al. (1965, Italy)	172	3	
Selikoff and Hammond (1965, U. S.)	307	4	6
	689	14	12

Study	**Cases of mesothelioma**	**Exposure to asbestos**
Wagner et al. (1960, South Africa)	33	28
McCaughey et al. (1962, Scotland)	15	12
Elmes et al. (1965, Ireland)	42	32

*From Freundlich, I. M., and Greening, R. R.: Radiology **89:**224, 1967.

The clinical presentation in these cases is characterized by dyspnea, chest pain, weight loss, and finger clubbing. The chest radiograph usually shows a mass with pleural effusion (Fig. 9-4), although the latter may be absent (Fig. 9-5). The presence of a "pleural peel" is a helpful sign.[13] Multiple pleural nodules may be seen following a pleural tap and are more clearly outlined in the presence of pneumothorax. Occasionally invasion of the chest wall with rib destruction or extension deep into the lung parenchyma may be seen.[13]

Distant metastases are not commonly apparent during life. When metastases do occur they may be seen in regional lymph nodes, as well as peritoneum, brain,[44] bone,[32] pancreas,[34] adrenals,[33] and spinal cord.[34] A single case of extensively calcified hepatic metastases has been reported, although this must be exceedingly rare.[32]

Examination of pleural fluid usually reveals blood, and cytologic examinations are positive for malignant disease in a high percentage of cases.[34] Some investigators have reported an increased hyaluronic acid content in the pleural fluid, and this may prove to be a more specific finding.[12] In most series needle biopsy has proved inadequate, and open thoracotomy is usually necessary for specific histologic diagnosis.

The prognosis for these patients is poor. Surgical resection is usually not feasible. Palliative radiotherapy has been used extensively, although it has not been very effective. The efficacy of various modes of therapy was reported by

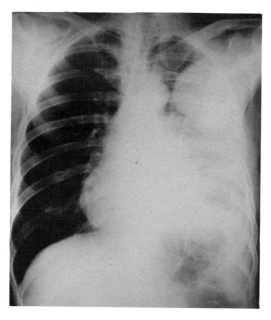

Fig. 9-4. Malignant pleural mesothelioma. Radiograph shows large left pleural mass with associated effusion. Patient had worked with asbestos for 6 months 15 years earlier.

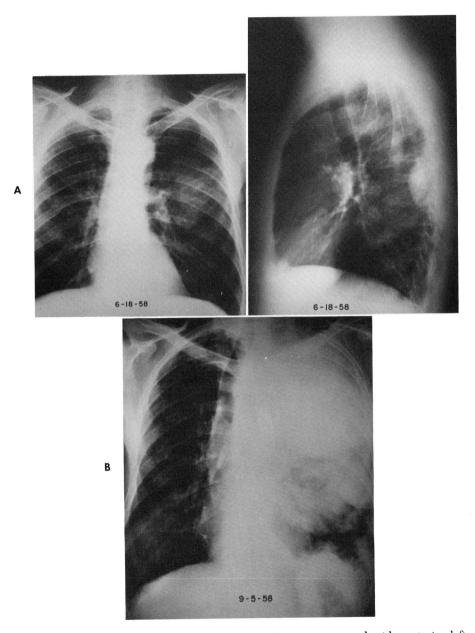

Fig. 9-5. Malignant pleural mesothelioma. **A,** Patient presented with posterior left pleural mass but no effusion. **B,** Characteristic rapid growth with secondary mediastinal shift has occurred within 3 months.

Ratzner et al.[34] in a series of 31 cases. The modalities used included surgery, radiation, and various forms of chemotherapy. They concluded that treatment failed in all cases.[34]

Peritoneal mesothelioma has not been described as frequently as the pleural variety. In a survey of 83 cases of malignant mesothelioma reported by Newhouse and Thompson,[31] 27 were peritoneal. The asbestos-exposure relationship held equally true for both pleural and peritoneal types of tumors.

Peritoneal mesothelioma frequently presents with diffuse abdominal pain and swelling. In the advanced stage of the disease, ascites is the rule. The pathologic appearance varies from multiple serosal implants to a single (often palpable) mass. Characteristically, the tumor encases the abdominal viscera, but intramural penetration is rare.[43] The radiographic appearances are non-specific. Multiple extrinsic pressure defects on the stomach, small intestine, and colon have been reported.[24] These findings could be produced by any intra-abdominal metastatic neoplasm. The histologic appearance may also be misleading, since highly undifferentiated adenocarcinoma or fibrosarcoma can have a similar appearance. The prognosis is no better than for pleural mesothelioma.

Bronchogenic carcinoma

The question of increased incidence of bronchogenic carcinoma in asbestosis was first raised in 1935.[25] In the period from 1961 to 1963, of 77 male death certificates in Britain that recorded asbestosis, no less than 42 had either carcinoma or malignant mesothelioma.[2] McVittie[27] performed a prospective study of 247 cases of asbestosis. Of 59 of these patients who had died prior to 1965, 42% had developed either bronchogenic carcinoma or malignant meso-

Table 9-4. Association of asbestosis and bronchogenic cancer*

Study	Deaths in asbestosis patients	Deaths due to bronchogenic carcinoma	Frequency (%)
Isselbacher et al. (compilation of literature to date) (1953)	603	83	13.8
Keal (1960)	30	14	46.4
Konig (1960)	36	11	30.5
Jones-Williams (1965)	52	10	19.2
	721	118	16.3
Deaths in asbestos workers			
Doll (1955)	105	18	17.1
Selikoff and Hammond (1965)	307	53	17.2

*From Freundlich, I. M., and Greening, R. R.: Radiology 89:224, 1967.

thelioma. The association of asbestos exposure and bronchogenic carcinoma is summarized in Table 9-4.

There appears to be a tendency for bronchogenic carcinoma to occur in the lower lobes in asbestos workers, as distinct from the normal upper lobe predilection.[19] This is consistent with the finding that asbestos fibers gravitate to the lung bases.[40] The average latent period between the first exposure to asbestos and development of bronchogenic carcinoma is about 30 years.[19]

Selikoff et al.[38] conducted a study to determine the effect of cigarette smoking in asbestos workers. Among 370 workers, 49 died of carcinoma of various types, as against the expected incidence of 8.6. Twenty-seven of these had either bronchogenic carcinoma or malignant mesothelioma, a 10-fold increase over the predicted incidence. Among 48 men who never smoked regularly and 39 who smoked only pipes or cigars, there were no deaths. All the deaths occurred among the remaining 282, who were regular cigarette smokers. Upon the basis of these figures, Selikoff et al. calculated that the incidence of death from bronchogenic carcinoma among asbestos workers who smoked was eight times that predicted for smokers in the general population. The question of a synergistic carcinogenic effect is therefore raised.

Gastrointestinal carcinoma

An increased rate of gastrointestinal malignancy has also been reported in numerous recent surveys among asbestos workers.[11] Carcinoma of the stomach, colon, and rectum have been specifically indicted. It should be stated that this relationship has not been conclusively proved as yet, although the common misdiagnosis of peritoneal mesothelioma (which can be histologically similar to undifferentiated cancer of other types) may contribute to the confusion on this point. The widely varying reported incidence of peritoneal mesothelioma tends to support this contention (Table 9-2).

SUMMARY

Significant asbestos exposure is widespread among certain occupational groups, and some exposure is probably universal among city dwellers. The theoretical danger to the general population is an increased incidence of various types of malignant disease. It would seem that the carcinogenic effect can result from brief exposure, and there is usually a long latent period before the tumor becomes manifest.

Fig. 9-6 shows the greatly increased rate of production of asbestos in recent years. Assuming a 30-year latent period for associated neoplasms, most patients that are presently being seen probably incurred critical asbestos exposure in the 1940s. World production has increased sixfold since then, and the trend is continuing. Industrial exposure is now better controlled, but air pollution is considerably worse.

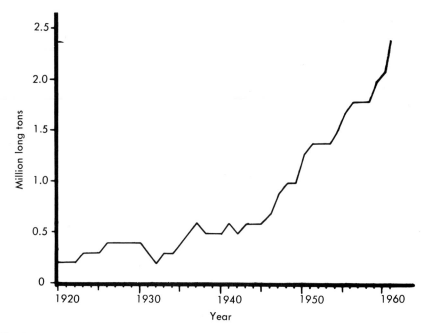

Fig. 9-6. Increasing world production of asbestos. (From Thomson, J. G.: Ann. N. Y. Acad. Sci. **132**:196, 1965.)

Table 9-5. Expected and observed deaths among 632 asbestos workers exposed to asbestos dust 20 years or longer*

	1943-1962	1963-1967	1943-1967 (totals)
Total deaths: all causes			
Expected	203.5	47.5	251
Observed	255	94	349
Total cancer: all sites			
Expected	36.5	8.6	45.1
Observed	95	49	144
Cancer of lung, trachea, pleura			
Expected	6.6	2.3	8.9
Observed	45	27	72
Cancer of stomach, colon, rectum			
Expected	9.4	1.8	11.2
Observed	29	8	37
Cancer of all other sites combined			
Expected	20.5	4.5	25
Observed	21	14	35
Asbestosis			
Expected	0	0	0
Observed	12	15	27
All other causes			
Expected	167	38.9	205.9
Observed	148	30	178

*From Selikoff, I. J., et al.: J.A.M.A. **204**:110, 1968.

Asbestos exposure may be manifested by characteristic pleural plaques, diffuse pulmonary fibrosis, or the secondary malignant processes such as mesothelioma, bronchogenic carcinoma, and gastrointestinal cancers (Table 9-5).

An awareness of the multiple potential effects of the asbestos fiber will enable the radiologist to play an increasingly important role in identifying these diseases.

Acknowledgment

We are indebted to Dr. Nicholas G. Demy of the Somerset Hospital, Somerville, New Jersey, who supplied much of the case material for this paper.

References

1. Auribault, M.: Observations regarding the hygiene and safety of workers in asbestos spinning and weaving mills, Bull. Insp. Travail, p. 196, 1906.
2. Buchanan, W. D.: Asbestos and primary intrathoracic neoplasms, Ann. N. Y. Acad. Sci. **132:**507, 1965.
3. Clinical Conference in Pulmonary Disease: Pulmonary complications of asbestos exposure, Chest **59:**77, 1971.
4. Cooke, W. E.: Pulmonary asbestosis, Br. Med. J. **2:**1024, 1927.
5. Demy, N. G., and Adler, H.: Asbestosis and malignancy, Am. J. Roentgenol. **100:**597, 1967.
6. Editorial: Action on asbestos, N. Engl. J. Med. **285:**1271, 1971.
7. Elmes, P. C., and Wade, O. L.: Relationship between exposure to asbestos and pleural malignancy in Belfast, Ann. N. Y. Acad. Sci. **132:**549, 1965.
8. Freundlich, I. M., and Greening, R. R.: Asbestosis and associated medical problems, Radiology **89:**224, 1967.
9. Gaze, R.: The physical and molecular structure of asbestos, Ann. N. Y. Acad. Sci. **132:**23, 1965.
10. Gross, P., deTreville, R. T. P., and Heller, M.: Pulmonary ferruginous bodies in city dwellers: a study of their central fibre, Arch. Environ. Health **19:**186, 1969.
11. Hammond, E. C., Selikoff, I. J., and Churg, J.: Neoplasia amongst insulation workers in the United States with special reference to intra-abdominal neoplasia, Ann. N. Y. Acad. Sci. **132:**519, 1965.
12. Harrington, G. S., Wagner, J. C., and Smith, M.: The detection of hyaluronic acid in pleural fluids of cases with diffuse pleural mesotheliomas, Br. J. Exp. Pathol. **44:**81, 1963.
13. Heller, R. M., Janower, M. L., and Weber, A. L.: The radiological manifestations of pleural mesothelioma, Am. J. Roentgenol. **108:**53, 1970.
14. Hendry, N. W.: The geology, occurrences, and major uses of asbestos, Ann. N. Y. Acad. Sci. **132:**12, 1965.
15. Hoffman, N. E., and Frederick, L.: Mortality from respiratory disease in dusty trades: inorganic dust, Bull. U. S. Bureau of Labor Statistics No. 231, Industrial Accidents and Hygiene Series No. 17, Washington, D. C., U. S. Government Printing Office.
16. Hourihan, D.: The pathology of mesotheliomata and an analysis of their association with asbestos exposure, Thorax **19:**268, 1964.
17. Hourihan, D., Lessof, L., and Richardson, P. C.: Hyaline and calcified pleural plaques as an index of exposure to asbestos: a study of radiological and pathological

features of 100 cases with a consideration of epidemiology, Br. Med. J. **1**:1069, 1966.

18. Hueper, W. C.: Occupational and non-occupational exposures to asbestos, Ann. N. Y. Acad. Sci. **132**:184, 1965.

19. Jacob, G., and Anspach, N.: Pulmonary neoplasia amongst Dresden asbestos workers, Ann. N. Y. Acad. Sci. **132**:536, 1965.

20. Jacob, G., and Bohlig, M.: The roentgenological complications in pulmonary asbestosis, Fortschr. Röntgenstr. **83**:575, 1955.

21. Kiviluoto, R.: Pleural calcification as a roentgenologic sign of non-occupational endemic anthophyllite-asbestos, Acta Radiol. suppl. 194:entire issue, 1960.

22. Kochberg, L. A.: Endothelioma (mesothelioma) of the pleura: review with report of seven cases, four of which were extirpated surgically, Am. Rev. Tuberc. **63**:150, 1951.

23. Langer, A. M., Selikoff, I. J., and Sastre, A.: Chrysotile asbestos in the lungs of persons in New York City, Arch. Environ. Health **22**:348, 1971.

24. Lazarus, H., Widrich, W. C., and Robbins, A. H.: Peritoneal mesothelioma with roentgenographic findings, Am. J. Roentgenol. **113**:171, 1971.

25. Lynch, K. M., and Smith, W. A.: Pulmonary asbestosis. III. Carcinoma of the lung in asbesto-silicosis, Am. J. Cancer **26**:56, 1935.

26. McCaughey, W. T. E., Wade, O. L., and Elmes, P. C.: Exposure to asbestos dust and diffuse pleural mesotheliomas, Br. Med. J. **2**:1397, 1962.

27. McVittie, J. C.: Asbestosis in Great Britain, Ann. N. Y. Acad. Sci. **132**:128, 1965.

28. Merewether, B. R. A., and Price, C. W.: Report on effects of asbestos dust on the lungs, and dust suppression in the asbestos industry, London, 1931, Her Majesty's Stationer's Office.

29. Murphy, R. L. H., et al.: Effects of low concentrations of asbestos: clinical, environmental, radiologic and epidemiologic observation in shipyard pipe workers and controls, N. Engl. J. Med. **285**:1271, 1971.

30. Murray, H. M.: Report of the Departmental Committee on Compensation for Industrial Diseases: minutes of evidence, appendices and index, London, 1907, Her Majesty's Stationer's Office, p. 127.

31. Newhouse, M. L., and Thompson, H.: Mesothelioma of pleura and peritoneum following exposure to asbestos in the London area, Br. J. Ind. Med. **22**:261, 1965.

32. Persaud, V., Bateson, E. M., and Bankay, C. D.: Pleural mesothelioma associated with massive hepatic calcification and unusual metastases, Cancer **26**:920, 1970.

33. Porter, J. M., and Cheek, G. M.: Pleural mesothelioma: review of tumor histogenesis and report of 12 cases, J. Thorac. Cardiovasc. Surg. **55**:882, 1968.

34. Ratzner, E. R., Pool, G. L., and Meramed, M. R.: Pleural mesotheliomas: clinical experience with 37 patients, Am. J. Roentgenol. **89**:863, 1967.

35. Selikoff, I. J.: The occurrence of pleural calcification amongst asbestos insulation workers, Ann. N. Y. Acad. Sci. **132**:351, 1965.

36. Selikoff, I. J., Churg, J., and Hammond, E. C.: Asbestos exposure and neoplasia, J.A.M.A. **188**:22, 1964.

37. Selikoff, I. J., Churg, J., and Hammond, E. C.: Relationship between exposure to asbestos and mesothelioma, N. Engl. J. Med. **272**:560, 1965.

38. Selikoff, I. H., Hammond, E. C., and Churg, J.: Asbestos exposure, smoking, and neoplasia, J.A.M.A. **204**:106, 1968.

39. Smith, A. R.: Pleural calcification resulting from exposure to certain dusts, Am. J. Roentgenol. **67**:375, 1952.

40. Thomson, J. G.: Asbestos and the urban dweller, Ann. N. Y. Acad. Sci. **132**:196, 1965.

41. Viikeri, M.: Ultrasound examination of pleural plaques, Acta Radiol. **301**(suppl.): 1970.

42. Wagner, J. C., Sleggs, C. A., and Marchand, P.: Diffuse pleural mesothelioma and asbestos exposure in northwestern Cape Province, Br. J. Ind. Med. **17**:250, 1960.

43. Winslow, O. J., and Taylor, M. B.: Malignant peritoneal mesotheliomas, Cancer **13**:127, 1960.

44. Zeckwer, I. T.: Mesothelioma of the pleura, Arch. Intern. Med. **34**:191, 1924.

10 Frontiers in gastrointestinal radiology

Martin W. Donner

A number of useful and, in some instances, significant clinical advances have been made in gastrointestinal radiology during the past few years. Some of them are the result of refined conventional methodology; others have emerged from the application of new radiographic and endoscopic techniques. Initial developments for much of this progress, now apparent, date back several years, while other advances are of more recent date. They reflect applied radiologic investigation, frequently in collaboration with gastroenterologists, and the progress made in radiologic imaging with the capability of recording dynamic events.

It is the purpose of this chapter to sample some of these advances, to convey their impact on clinical medicine, and to suggest future developments in the field.

NORMAL AND DISTURBED MOTILITY OF PHARYNX

Until the advent of image-intensified fluoroscopy, radiographic evaluation of the pharynx was limited to the detection of changes in structure, as, for example, those changes caused by tumors, inflammatory disease, or postoperative deformity. Disordered motility in the absence of organic disorders has been difficult to recognize due to technical limitations in recording functional sequences. Spot films obtained during fluoroscopic examinations were invariably inadequate, as patients with dysphagia are unpredictable in terms of the timing of individual swallows.

In order to analyze and interpret in more detail the radiographic changes seen in abnormal pharyngeal deglutition, a brief discussion of the *normal swallowing sequence* is presented.[5]

1. The tongue transports the food bolus toward the pharynx, where an involuntary swallowing reflex is initiated by sensory receptors in the mucous membrane that covers, in a circular fashion, the anterior and posterior pillars of the fauces, the tonsils, the soft palate, the base of the tongue, and the posterior pharyngeal wall. Transmitted by the seventh, ninth, and tenth cranial nerves to the swallowing center in the brain stem, these sensory signals are transformed into motor responses

230

relayed by the ninth, tenth, and twelfth cranial nerves. The tongue is elevated, and the food bolus is thrust against the inferior margin of the palate.

2. The root of the tongue is then pressed against the posterior pharyngeal wall.
3. Subsequently, elevation of the soft palate occurs in a characteristic triangular fashion with the structure extending well above the level of the hard palate.
4. The larynx is then elevated and the hypopharynx is narrowed by the action of the middle and inferior pharyngeal constrictors. This elevation

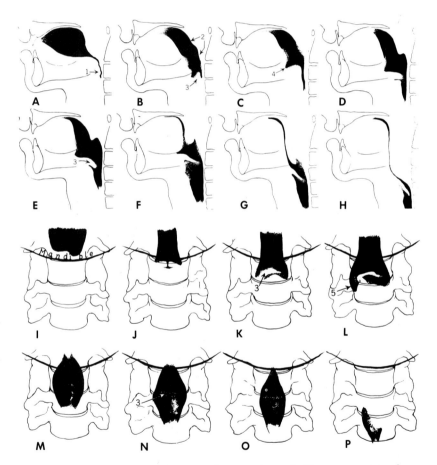

Fig. 10-1. Normal barium swallow (oropharyngeal stage). Note symmetric pharyngeal constriction and absence of pharyngeal retention. Selection of cine frames in lateral, **A** to **H,** and PA, **I** to **P,** projections. *1,* Posterior surface of tongue; *2,* soft palate; *3,* epiglottis; *4,* valleculae; *5,* piriform sinus. (From Donner, M. W., and Silbiger, M. L.: Am. J. Med. Sci. **251:**134, 1966.)

of the larynx represents the most important movement in the swallowing sequence, for it avoids the entry of bolus into the airway.

5. Musculature of the floor of the mouth contracts, resulting in a tilt of the epiglottis, which moves from an upright position to a horizontal and downward position (Fig. 10-1).

Three major functions should be carried out during the involuntary stage of pharyngeal swallowing: (1) rapid propulsion of food into the esophagus, (2) simultaneous protection of the airway, and (3) opening of the cricopharyngeal sphincter. Because of the crossing between the alimentary and respiratory tract in the region of the pharynx, the cricopharynx must open and the trachea must be closed as soon as the bolus passes the pharynx. On the other hand, the pharynx must be free from liquids or food particles when the airway re-opens. As long as these important functions are maintained, unobstructed and rapid passage of food from the mouth to the esophagus, clearance of the food channels, and protection of the airway will be guaranteed.

Abnormal deglutition

Deviation from either the order or character of the physiologic movements during the oropharyngeal state of swallowing will invariably lead to abnormal deglutition and may give rise to dysphagia.

Radiologic studies begin with the attempt to rule out the presence of mechanical obstruction, because not infrequently functional disturbances are associated with organic disease. As soon as abnormal oropharyngeal swallowing has been recognized as functional in nature, the following characteristic radiographic signs may be useful.

Disturbance of motility. This is the most frequent sign of abnormal deglutition, ranging from slight impairment to complete loss of certain movements with or without disordered sequence of functional activity. The latter may be due to a delayed initiation or prolonged direction of muscular activity or to a disturbance in the sequential order of the swallowing process. Repeated attempts at swallowing may be made, and the tongue may move backward several times until the swallowing reflex is initiated. Auxiliary movements of the head and jaws may be present to aid the transfer of food to the esophagus. These movements are usually accompanied by additional manifestations of abnormal deglutition, including stasis and aspiration.

Residual filling of pharyngeal recesses. This is most widely known as a sign of altered sensitivity of adjacent mucosa, decreased muscular tone, mechanical obstruction, changes in recess shape, and neuromuscular disturbance. Atrophy of fat tissue, normally found below the valleculae and supporting the epiglottis, may be responsible for the dilatation of these pouches and subsequent retention of food. Residual filling of the pharyngeal recesses is invariably present in patients with peripheral or central motor nerve paralysis. This sign of vallecular retention, frequently associated with a swallowing disorder, is valuable as a differential sign only if additional roentgenographic changes are observed.

Pharyngeal stasis. This is a reliable sign of pharyngeal motor disturbance seen in pharyngeal paralysis or in mechanical obstruction produced by intrinsic or extrinsic tumors. Dilatation of the pharyngeal cavity is frequently associated with lateral pharyngeal pouches or diverticula.

Aspiration. Due to misdirected swallowing, this is one of the most striking abnormalities when the bolus deviates from its normal pathway and proceeds either into the nasal cavity or the trachea. This phenomenon occurs when there is impairment of the closing mechanism or pathologic communication to the nasopharynx and the trachea. Retained pharyngeal contents may be aspirated during respiration without swallowing. Uni- or bilateral paresis of the soft palate, morphologic defects of the hard palate, or tumors of the epipharynx will lead to reflux into the nasopharynx. Paralysis of muscles of the floor of the mouth and interference with the function of the recurrent laryngeal nerve also result in suppression of important safety mechanisms. Examples of interference with motor function are seen in myasthenia gravis and postresectional alterations of pharyngeal anatomy and innervation; examples of interference with sensory perception are peripheral toxic injuries such as diphtheria or anesthesia of the pharynx.

· · ·

While motor disturbances almost invariably accompany organic disease of the pharynx, they are seen most prominently in neuromuscular disorders affecting the pharynx.* Hence this discussion will be limited to disorders involving either neurologic or muscular diseases of this area.

Brain stem lesions. Pseudobulbar palsy, poliomyelitis, and the posterior-inferior cerebellar artery syndrome are the more common representatives in this group of disorders. Brain stem involvement with pharyngeal dysphagia is also observed in several of the congenital and degenerative processes such as hereditary spastic paralysis. The type of pathologic change involving the brain stem is less important than the anatomic area of destruction.

The most striking abnormality of pharyngeal swallowing in many patients with brain stem lesions is the failure of the cricopharyngeal sphincter to relax normally (Fig. 10-2). Pharyngeal retention, stasis, nasal regurgitation, and aspiration into the trachea occur as the result of this incoordinated motor activity.

In normal subjects, deviation of the food column to either or both lateral food channels occurs infrequently. In patients with unilateral brain stem disease this deviation is quite common due to asymmetric weakness of the pharyngeal constrictors. Under these conditions, the barium usually outlines

---

*For further information, see Donner and Siegel,[9] Donner and Silbiger,[10] and Silbiger et al.[29]

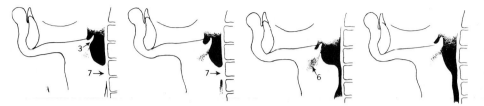

Fig. 10-2. Posterior inferior cerebellar artery syndrome. Note tightness and elongation of cricopharyngeal sphincter, 7; retention of barium in pharyngeal recesses; and aspiration into laryngeal vestibule, 6. Epiglottis, 3. (From Donner, M. W., and Silbiger, M. L.: Am. J. Med. Sci. **251:**134, 1966.)

the epiglottis, which progressively tilts toward the affected side during a swallow. A representative example of a patient with a brain stem lesion, namely, thrombosis of the posterior-inferior cerebellar artery, has been traced in Fig. 10-2. In addition to vascular disease and hemorrhage, disorders such as syphilis, bulbar paralysis, syringobulbia, tumors, and multiple sclerosis may produce this syndrome.

Myoneural junction disorders. Myasthenia gravis patients are a group with impaired conduction at the myoneural junction of striated muscles. Fatigability is usually first observed in the ocular muscles, but as soon as the bulbar muscles are involved, dysphagia occurs. Swallowing becomes more difficult in the evening and during the course of a meal that the patient may begin to swallow without noticeable distress. Remissions and exacerbations are characteristic but are not found in all cases. The easy fatigability of the pharyngeal motor activity is a characteristic feature of myasthenia gravis. Radiologically, during the pharyngeal stage, prolonged coating of the walls and pooling of barium in the pharyngeal recesses are associated with loss of tone and ballooning of the pharyngeal cavity (Fig. 10-3, *A* to *D*). There may be nasal regurgitation during successive swallows due to a diminishing ability to raise the pharynx, to close the epipharynx, and to approximate the posterior pharyngeal wall and the palate effectively to the base of the tongue. In the PA projection, passage of the bolus through the pharynx is symmetric by virtue of the generalized muscle involvement. Never is there any spasm or hypertrophy of the cricopharyngeal sphincter as seen in brain stem lesions, sideropenic dysphagia, or pharyngoesophageal incoordination. As shown in Fig. 10-3, *E* to *H*, the subcutaneous injection of prostigmine helps to establish the diagnosis of myasthenia gravis with principal involvement of the muscles of deglutition. Documentation and quantitation of improvement with prostigmine therapy has helped to ascertain the adequacy of therapy by the return of motor function to normal.

Primary muscle disorders. Many diseases in the category of primary muscle disorders show involvement of the pharyngeal musculature. While the

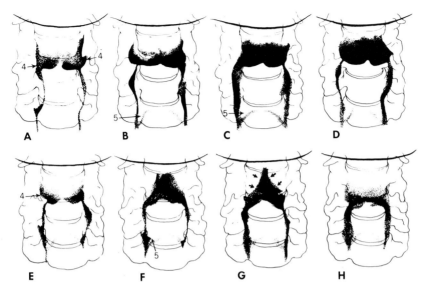

Fig. 10-3. Myasthenia gravis. Tracings of barium swallow studies before, **A** to **D**, and 30 minutes following subcutaneous injection of 1 mg prostigmine, **E** to **H**. Note persistent retention of barium in valleculae, *4*, and piriform sinuses, *5*; moderate distention of pharyngeal cavity, **A** to **D**; improved pharyngeal contraction (arrows); and small amount of retained barium in pharyngeal recesses, **E** to **H**. (From Donner, M. W., and Silbiger, M. L.: Am. J. Med. Sci. **251**:134, 1966.)

etiology and cause of the disorder are often unknown, pathologically they are characterized by degenerative or inflammatory changes in the muscle itself. Prolongation of muscular activity and weakened or even shallow pharyngeal contractions are observed. There may be retention of the bolus in the pharyngeal recesses, and stasis may develop in advanced cases. The cricopharyngeal sphincter is usually not affected and opens normally.

An example in this category of myopathies is *myotonia dystrophica*, a hereditary disorder in which prolonged contraction of striated muscle is associated with gastrointestinal motility disturbance in addition to muscle wasting, frontal baldness, and Raynaud's phenomenon. The myotonia is intensified by emotion and cold temperatures. It may be diminished by repetition of the movement and distinguishes itself from myasthenia gravis, in which increasing fatigability occurs with continued use of the afflicted muscle. The impairment of pharyngeal swallowing in this disease may range from slight dysfunction to complete paralysis with nasal and tracheal aspiration (Fig. 10-4). Successive swallows frequently show improvement and decreased duration in pharyngeal contraction. The motility disturbance can be produced or exaggerated by chilled barium. An interesting radiologic phenomenon seen occasionally in myopathies is the so-called pseudotumor effect. The larynx, whose supporting musculature is involved in the disease process, is displaced posteriorly

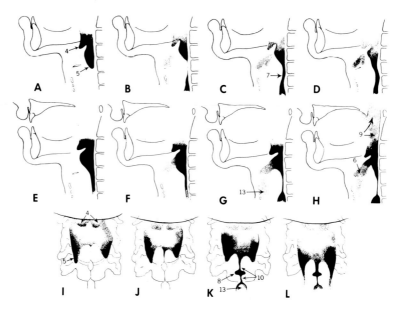

Fig. 10-4. Myotonia dystrophica. Note retention and stasis of barium in pharyngeal recesses, *4* and *5*, and cavity; aspiration into laryngeal vestibule, *6*, and ventricle, *8*; and reflux of contrast material into epipharynx, *9*. **A** to **H**, Lateral projections. **I** to **L**, PA studies. *7*, Cricopharyngeal sphincter; *10*, vocal cords; *13*, trachea. (From Donner, M. W., and Silbiger, M. L.: Am. J. Med. Sci. **251**:134, 1966.)

and causes an impression on the barium column at the appropriate level of the pharynx. The entire hypopharynx may show evidence of extrinsic pressure impinging upon the piriform sinuses and narrowing the lumen of the cricopharyngeal sphincter segment. The structural deformity of the pharynx often suggests a mass lesion on conventional roentgenograms. During fluoroscopy or cine recordings there is no tumor fixation seen, and free movability of the pharyngeal structures during swallowing prevails. The cricopharyngeal sphincter segment often distends only briefly but adequately during the examination.

Swallowing disorders of unknown pathogenesis. Among the many disorders in this category, cricopharyngeal hypertrophy (bar) and sideropenic dysphagia are two disorders with "high dysphagia," in which the pathogenesis is undefined.

In *cricopharyngeal hypertrophy* the cricopharyngeal sphincter protrudes as a posterior indentation into the barium column, usually at the level of the fifth or sixth cervical vertebral body. It is occasionally seen in normal subjects in older age groups. In younger individuals, however, an indentation by the cricopharyngeal sphincter is not visible. In patients with cricopharyngeal hypertrophy, partial or almost complete obstruction at the pharyngoesophageal

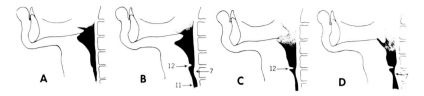

Fig. 10-5. Sideropenic dysphagia. Frame sequence obtained in lateral projection. Note anterior hypopharyngeal web, *12*, and posterior indentation caused by cricopharyngeal sphincter, *7*. *11*, Esophagus. (From Donner, M. W., and Silbiger, M. L.: Am. J. Med. Sci. **251:**134, 1966.)

junction is observed. The defect is usually associated with pharyngeal dilatation, weakness of pharyngeal contraction, and aspiration.

Atrophy and morphologic changes of the pharyngeal mucosa may be responsible for difficulty in swallowing, as seen in *sideropenic disturbance of deglutition.* Iron deficiency anemia associated with difficulty of swallowing, better known as the Plummer-Vinson syndrome, has been observed with relatively high frequency in the Scandinavian countries. In these patients the dysphagia is usually localized at the level of the hypopharynx, where a characteristic radiographic finding is a web indenting the anterior wall of the hypopharynx, usually close to the cricopharyngeal sphincter. More than one web may be seen, and occasionally a web may indent the esophagus as far distally as the level of the aortic arch. The web is pointed, semicircular, and occasionally produces obstruction. A posterior indentation at the level of the sixth cervical vertebral body indicates spasm of the cricopharyngeal sphincter, a frequent if not obligatory companion sign of this disorder. The web is best seen with large swallows of barium when patients are examined in the prone lateral position (Fig. 10-5). Endoscopically, a protruding mucosal fold usually confirms the radiographic findings, but biopsies have shown normal mucosa. Within hours following the administration of iron medication, both the web and spasm of the upper esophageal sphincter may disappear. Radiographic improvement and symptomatic relief usually coincide, but sometimes dysphagia persists. A high incidence of cancer involving the larynx or pharynx in patients with persistent sideropenic webs has been reported in Scandinavian countries. Asymptomatic webs are occasionally seen in children without associated disorders and in adults proximal to carcinomatous lesions of the esophagus or secondary to scarring following radiation therapy to the mediastinum.

Method of examination

Patients undergoing radiographic evaluation of pharyngeal deglutition require examination in both the prone and erect positions. Patients with "high dysphagia" usually have more difficulty swallowing when prone than when in the erect position. However, roentgenographic abnormalities such as webs, cricopharyngeal sphincter defects, and motor weakness of pharyngeal contraction are exaggerated in this position and are therefore easier to detect. The disturbing effect of gravity on swallowing is eliminated. With the patient standing erect, barium swallow studies are made in the PA and lateral projections. This part of the examination provides valuable information concerning tone of the pharynx and pooling of contrast material in the pharyngeal recesses. In addition, the PA projection is useful in cases of paralysis of specific groups of muscles to demonstrate asymmetric contraction of the constrictors and deflection of the bolus to either food channel as it passes through the pharynx.

A conventional barium suspension is given unless the patient's history strongly suggests aspiration. Under these conditions, bronchographic contrast media are of equal value. Studies of pharyngeal deglutition are never begun with barium paste. The patient with paralysis of the constrictor muscles, unable to force the material into the esophagus, may obstruct his airway and suffer considerable respiratory distress. In an attempt to obtain films with optimal definition of the soft tissue structures of the pharynx and larynx in lateral projection, a bag filled with rice flour is recommended for use during these examinations. The flour bag may be attached to the jaw and the medial end of the clavicle, making up for the lack of soft tissue mass in the neck with resultant uniform radiographic detail of the entire area.

NORMAL AND ABNORMAL MOTILITY OF ESOPHAGUS

Progressive peristaltic movements of the esophagus are well coordinated with the movements of the pharynx and, under *normal* conditions,[15] both structures function as a single unit. As elsewhere in the gastrointestinal tract, the esophagus is separated from adjacent segments of the alimentary canal by sphincters with a resting tone greater than that of adjacent segments. These sphincters relax in response to the stimulus of swallowing. The upper esophageal sphincter prevents air from filling the esophagus during inspiration, and the lower sphincter prevents reflux of gastric contents into the esophagus.[14] After relaxation of the upper esophageal sphincter, which is accomplished well ahead of the bolus, a moving ring of contraction propels the bolus from the pharynx into the lower portion of the esophagus. This peristaltic wave is uninterrupted unless a subsequent swallow prematurely suspends the preceding peristaltic wave. Prior to the arrival of the bolus in the distal esophagus, the lower esophageal sphincter relaxes.

Two types of peristalsis are identified in the esophagus, primary and secondary. Primary peristaltic waves, initiated by swallowing, sweep over the entire length of the esophagus at a rate of 2 to 4 cm/sec. These waves cease at the junction between the tubular esophagus and the phrenic ampulla, where they are followed without delay by a concentric contraction of the lower sphincter. From there the bolus is passed into the stomach at the point of the cardia. Secondary peristaltic waves are initiated when local esophageal stimulation occurs. The most common stimulus is intraluminal esophageal distention secondary to food particles left behind in the esophagus after the primary peri- staltic wave has passed or as the result of material regurgitated from the stomach into the esophagus. The waves are considered to be a protective ac- tion of the esophagus against material that is retained in the lumen and is po- tentially harmful to its wall in terms of inflammation and perforation. Primary and secondary waves are progressive in nature and are hence peristaltic. So- called tertiary waves represent stationary ringlike contractions that appear simultaneously at various levels of the lower esophagus; they have an undulat- ing or curling delineation. Shallow tertiary waves are frequently seen in elderly individuals but are also associated with such disorders as achalasia. Deep local contractions are present in diffuse esophageal spasm.

Abnormal esophageal motility

The most frequent type of nonperistaltic esophageal contraction is seg- mental spasm associated with a variety of local or more generalized disorders. Spasm may occur in response to gastroesophageal reflux, in inflammatory or chemical irritation of the esophageal wall, and as a reaction to pharmacologic agents, for example, methacholine (Mecholyl) in achalasia.

Another type of neuromotor dysfunction of the esophagus is aperistalsis. It is observed in systemic diseases and in achalasia. In systemic diseases such as scleroderma, muscle tissue in the esophageal wall is replaced by fibrotic material, and in achalasia, intramural nerve cells are defective or completely missing. Both disorders prevent the esophagus from contracting in a coordi- nated fashion. Manometric recordings of normal and abnormal motility pat- terns of the most frequent disorders involving the pharynx and esophagus are shown in Fig. 10-6.

Esophageal motility is affected by chilled liquids that slow or abolish esoph- ageal peristalsis and by hot liquids that accelerate the peristaltic response to a swallow. The following are among the pharmacologic agents having diag- nostic or therapeutic indications:

Methacholine (Mecholyl)	2.5 to 7.5 mg (total) given subcutaneously; produces strong segmental contractions of the esophagus in achalasia
Atropine	1 mg given intravenously; relieves spasm in positive methacholine (Mecholyl) test for achalasia and im- proves "diffuse esophageal spasm"
Nitroglycerin	1.2 mg given orally to patients with idiopathic eso- phageal spasm
Hydrochloric acid	As "acid barium" to study sensitivity of the esopha- gus to acid
Propantheline (Pro-Banthine)	For relaxation of the distal esophagus during search for varices
Nystatin (Mycostatin)	To treat fungus disorders of the esophagus that are invariably associated with episodes of spasm

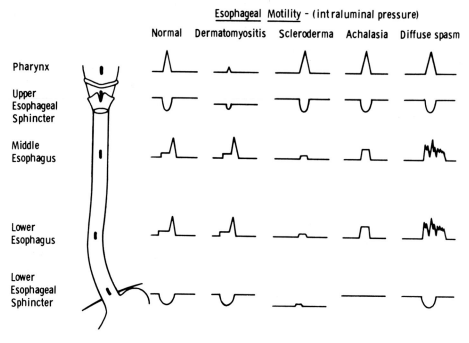

Fig. 10-6. Positions of manometric recording sites are indicated in diagram at left and characteristic intraluminal pressure changes are indicated at right. In normal subject, upper esophageal sphincter relaxes prior to appearance of pharyngeal peristalsis, which propels bolus into the esophagus. Entrance of bolus into esophagus produces simultaneous rise in intraluminal pressure in all intraesophageal recording sites. Lower esophageal sphincter relaxes to allow bolus to pass into stomach. Peristaltic wave sweeps down esophagus, pushing bolus ahead of it. When peristaltic wave enters lower sphincter, sphincter regains its resting tone. In dermatomyositis, involvement of striated muscle portion of swallowing apparatus leads to weak pharyngeal peristalsis and decreased tone in upper esophageal sphincter. In scleroderma, which involves smooth muscle, no peristalsis is seen in body of the esophagus, and lower esophageal sphincter is atonic. Elevation of pressure recorded in body of esophagus is due to pharynx propelling bolus into esophagus. In achalasia there is also no peristalsis in body of esophagus; in contrast to scleroderma, lower esophageal sphincter maintains normal resting tone but does not relax in response to swallowing. In diffuse spasm, entrance of bolus into esophagus is associated with multiple simultaneous segmental contractions rather than single peristaltic wave. (From Hendrix, T. R.: In Harvey, A. M., et al., editors: The principles and practice of medicine, ed. 18, New York, 1972, Appleton-Century-Crofts.)

Physiologically, the hormone gastrin affects lower esophageal sphincter pressure. With increased production of gastrin (food intake, gastric distention, and administration of bicarbonate), lower esophageal sphincter pressure increases. With diminished production, as in peptic ulcer disease of the stomach or duodenum, lower esophageal sphincter pressure diminishes.

The sensitivity of the esophagus to acid is of particular interest since it enables radiologists to employ a simple test in an attempt to distinguish symptoms originating in the esophagus from cardiovascular or musculoskeletal complaints.* Symptoms having these origins in the esophagus are often caused by motor disturbances,[28] which are responses to gastrointestinal reflux.

When gastroesophageal reflux occurs, impaired lower esophageal sphincter pressure is in large measure responsible for heartburn, substernal discomfort, and chest pain. In the past, radiologic identification of gastroesophageal reflux has often been difficult unless a scarred, deformed, and ulcerated esophagus demonstrated the end stage of chronic esophagitis or unless frequent episodes of free gastroesophageal reflux were observed during fluoroscopy. In our experience the observation of gastroesophageal reflux under fluoroscopic control and employing methods to increase intra-abdominal pressure has only been partially successful. For all patients eventually determined by other techniques to have gastroesophageal reflux, only 40% showed reflux during fluoroscopy. Moreover, one of the most crucial questions in this regard has been the clinical significance of a small sliding hiatus hernia or a lower esophageal ring detected radiologically. Previous manometric studies have shown that acid perfusion of the esophagus induces abnormal esophageal motility in patients with reflux symptoms.[4,28] This information has been used to develop a simple, effective method for the radiologic diagnosis of symptoms most likely related to an acid-sensitive esophagus, namely, the *acid barium test*.

Method of examination

Each patient receives conventional barium suspension (pH 6.0 to 7.0) as well as an acid barium mixture. The acid barium is made by mixing well 100 ml of standard barium sulfate suspension and 0.5 ml of concentrated hydrochloric acid (37%), resulting in a pH of 1.6 to 1.7. To obtain constant pH values, acid barium should be prepared prior to each examination. Moreover, it is conceivable that different barium mixtures may require more or less hydrochloric acid to reach the desired pH level. To confirm the critical value of pH 1.6 to 1.7, a pH meter should be employed initially. Acid barium with pH values lower than 1.6 (for example, pH 1.2) may set off motility disturbances in asymptomatic patients (false positive test), whereas barium mixtures with pH values above the desired level (for example, pH 2.5) may result in a false negative test in which the results indicate normal esophageal motility.

Patients are examined in prone right anterior oblique position to evaluate the strength of each peristaltic wave without the disturbing effect of gravity on swallowing. It is important to observe each progressive peristaltic contraction responding to a single barium swallow as it traverses the entire length of the esophagus because subsequent swallows, if initiated prematurely, result in interruption of the peristaltic wave. Such interruption may be mistaken for segmental spasm. One or several swallows of conventional barium suspension

---

*For further information, see Donner,[8] Donner et al.,[11] and McCall et al.[21]

are studied in this fashion fluoroscopically and then recorded on motion picture film, videotape, or rapid sequential spot films. The same procedure is repeated with acid barium with delay in cine recording until two or three swallows have provided adequate contact of the acid with esophageal mucosa. Parenthetically, it is our experience that normal peristalsis follows the first two swallows of acid barium in a few patients with reflux symptoms in whom a subsequent test was positive. After recording the findings for several acid barium swallows, the patient receives 1 tablespoon of antacid medication to

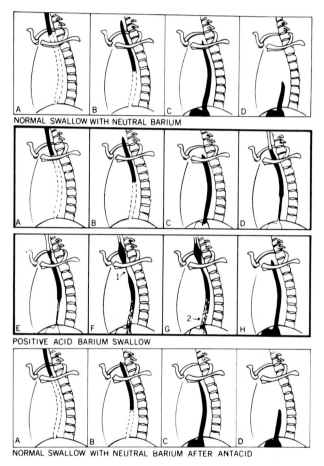

Fig. 10-7. Animated cine frame sequence in symptomatic patient with esophagitis (acid-perfusion positive). Upper row: Neutral barium swallow. Note progressive peristaltic wave with normal emptying of esophagus. Middle rows: Acid barium swallow. Note aperistalsis with stasis of barium; segmental nonperistaltic contractions, 1; and gastroesophageal reflux, 2. Lower row: Neutral barium swallow after antacid medication; normal progressive peristalsis. (From Katz, D., and Hoffman, F.: The esophagogastric junction, Amsterdam, 1971, Excerpta Medica Foundation.)

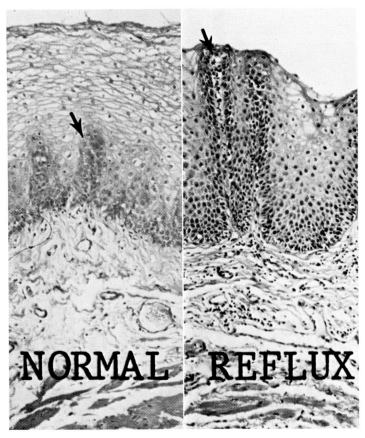

Plate I. Esophageal mucosa in symptom-free individual compared to mucosa of patient with reflux symptoms. Epithelial layer of tissue from patient with history of reflux contains many darkly stained immature cells. Note vascular papillae (arrow) approach epithelial surface in biopsy specimen of patient (right); papillae of normal individual penetrate epithelium less than halfway (arrow). (Hematoxylin-eosin stain; ×150.) (From Donner, M. W.: Radiologe 13:372, 1973.)

neutralize residual barium in the esophagus. Then esophageal motility is once more evaluated with conventional barium.

The normal esophagus in asymptomatic patients is insensitive to acid barium and peristaltic waves traverse the esophagus as they do when neutral barium is used. Only occasionally does the esophagus show a slight delay in the initiation of peristaltic waves.

Most patients with reflux symptoms respond to neutral barium with normal progressive peristalsis (Fig. 10-7, upper row). On the other hand, acid barium results in aperistalsis and segmental spastic contractions lasting 20 to 30 seconds. During this time, reflux of gastric contents into the lower esophagus can be observed until a secondary peristaltic wave sweeps the retained barium from the lower esophagus into the stomach (Fig. 10-7, middle rows). In patients with such motility disturbances as a result of acid barium, esophageal function returns to normal or almost normal when antacid medication is given and when the radiologic examination is completed with neutral barium (Fig. 10-7, lower row).

In patients whose acid barium test is positive, symptoms may be reproduced during the procedure. In most cases, however, the amount of acid barium given is too small and the time during which the esophageal mucosa is exposed to acid is too short to produce heartburn or retrosternal discomfort. In our experience the test is positive in 85% of patients with reflux symptoms; that is, normal peristalsis with neutral barium reverts to a motility disturbance in response to acid barium. An additional 12.5% of patients have abnormal motility even with neutral barium. Among asymptomatic patients, 3.8% exhibit a positive response to the test with acid barium (false positive). Several subjects with hiatus hernia that were asymptomatic had negative acid barium tests and subsequently proved to have no evidence of gastroesophageal reflux.

Histologic examination of specimens from patients with reflux symptoms reveals a diminished layer of stratified squamous epithelium with many immature cells. In addition, the vascular papillae often reach the surface of the epithelium, whereas in normal individuals, these papillae penetrate the epithelial layer to less than half its thickness (Plate I). The development of symptoms in patients with gastroesophageal reflux is shown in Fig. 10-8.

DOUBLE-CONTRAST EXAMINATION OF STOMACH

Recent advances in the diagnosis of gastric and duodenal disease using fiber optic endoscopes have stimulated the refinement of radiographic techniques in an attempt to improve the demonstration of morphologic detail. Among these techniques, double-contrast examination is of particular value. It allows a see-through look at the stomach and duodenum with delineation of mucosal architecture and, by means of gaseous distention, enables the examiner to evaluate satisfactorily such "difficult" areas as the gastric fundus and antrum. Gastric segments of questionable fixation, small mucosal ulcerations,

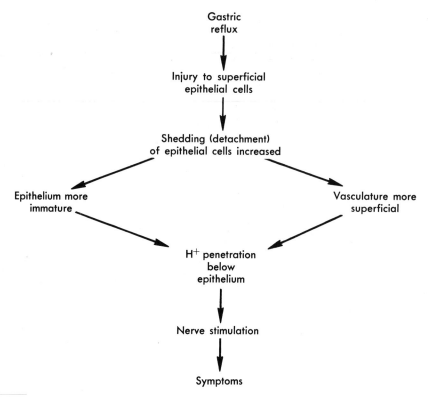

Fig. 10-8. Yardley's schema of development of symptoms in patients with reflux esophagitis. (From Donner, M. W.: Radiologe **13:**372, 1973.)

early carcinomas, and pathology of anastomoses resulting from partial or subtotal gastric resection are more easily detected by this technique, as is pathology in the lower esophagus, including varices.

In the past the major disadvantage of double-contrast examinations using effervescent compounds has been the formation and retention of excessive foam and air bubbles. To counteract this undesirable effect, gas-producing granules and tablets composed of sodium bicarbonate, tartaric acid, and a silicone antifoaming agent have been used. The granules or tablets are placed on the patient's tongue and swallowed down with 1 ounce of barium suspension, releasing several hundred milliliters of carbon dioxide without delay.[13,18] More recently simethicone, a surface-active agent, has been added to barium preparations.[23]

Films are usually taken with the patient in the supine and erect positions. In the supine position, exposures are made with the patient rotated to the left (LPO) and to the right side (RPO). With the table raised 45°, additional films may be useful to visualize duodenal bulb, C-loop, and greater curvature of the stomach. During the change in positions, the air moves from the body of the

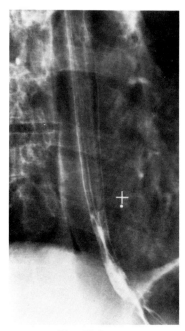
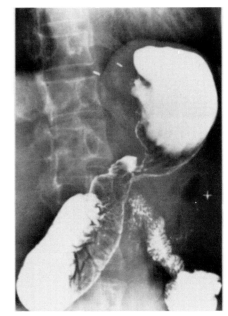

Fig. 10-9   Fig. 10-10

Fig. 10-9. Double-contrast examination of esophagus. Normal study. Note delineation of mucosal detail. (Courtesy Dr. Atsuko Heshiki, Baltimore, Md.)

Fig. 10-10. Gastric resection (Billroth I). Study of gastroduodenal anastomosis. Barium-coated walls and mucosal folds moderately distended by air. (Courtesy Dr. Atsuko Heshiki, Baltimore, Md.)

stomach into the gastric antrum, duodenal bulb, and C-loop. In the upright position the air outlines and distends the gastric fundus. This allows evaluation of the relationship between fundus, distal esophagus, and left diaphragm. Figs. 10-9 to 10-11 demonstrate the advantage of double-contrast studies in a number of cases.

ANGIOGRAPHIC LOCALIZATION AND PHARMACOLOGIC CONTROL OF GASTROINTESTINAL BLEEDING

The overall diagnostic accuracy of conventional radiographic techniques (barium studies) for the demonstration of a bleeding site ranges from 20% to 80%, depending upon patient selection and upon the radiologist's experience with such procedures. In many instances, acute gastrointestinal blood loss originates from shallow mucosal erosions in the distal esophagus or as in erosive gastritis from one or more sites in the stomach. These lesions may not produce sufficiently large defects to be appreciated on barium studies. Moreover, the frequent presence of blood clots in the stomach and the inability of the acutely ill patient to cooperate during the fluoroscopic examination are

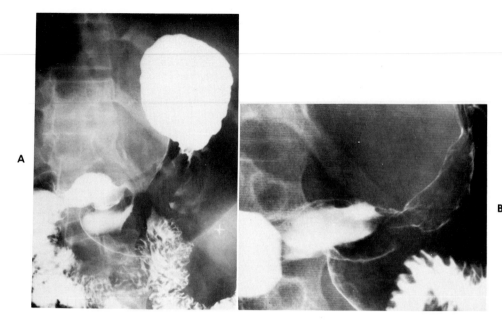

Fig. 10-11. Adenocarcinoma of stomach with atrophic gastritis. **A,** Absence of mucosal folds in body and antrum of stomach; lesser curvature mass lesion displacing intragastric air. **B,** Close-up view of gastric tumor showing extent of lesion. (Courtesy Dr. Atsuko Heshiki, Baltimore, Md.)

some of the reasons for these difficulties. But even the use of barium meals to demonstrate gastrointestinal pathology provides no assurance that a lesion seen radiographically represents the bleeding source.

Hence abdominal arteriography, with selective injection of contrast material into the celiac or superior and inferior mesenteric arteries, has become a valuable radiographic technique and already is well established in the diagnosis of acute gastrointestinal hemorrhage.* In patients with chronic unexplained blood loss from the gastrointestinal tract, correlation between the angiographic findings and the pathologic diagnosis approaches 75%.[19] Before angiography is performed, endoscopy should be employed for acutely hemorrhaging patients and conventional barium studies should be done for patients with chronic gastrointestinal blood loss.

Active arterial bleeding is localized by observing extravasation of contrast material into the intestinal lumen (Figs. 10-12 and 10-13). This observation usually requires a bleeding rate of at least 1.5 ml/min and has been reported experimentally at rates as low as 0.5 ml/min. In chronic bleeders, tumor vessels, early venous filling in the area of involvement, and hypervascularity may be seen in carcinomas of the colon or small bowel sarcomas (Fig. 10-14). Vascular malformations usually demonstrate a large collection of irregular blood

---

*For further information, see Baum et al.,[2,3] Klein et al.,[19] and Koehler and Salmon.[20]

Fig. 10-12. Active lower gastrointestinal bleeding in patient with extensive diverticulosis of colon. Superior mesenteric arteriogram showing extravasation of contrast material in region of the cecum. **A,** Bleeding point in early arterial phase can be identified. **B,** Large amount of contrast substance fills lumen of colon. **C,** Persistent extravasation of contrast material after most blood vessels and tissues are cleared of contrast medium. (Courtesy Dr. Robert White, Baltimore, Md.)

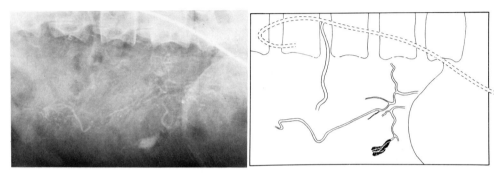

C

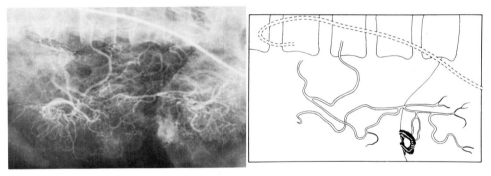

B

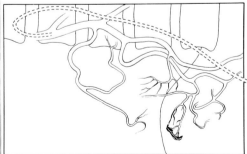

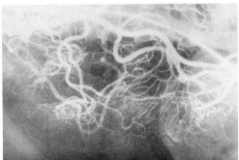

A

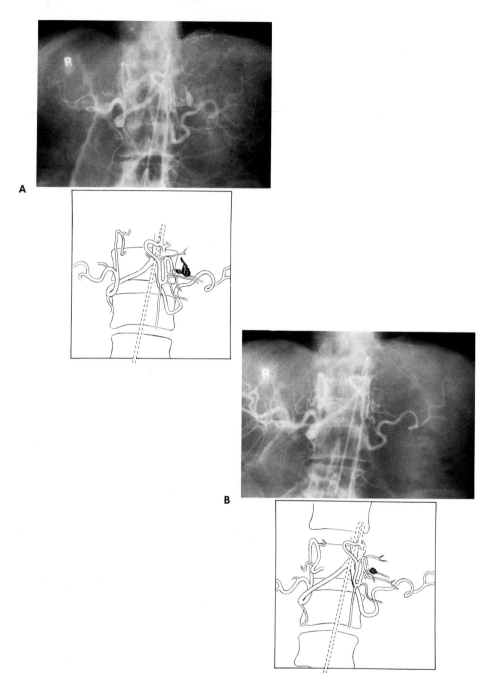

Fig. 10-13. Active upper gastrointestinal bleeding in stress gastritis. Left gastric arteriograms. **A,** Teardrop (hemorrhage) extravasation of contrast material into stomach from branch of left gastric artery. **B,** Bleeding considerably reduced following intra-arterial infusion using vasopressin (Pitressin), 0.2 unit/min for 3 hours. (Courtesy Dr. Robert White, Baltimore, Md.)

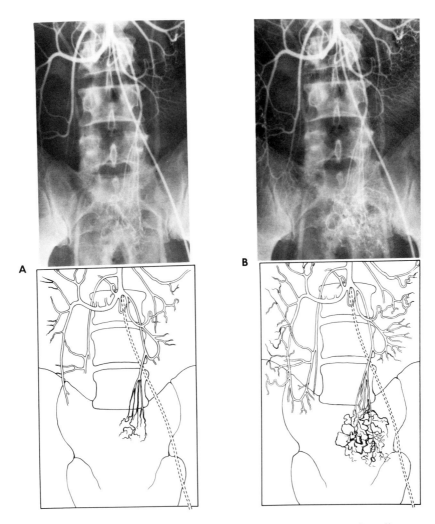

Fig. 10-14. Chronic gastrointestinal bleeding from leiomyosarcoma of small intestine. Patient had four bleeding episodes over 2 years; results of upper gastrointestinal and small bowel radiographic series were negative. Superior mesenteric arteriograms. **A,** Early arterial phase. Note feeding vessels from ileal branch. **B,** Late arterial phase. Tumor vessels and early venous filling are seen. (Courtesy Dr. Robert White, Baltimore, Md.)

vessels with early filling of veins or early filling of a small vein without other small vessel abnormality, as in telangiectasia.[19]

Aside from the identification of gastrointestinal bleeding sites, intra-arterial catheters have been used to administer vasoactive substances for the control of hemorrhaging.* This concept of infusing selective vasoconstrictors has

---

*For further information, see Baum and Nusbaum,[1] Conn et al.,[7] Murray-Lyon et al.,[22] Rosch et al.,[25-27] and White et al.[32]

yielded particularly convincing results in patients with esophageal varices and hemorrhagic gastritis. For example, vasopressin may be infused into the superior mesenteric artery in the treatment of patients with *bleeding esophageal varices.* At rates ranging from 0.1 to 0.4 unit/min for periods of several hours,[7] the bleeding may be controlled in 80% of all cases. It is accomplished by reducing blood flow in the superior mesenteric vein with a subsequent drop of pressure in the portal vein. In patients with *hemorrhagic gastritis,* success rates of intra-arterial application of epinephrine, 10 to 30 μg/min, into the celiac artery or vasopressin (Pitressin), 0.1 to 0.3 unit/min, into the left gastric artery are equally encouraging. In one series the bleeding in five of eight patients was controlled by either drug.[32] Treatment failures are likely to occur when superselective positioning of the catheter cannot be achieved or when severe thrombocytopenia or any established bleeding diathesis exist.

In cases in which bleeding cannot be controlled after a period of 3 hours, infusion is terminated. However, if some response has occurred during the first treatment or if bleeding recurs after it had ceased temporarily, infusion may be resumed for a second period of 24 hours. The chances of pharmacologic control by arterial infusion are poor in patients with peptic ulcer disease and malignant gastric and small bowel tumors. Recently, selective arterial embolization with an autologous blood clot has been tried in patients with duodenal ulceration[31] and with pelvic fractures causing bleeding from larger arteries.

ENDOSCOPIC RETROGRADE CHOLANGIOPANCREATOGRAPHY

The perfection of fiber optic endoscopes has provided a new approach to the evaluation of upper and lower gastrointestinal disorders. The endoscope, designed specifically for duodenal observation and cannulation of the papilla of Vater, has been used to develop an effective technique for the contrast visualization of the pancreatic as well as the biliary duct systems.*

Recent improvements in instrumentation and in the skill of the examiners have made this procedure reliable and safe. It has become an accepted clinical examination yielding information heretofore obtainable only by percutaneous cholangiography, laparoscopy, or abdominal exploratory surgery.

Method of examination

The fasting patient is sedated in the radiology department using an intravenous drip of diazepam (Valium). A level of cooperative somnolence is attained by the slow administration of 5 to 30 mg. In addition to 0.6 mg of atropine, 0.5 to 1.0 mg of glucagon is given intravenously periodically throughout the procedure (0.5 mg every 20 minutes) to achieve duodenal atony and papil-

---

*For further information, see Burwood et al.,[6] Doubilet et al.,[12] Kasugai et al.,[16,17] Ogoshi et al.,[24] and Silvis et al.[30]

lary smooth muscle relaxation. The patient is examined on a padded x-ray table, and the instrument is gently passed through the stomach and duodenal bulb into the descending duodenum. The patient is then turned from an initial left lateral position into prone position, permitting the observers a more panoramic view of the descending duodenum and proper air distribution about the papilla of Vater. Air may have to be insufflated for visualization of the papilla. The papilla is usually seen as a raised structure on the posterior medial wall about 6 to 8 cm beyond the bulb.[12,30] The cannula is engaged with its tip into the ductal orifice and advanced into the ductal lumen proper. Usually 2 to 5 ml of contrast material (Renografin 50%) is cautiously injected under close fluoroscopic control. If visualization of the pancreatic duct alone occurs, injection should be slow to avoid overdistention. However, it may be desirable to increase the injection pressure slightly to fill branches of the first and second order, in which early signs of chronic inflammatory disease are frequently observed. One radiograph may be taken at this time, while additional films are obtained after withdrawal of the cannula. While the normal duct system empties in a matter of a few minutes, delayed emptying indicates the presence of a pathologic condition. Attempts are usually also made to visualize the biliary duct system; the scope is repositioned with the patient in either a prone or left lateral position, and as much as 40 ml of Renografin is needed. The common bile duct requires entry of the cannula with the tip oriented in a cephalad direction. Frequently both ductal systems are filled simultaneously; again, slow filling should be attempted to avoid overdistention of the more fragile pancreatic duct. In the presence of a patent cystic duct the gallbladder may be visualized. Spot films of the ductal system and the gallbladder should be taken throughout the procedure as these structures fill with contrast material.

Films of the pancreatic duct can usually be taken up to 1 minute after completion of the injection, at which time emptying occurs rapidly. Biliary tree visualization in most instances is satisfactory up to 10 minutes following injection. Spot films from a high-resolution image intensifier provide the desirable detail of secondary branches from the pancreatic and biliary ducts (Fig. 10-16). Average examination time varies between 15 and 45 minutes. Successful cannulation is achieved in 75% to 85% of all cases, with filling of the desired duct in 60% to 70%.

Indications

Retrograde examination of the biliary tract should be considered in patients with jaundice of more than 3 weeks' duration in the absence of a specific diagnosis. The study is particularly helpful in those patients in whom there is doubt as to whether jaundice is due to biliary tract obstruction or hepatocellular disease. Patients with undiagnosed upper abdominal pain after cholecystectomy usually benefit by transduodenal cholangiography. Furthermore, it

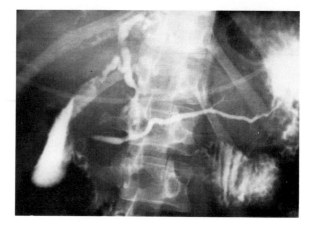

Fig. 10-15. Normal pancreatocholangiogram after withdrawal of endoscope. Note horizontal course of main pancreatic duct with visualization of some branches. Biliary ducts and gallbladder partly opacified. Some contrast material in stomach and small intestine. (Courtesy Dr. Francis B. Milligan and Dr. Bob W. Gayler, Baltimore, Md.)

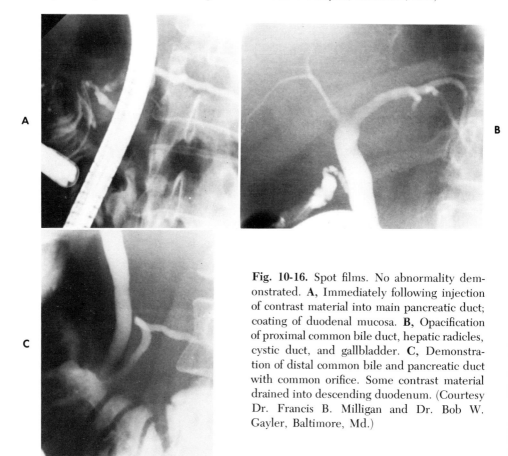

Fig. 10-16. Spot films. No abnormality demonstrated. **A,** Immediately following injection of contrast material into main pancreatic duct; coating of duodenal mucosa. **B,** Opacification of proximal common bile duct, hepatic radicles, cystic duct, and gallbladder. **C,** Demonstration of distal common bile and pancreatic duct with common orifice. Some contrast material drained into descending duodenum. (Courtesy Dr. Francis B. Milligan and Dr. Bob W. Gayler, Baltimore, Md.)

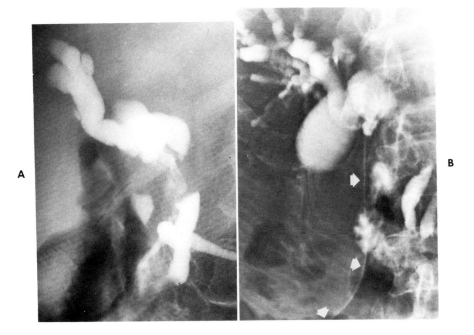

Fig. 10-17. Carcinoma of common bile duct. **A,** Large filling defect of duct involving ductal bifurcation. Considerable dilatation of hepatic ducts. **B,** Huge gallbladder (Courvoisier's sign) indicated by arrows. Also note marked dilatation of cystic duct. (Courtesy Dr. Francis B. Milligan and Dr. Bob W. Gayler, Baltimore, Md.)

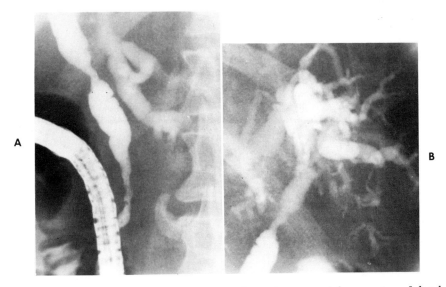

Fig. 10-18. Carcinoma of gastric antrum. **A,** Stenotic, segmental narrowing of distal common bile duct with proximal dilatation due to invading tumor tissue. Second short segment of narrowing in region of cystic duct, not opacified due to obstruction (tumor extension). **B,** View of dilated hepatic ducts and branches. Patient in left posterior oblique position. (Courtesy Dr. Francis B. Milligan and Dr. Bob W. Gayler, Baltimore, Md.)

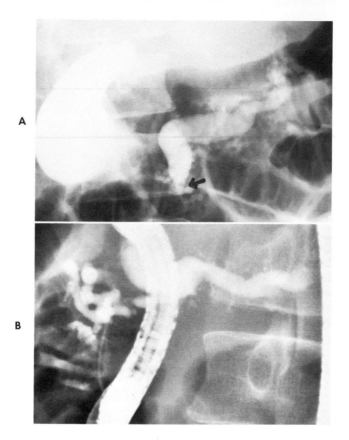

Fig. 10-19. Chronic pancreatitis. **A,** Dilated tortuous main pancreatic duct with proximal tapering (arrow) due to stenosis. Gallbladder opacified. Patient in left posterior oblique position. **B,** Small branch ducts dilated and distorted; partial filling of distal biliary duct and duodenum. Patient in right posterior oblique position. (Courtesy Dr. Francis B. Milligan and Dr. Bob W. Gayler, Baltimore, Md.)

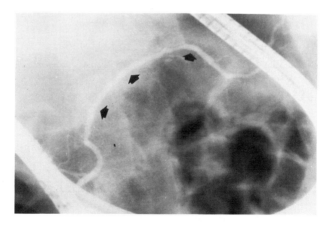

Fig. 10-20. Pseudocyst of pancreas. Marked displacement and deformity of main pancreatic duct (arrows). (Courtesy Dr. Francis B. Milligan and Dr. Bob W. Gayler, Baltimore, Md.)

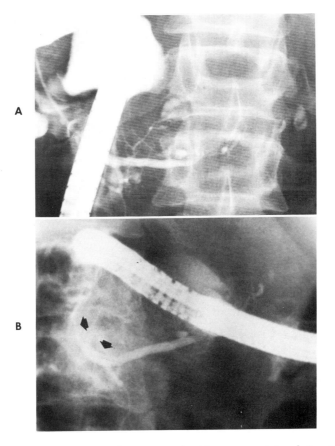

Fig. 10-21. Adenocarcinoma of pancreas. **A,** Almost complete obstruction of main pancreatic duct. Cystic dilatation of several branches. **B,** Curvilinear downward displacement of main pancreatic duct due to tumor mass in head of pancreas (arrows). (Courtesy Dr. Francis B. Milligan and Dr. Bob W. Gayler, Baltimore, Md.)

is indicated in suspected chronic pancreatitis and ductal and stenosing carcinoma of the pancreas. Whenever a pseudocyst of the pancreas fills with contrast material, surgical intervention is usually required within a period of 6 hours.

In the absence of convincing results using scintigraphy, ultrasound B scanning, and angiography, endoscopic retrograde cholangiopancreatography promises to be a useful diagnostic technique for radiologists and gastroenterologists alike. Examples of normal studies and those with pancreatic and biliary duct abnormalities show characteristic radiologic findings (Figs. 10-15 to 10-21).

References

1. Baum, S., and Nusbaum, M.: The control of gastrointestinal hemorrhage by selective mesenteric arterial infusion of vasopressin, Radiology **98:**497, 1971.

2. Baum, S., et al.: The preoperative radiographic demonstration of intra-abdominal bleeding from undetermined sites by percutaneous selective celiac and superior mesenteric arteriography, Surgery **58**:797, 1965.

3. Baum, S., et al.: Angiography in the diagnosis of gastrointestinal bleeding, Arch. Intern. Med. **119**:16, 1967.

4. Bernstein, L. M., and Baker, L. A.: A clinical test for esophagitis, Gastroenterology **34**:760, 1958.

5. Bosma, J. F.: Deglutition—pharyngeal stage, Physiol. Rev. **37**:275, 1957.

6. Burwood, R. J., et al.: Endoscopic retrograde choledocho-pancreatography: a review with a report of a collaborative series, Clin. Radiol. **24**:397, 1973.

7. Conn, H. O., Ramsby, G. R., and Storer, E. H.: Selective intraarterial vasopressin in the treatment of upper gastrointestinal hemmorrhage, Gastroenterology **63**:634, 1972.

8. Donner, M. W.: Der Schluckvorgang mit saurem Barium: ein neuartiger Röntgentest bei Patienten mit Refluxbeschwerden, Radiologe **9**(suppl.): 372, 1973.

9. Donner, M. W., and Siegel, C. I.: The evaluation of pharyngeal neuromuscular disorders by cinefluorography, Am. J. Roentgenol. **94**:299, 1965.

10. Donner, M. W., and Silbiger, M. L.: Cinefluorographic analysis of pharyngeal swallowing in neuromuscular disorders, Am. J. Med. Sci. **251**:134, 1966.

11. Donner, M. W., Silbiger, M. L., Hookman, P., and Hendrix, T. R.: Acid-barium swallows in the radiographic evaluation of clinical esophagitis, Radiology **87**:220, 1966.

12. Doubilet, H., Poppel, M. H., and Mulholland, J. H.: Pancreatography: technics, principles and observations, Radiology **64**:325, 1955.

13. Gelfand, D. W., and Hachiya, J.: The double-contrast examination of the stomach using gas-producing granules and tablets, Radiology **93**:1381, 1969.

14. Hendrix, T. R.: Dysphagia and heartburn. In Harvey, A. M., Johns, R. J., Owens, A. H., and Ross, R. S., editors: The principles and practice of medicine, ed. 18, New York, 1972, Appleton-Century-Crofts.

15. Ingelfinger, F. J.: Esophageal motility, Physiol. Rev. **38**:533, 1958.

16. Kasugai, T., Kuno, N., Kobayashi, S., and Hattori, K.: Endoscopic pancreatocholangiography. I. The normal endoscopic pancreatocholangiogram, Gastroenterology **63**:217, 1972.

17. Kasugai, T., et al.: Endoscopic pancreatocholangiography. II. The pathological endoscopic pancreatocholangiogram, Gastroenterology **63**:227, 1972.

18. Kawai, K., et al.: Double-contrast radiograph on routine examination of the stomach, Am. J. Gastroenterol. **53**:147, 1972.

19. Klein, H. J., Alfidi, R. J., Meaney, T. F., and Poirier, V. C.: Angiography in the diagnosis of chronic gastrointestinal bleeding, Radiology **98**:83, 1971.

20. Koehler, P. R., and Salmon, R. B.: Angiographic localization of unknown acute gastrointestinal bleeding sites, Radiology **89**:244, 1967.

21. McCall, I. W., Davies, E. R., and Delahunty, J. E.: The acid-barium test as an index of intermittent gastro-oesophageal reflux, Br. J. Radiol **46**:578, 1973.

22. Murray-Lyon, I. M., et al.: Treatment of bleeding oesophageal varices by infusion of vasopressin into the superior mesenteric artery, Gut **14**:59, 1973.

23. Obata, W. G.: A double contrast technique for examination of the stomach using barium sulfate with simethicone, Am. J. Roentgenol. **115**:275, 1972.

24. Ogoshi, K., Niwa, M., Hara, Y., and Nebel, O. T.: Endoscopic pancreatocholangiography in the evaluation of pancreatic and biliary disease, Gastroenterology **64**:210, 1973.

25. Rosch, J., Dotter, C. T., and Antonovic, R.: Selective vasoconstrictor infusion in

the management of arterio-capillary gastrointestinal hemorrhage, Am. J. Roentgenol. **116:**279, 1972.

26. Rosch, J., Dotter, C. T., and Rose, R. W.: Selective arterial infusions of vasoconstrictors in acute gastrointestinal bleeding, Radiology **99:**27, 1971.

27. Rosch, J., et al.: Selective arterial drug infusions in the treatment of acute gastrointestinal bleeding: a preliminary report, Gastroenterology **59:**341, 1970.

28. Siegel, C. I., and Hendrix, T. R.: Esophageal motor abnormalities induced by acid perfusion in patients with heartburn, J. Clin. Invest. **42:**686, 1963.

29. Silbiger, M. L., Pikielney, R., and Donner, M. W.: Neuromuscular disorders affecting the pharynx: cineradiographic analysis, Invest. Radiol. **2:**442, 1967.

30. Silvis, S. E., Rohrmann, C. A., and Vennes, J. A.: Diagnostic criteria for the evaluation of the endoscopic pancreatogram, Gastrointest. Endosc. **20:**51, 1973.

31. White, R. I., Jr., Giargiana, F. A., Jr., and Bell, W.: Bleeding duodenal ulcer control. Selective arterial embolization with autologous blood clot, J.A.M.A. **229:**546, 1974.

32. White, R. I., Jr., et al.: Pharmacologic control of hemorrhagic gastritis—clinical and experimental results, Radiology **111:**549, 1974.

11 Emergency nuclear medicine

A. Everette James, Jr., Atsuko Heshiki, Ralph E. Coleman,
and Barry A. Siegel

GENERAL CONSIDERATIONS

In this chapter we will discuss the use of tracer quantities of radioactive material to detect and measure altered physiologic processes. Nuclear medicine procedures performed in emergency situations do not represent different tests but involve a different emphasis of the diagnostic technique and clinical considerations that make the performance of emergency nuclear medicine studies unique in their application.[64,107]

Because of the complexity, size, and expense of the imaging devices employed in nuclear medicine, most hospitals commonly have these facilities in a central location that is often not in immediate proximity to the emergency care area. However, with renewed interest in the delivery of health care in emergencies, small nuclear medicine units are being placed in the emergency areas of certain hospitals. Instrument manufacturers have become interested in the possibilities of compact, self-contained, mobile nuclear medicine imaging devices. These probably will be developed in the next few years and will provide the flexibility necessary to perform studies in the primary emergency treatment area.

In general, nuclear medicine studies require little in the way of patient cooperation, are not hazardous to the patient, and employ such small amounts of injected radiopharmaceuticals that they do not alter body functions or impose stress upon what may be a compromised physiologic situation. These procedures are also subject to accurate quantification and are not as time consuming as many other types of diagnostic tests.[28,50]

The noninvasive nature and simplicity of performing nuclear medicine studies is particularly appealing in emergency situations.[7] Radiopharmaceuticals may well be injected intravenously and other diagnostic tests performed or treatment instituted prior to the initiation of the imaging portion of the nuclear medicine study. Except for dynamic imaging, there is considerable latitude with regard to the time between injection of the radiopharmaceutical and the point at which diagnostic images may be obtained.

Throughout this chapter we will not only emphasize the value of nuclear medicine studies in emergency clinical situations but intend also to point out areas in which nuclear medicine studies are unlikely to provide additional data that are definitive enough to be clinically useful. Thus we hope to identify those circumstances in which nuclear medicine techniques would not be profitably employed but would represent only another diagnostic test. If there is an alternative diagnostic study that provides greater specific information with as little risk to the patient, we recommend that the clinician decide in favor of this study.

PULMONARY PROCEDURES

Patients with chest disease often present difficult diagnostic problems. Pulmonary thromboembolism can manifest a variety of signs and symptoms. In a large study, only approximately 25% of patients with pulmonary thromboembolism had characteristic signs and symptoms of this disorder. Hemoptysis has been considered a common manifestation of pulmonary embolism; yet in a large series of patients with embolism this sign was present in only 11%.[66] Serum enzyme studies are also not very sensitive and certainly are not specific for pulmonary embolism. An elevated serum LDH may be helpful in confirming the diagnosis, but a normal result does not exclude the diagnosis of pulmonary emboli.[96] Of the laboratory determinations, the pO_2 is probably the most reliable in diagnosing pulmonary emboli. A normal arterial pO_2 makes the diagnosis of pulmonary emboli most unlikely.[66,102]

Patients may arrive in the emergency care area with symptoms of vague chest pain, shortness of breath, cough, low-grade fever, and a questionable history of hemoptysis. Chest trauma can usually be excluded by history and physical examination; the differential diagnosis usually includes pulmonary thromboembolism, myocardial infarction, and inflammatory lung disease. If the patient has recently been confined to bed or undergone surgery, then atelectasis, pneumonia, and pulmonary embolism are all reasonable possibilities. If shortness of breath is accompanied by wheezing, asthma must also be excluded.

Perfusion studies using labeled albumin macroaggregates or microspheres to examine regional blood flow are the most commonly performed emergency nuclear medicine procedure.[82,104] Inhalation of a gas such as ^{133}Xe or an aerosol mist are procedures used to detect airway pathology.[80] The usual indication is to exclude pulmonary emboli as the cause of the patient's respiratory symptoms (Fig. 11-1).

Perfusion lung scans accurately reflect regional distribution of pulmonary blood flow and are sensitive but not specific for the presence of major pulmonary emboli.[71] Characteristically, pulmonary emboli produce multiple segmental defects on the lung scan that are peripheral in location[107] (Fig. 11-2). A concomitant good-quality upright chest radiograph should be obtained. Generally in cases of pulmonary embolism the chest radiograph is normal, although pleural effusion, atelectasis, areas of diminished vascularity, elevation of the diaphragm, or signs of pulmonary edema may be present.[51,53,55] If per-

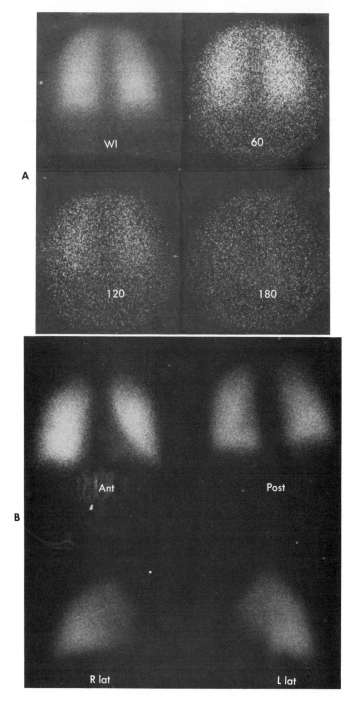

Fig. 11-1. Normal ventilation-perfusion study. **A,** Ventilation images were obtained in posterior projection. Following 3- to 4-minute wash-in period (*WI*) of ^{133}Xe, there is uniform distribution of radioactivity throughout both lungs. Images obtained during washout phase at 60, 120, and 180 seconds demonstrate rapid, symmetric clearance of activity from lungs that is essentially complete by 3 minutes. **B,** Four-view perfusion lung scan obtained on same patient with ^{99m}Tc-human albumin microspheres demonstrates uniform distribution of activity throughout lung fields. Note on anterior and left lateral views that diminished activity is in region of cardiac impression on left lung.

fusion abnormalities are present in areas that are normal on the chest radiograph, then the probability that these defects are due to pulmonary emboli is increased (Fig. 11-3). However, the chest radiograph may not detect areas of lung with abnormal ventilation (due to asthma or chronic obstructive pulmonary disease, for example) that can also be associated with perfusion defects. These perfusion defects often cannot be differentiated from those of pulmonary emboli, although the defects associated with ventilatory abnormalities are usually diffuse, irregular, and nonsegmental.[33] Alderson et al.[2] found that approximately 50% of patients with obstructive pulmonary disease diagnosed by a ^{133}Xe ventilation study exhibit no radiographic evidence of this disorder. Of the patients with normal chest radiographs, 80% had perfusion defects in areas of abnormal ventilation with prolonged ^{133}Xe retention. Thus the emer-

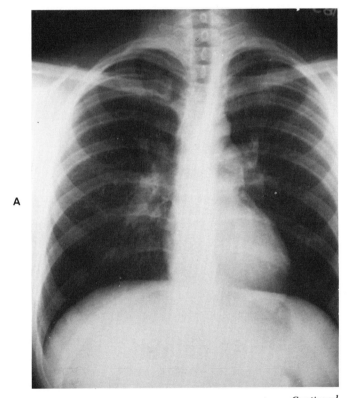

A

Continued.

Fig. 11-2. Multiple pulmonary emboli. This 22-year-old male presented with shortness of breath. **A,** Chest radiograph was normal. **B,** [133]Xe ventilation study demonstrates uniform distribution of activity at end of wash-in period (*WI*) with symmetric clearance of activity at normal rate during washout phase of study. **C,** Perfusion lung scan demonstrates multiple segmental perfusion defects throughout both lungs. Presence of multiple pulmonary emboli was confirmed by pulmonary angiogram.

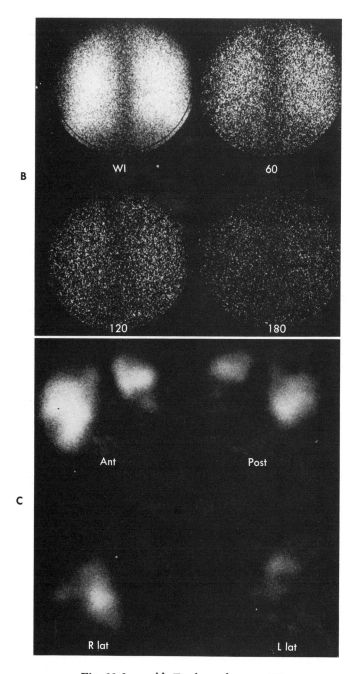

Fig. 11-2, cont'd. For legend see p. 261.

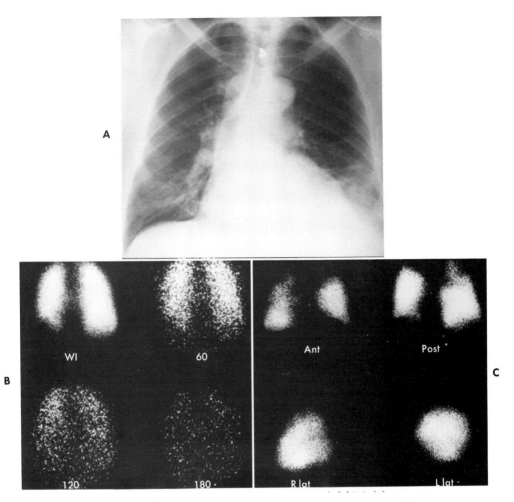

Fig. 11-3. Pulmonary embolism with infarction. **A,** Chest radiograph demonstrates left lower lobe infiltrate in 55-year-old man with recent onset of pleuritic chest pain. **B,** Xenon ventilation study demonstrates no wash-in of radioactivity at left base in area of infiltrate. Wash-in to other portions of lungs is uniform and washout is normal. **C,** Perfusion lung scan shows absence of perfusion to left base in area of radiographic infiltration. Other perfusion defects are also present in both upper lobes and at right lung base. Finding of additional perfusion defects in regions that are normally ventilated and appear normal radiographically supports diagnosis of multiple pulmonary emboli and suggests that most likely etiology of left lower lobe infiltrate is associated infarction.

gency lung scanning procedure should optimally include an evaluation of both pulmonary ventilation and perfusion for greater diagnostic specificity.

If after a review of the chest radiograph, ventilation-perfusion study, patient history, and laboratory findings the diagnosis of pulmonary thromboembolism is still in doubt, or if embolectomy is contemplated, contrast angiography studies should be performed. Pulmonary angiography is a very specific but somewhat insensitive method of diagnosing pulmonary emboli.[9] The sensitivity of this study can be increased by selective catheterization of those segmental arteries supplying the areas of perfusion defects seen on the lung scan and by the use of magnification techniques in the diagnosis of small emboli.

Obstructive pulmonary disease can be diagnosed by characteristic ventilation abnormalities (Fig. 11-4). Irregular areas of ventilation seen on the wash-in (inhalation) image with retention of ^{133}Xe seen on washout (exhalation) images are noted with obstructive airway disease. Of these patients, 90% have associated perfusion abnormalities.[2] Patients with bronchiectasis (Fig. 11-5) and acute bronchitis may also have large perfusion defects that will correspond to areas of abnormal ventilation.[3,48] Patients with pulmonary embolism alone have a normal xenon ventilation study. Although animal studies have shown increased airway resistance after pulmonary emboli, this is short lived and is not often present at the time of the ventilation study.[100]

If a patient enters the emergency room with respiratory distress and wheezing is present on physical examination, an asthmatic attack must be excluded, since segmental perfusion defects can be seen on the lung scan in asthma.[116]

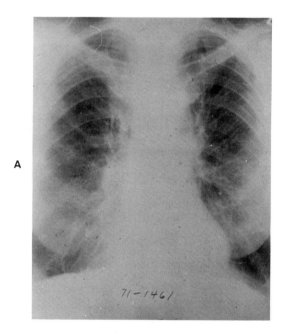

Fig. 11-4. Chronic obstructive pulmonary disease. **A,** Chest radiograph of 66-year-old man with known alpha-1 antitrypsin deficiency showing flattened diaphragm and peripheral pulmonary vascular attenuation. **B,** Ventilation study demonstrating incomplete ^{133}Xe wash-in at right lung base and delayed washout of xenon from right base and midzone and left base. **C,** Perfusion lung scan showing irregular perfusion defects of both lower lobes.

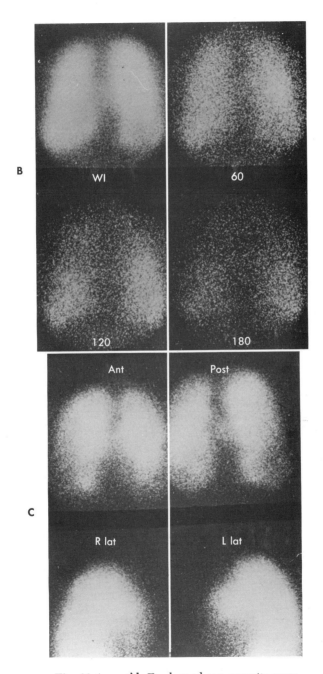

Fig. 11-4, cont'd. For legend see opposite page.

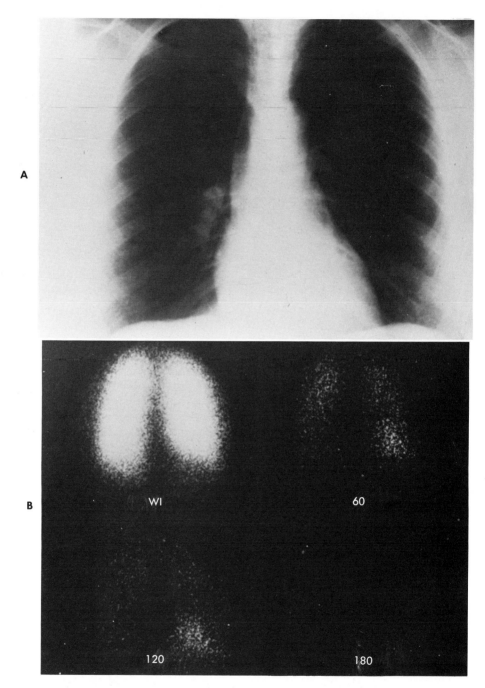

Fig. 11-5. Bronchiectasis. **A,** Normal chest radiograph of 58-year-old woman with right pleuritic chest pain. **B,** Ventilation study showing diminished wash-in at right lung base and delayed clearance from same region. **C,** Perfusion lung scan demonstrating single defect in right posterior basal segment. **D,** Bronchogram demonstrating localized bronchiectasis in right lower lobe.

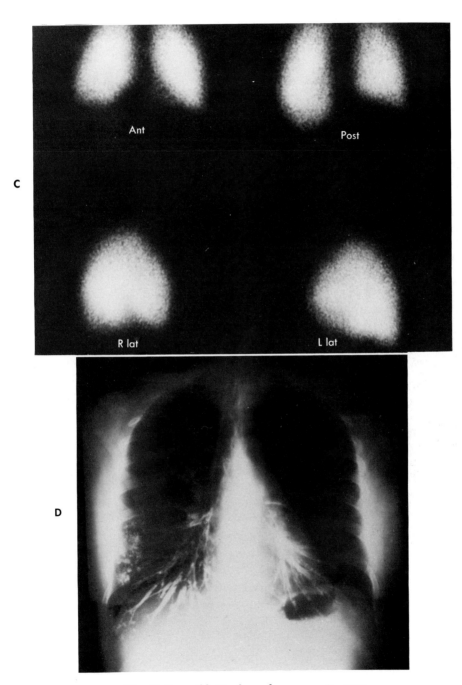

C

Ant

Post

R lat

L lat

D

Fig. 11-5, cont'd. For legend see opposite page.

Often the patient's clinical history is helpful in differentiation, but recurrent episodes of pulmonary emboli can be manifest clinically in a manner similar to episodes of asthma.[110] Ventilation studies with ^{133}Xe may be helpful in differentiating the perfusion defects of pulmonary emboli from those of asthma. If the perfusion defects occur only in regions of abnormal ventilation, pulmonary embolism is unlikely. However, if there are perfusion defects in regions of normal ventilation, pulmonary embolism becomes a more likely diagnosis. After treatment of asthmatic patients with relief of bronchospasm, the ventilation and perfusion studies usually return to normal.

Patients with acute myocardial infarction may have respiratory distress from pulmonary edema. The accompanying chest pain often is not characteristic of infarction. Perfusion lung scans may demonstrate multiple small, nonsegmental defects.[54] If alveolar edema is present, focal defects corresponding to the location of the edema fluid will be seen.[51] Chest radiographs of sufficient quality to assess the pulmonary vessel wall-air interface and electrocardiograms will greatly aid in differentiation of myocardial infarction from pulmonary embolism. A ventilation study generally will not be of much help in this differential problem unless underlying obstructive lung disease is also present. In patients with myocardial infarction, further evaluation by contrast angiography is to be avoided.

Trauma to the chest wall can result in perfusion and ventilation changes that are primarily the result of the destruction of underlying lung parenchyma or that occur secondary to pathophysiologic alterations accompanying splinting, atelectasis, mucus plugs, elevation of the diaphragm, or intrapulmonary shunting of blood. In patients with rib fractures, perfusion defects in the areas of the fracture (often larger than might be expected) are generally noted. With closed chest trauma it is well known that the trauma to the lung due to rapid deceleration and shearing forces is not manifested on chest radiographs for several hours;[8] alveolar densities may occur days later. Perfusion lung scans will usually be abnormal immediately. In a series on experimental animals subjected to closed chest trauma, Rutherford et al.[93] found that those animals with perfusion defects on lung scans subsequently developed respiratory difficulty, and alveolar densities became apparent on chest radiographs.

It is well known that pleural reactions occur secondary to chest trauma. With the patient lying prone or supine, the pleural effusion will be spread over a large surface area and will cause a generalized diminished perfusion to an entire lung, which will change with alteration of patient position.[53,55,69,105] If the pleural fluid extends into the major interlobar fissure, a linear perfusion defect, the so-called fissure sign, may be seen.[53]

Lung contusions are infrequently studied by means of nuclear medicine procedures (Fig. 11-6). In opacification of the lung due to trauma it is often important to establish whether or not perfusion is present to the affected side (Fig. 11-7). Lung scans can provide this information in a noninvasive manner.

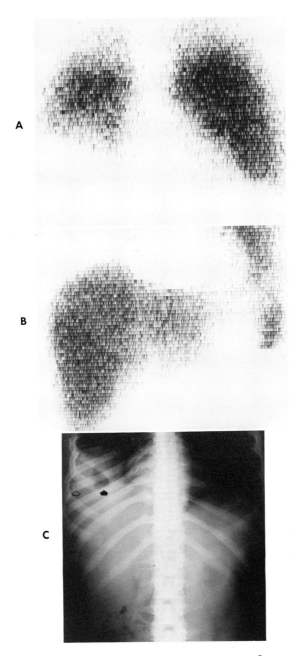

Fig. 11-6. Pulmonary contusion with abscess. **A,** Anterior perfusion scan obtained with 99mTc-human albumin microspheres showing large perfusion defect in right lower lobe. **B,** Anterior view of liver-lung study obtained immediately after lung scan by administering 99mTc-sulfur colloid, again showing perfusion defect in right lower lobe and normal superior border of liver. This localizes abnormality to right lower lobe. **C,** Abdominal radiograph shows loss of definition of right diaphragm with elevation, rib fractures (open arrow), and collection of air (closed arrow) either within area of right lower lobe or pleural space. Patient had suffered trauma to right chest, with multiple rib fractures and contusion of right lower lobe with subsequent abscess formation. (From Sanders, R. C.: Am. J. Surg. **124:**346, 1972.)

Localized hematomas are probably more accurately studied by means of serial chest radiographs and fluoroscopy.

Trauma or infection within the abdomen can cause perfusion abnormalities in the lower lobes without the appearance of concomitant abnormalities on the chest radiograph. Subdiaphragmatic infectious processes often are manifested by pain, fever, and respiratory distress. If the chest radiograph is normal, a combined lung-liver scan will often aid in the exact localization of the

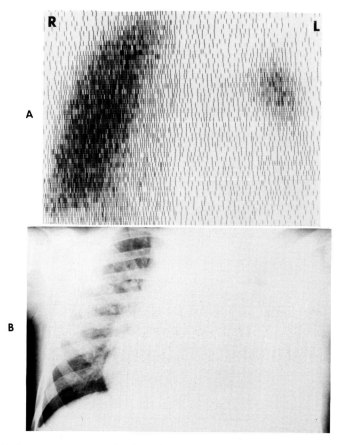

Fig. 11-7. Lung contusion with pleural effusion. **A,** Anterior perfusion scan showing nearly complete absence of perfusion to left lung. **B,** Chest radiograph shows opacification of entire left hemithorax due to contusion and pleural effusion following trauma in automobile accident. **C,** Anterior perfusion scan 5 days later shows no change in perfusion to left lung. **D,** Chest radiograph after partial lobectomy, again showing opacification of left chest. As there was no improvement in perfusion to left lung, it was decided to resect large contusion as well as to remove pleural fluid to improve respiratory status. (From James, A. E., and Squires, L. F.: Nuclear radiology, Philadelphia, 1973, W. B. Saunders Co.)

disease process. This will be subsequently considered in the discussion of gastrointestinal procedures.

Diaphragmatic ruptures, herniations, and congenital absence of the muscular portion must be differentiated from eventrations. These abnormalities often produce acute respiratory difficulty due to compression of normal lung tissue. Chest radiographs obtained in various positions and fluoroscopic examination should be employed initially, for they can be performed rapidly and

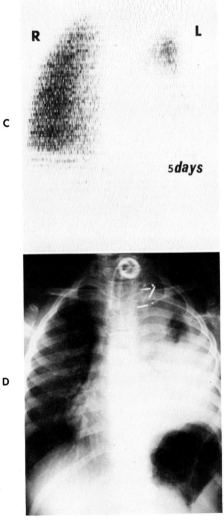

Fig. 11-7, cont'd. For legend see opposite page.

usually result in a correct diagnosis. Rarely, the location of the liver cannot be established by these means. In this clinical circumstance, correlation of liver scans with chest radiographs, a combined lung-liver scan, or dynamic imaging of pulmonary and hepatic blood flow will often accurately depict the location and position of the liver.

Thus lung scanning is a deservedly popular emergency nuclear medicine procedure. The use of emergency lung scans in cases of suspected pulmonary embolism has recently been evaluated in a prospective study by Tetalman et al.[104] In a series of 224 patients undergoing lung scanning, anticoagulation therapy was originally contemplated in 211. As a result of the scan findings, only 83 patients received anticoagulation therapy and only 18 of 50 patients with some contraindication to such therapy were so treated. Similarly, the need for arteriography was often obviated by the results of the lung scan and unnecessary hospitalization was prevented. In summary, the specificity of the lung scan procedure can be increased with an accompanying ventilation-imaging procedure. Correlation with a good quality upright chest radiograph is also necessary for correct interpretation of the lung scan.

NEUROLOGIC PROCEDURES

Nuclear medicine procedures now play a major role in the early evaluation of the patient with acute neurologic disease. Not uncommonly, patients arrive unconscious at the emergency room; often no relevant history can be obtained. Intracranial trauma may be suspected even without external physical signs. Skull radiographs provide a very insensitive screening test for underlying intracranial disease. Cerebral radionuclide angiograms and brain scans are of great value in these circumstances.[68]

Superficial lesions of the scalp and cranial vault can yield abnormal brain scans (Fig. 11-8). Alteration of the permeability of the walls of small blood vessels in the area, an increase in regional blood flow, and other explanations have been proposed to account for the abnormalities on the brain scan.

Often requests are made for radionuclide brain imaging in patients with known cranial trauma.[35,45] Even in this situation brain scans may be invaluable in establishing the presence of an underlying cerebral contusion or hematoma.[65] Multiple views of the brain should be obtained to characterize the size and depth of any abnormalities. Dynamic studies of the transit of a bolus injection of the radiopharmaceutical will increase the scan specificity in subdural hematomas by documenting the effect of the lesion upon regional cerebral blood flow.[44]

Subdural and epidural fluid collections pose a particularly interesting problem.[43,79] Chronic collections with a well-defined membrane will almost always be accurately delineated on a brain scan, even in infants and young children.[4,12,34] Indicators such as ^{99m}Tc-pertechnetate and ^{131}I-serum albumin are present in high concentrations in the limiting membrane and in the fluid it-

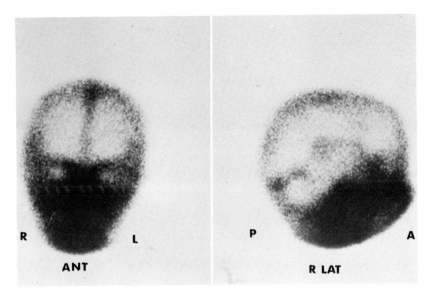

Fig. 11-8. Scalp laceration. Brain scan with superficial area of increased activity in right temporoparietal region apparent only on right lateral view; location corresponded to site of recent scalp laceration.

self. Cowan et al.[14] found an increased accuracy in the detection of subdural hematomas after 10 days. They attributed this to formation of a membrane. Conway and Vollert[12] found an accuracy level of 60% in radionuclide images in detecting dural collections in children, while an 80% accuracy level is reported in adults. The significantly lower detectability in pediatric patients relates to the higher incidence of bilateral subdural hematomas, which are often difficult to diagnose by the brain scan due to the symmetry of the lesions.

Epidural hematomas may be of arterial or venous origin. Those secondary to rupture of the middle meningeal artery usually require immediate definitive therapy. Thus these patients should not undergo nuclear medicine studies unless they can be performed immediately in the emergency treatment area. Epidural hematomas of venous origin may be studied in a routine fashion.

Subdural hematomas typically present with a peripheral band of increased activity seen on the anterior and posterior images, the so-called crescent sign (Fig. 11-9). Large subdural collections may have a rim of increased activity seen on the static images with the adjacent regions filling in on delayed views. This has been described as the "rim sign" and probably represents activity within the subdural membrane.[78] The dynamic study increases the accuracy of detecting subdural hematomas.[44,95] Scalp trauma can produce a crescent sign but would show no displacement of the vessels over the convexity on the dynamic study unless the trauma were accompanied by a subdural hematoma. Also, acute subdural hematomas may exhibit normal static images, whereas

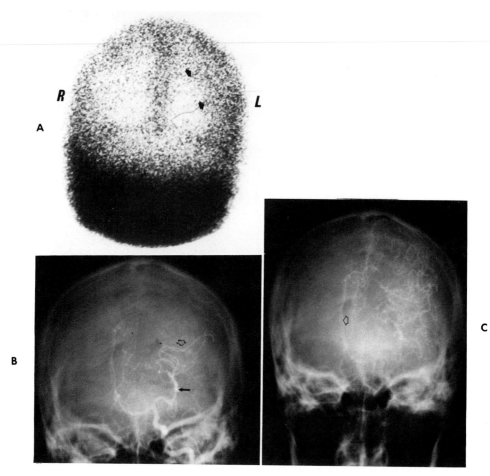

Fig. 11-9. Subdural hematoma. **A,** Posterior view of ^{99m}Tc-pertechnetate brain scan in patient with known trauma to left side of skull. There is increased radioactivity peripherally over left convexity. **B** and **C,** Arterial and delayed arterial phases of cerebral angiogram demonstrate that middle cerebral artery branches are displaced from inner table of calvarium; both middle and anterior cerebral vessels are shifted to the right. Study shows not only presence of subdural hematoma but its effect on intracranial structures.

the dynamic study shows displacement of the convexity vasculature.[78] In addition, cisternographic imaging after subarachnoid radiopharmaceutical injection has been advocated as a method of diagnosing subdural hematomas. Radiopharmaceuticals may on occasion accumulate in the hematoma fluid, but the most common finding is a localized area of diminished radioactivity that indicates arrested or reduced flow in the subarachnoid spaces of the cerebral convexity underlying the hematoma.[86]

Patients brought to an emergency care area often have a history and phys-

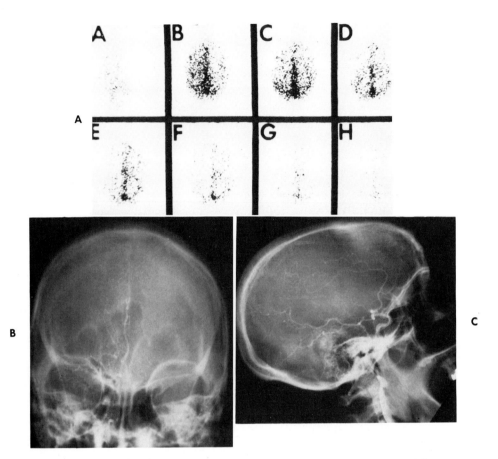

Fig. 11-10. Right middle cerebral artery infarction. **A,** Intravenous radionuclide angiogram in vertex projection from arterial to late venous phases. In early phase of radionuclide transit there is diminished radioactivity on right side, *A* to *C*, with a later increase of activity on that side during the venous phase, *D* to *F*. This type of pattern is often noted with cerebral infarctions and has been termed the "flip" sign. Delayed arrival of activity in infarcted hemisphere is result of collateral circulation. **B** and **C,** Anterior and lateral views of cerebral angiogram showing lack of opacification of middle cerebral artery due to complete occlusion. (Courtesy Dr. David C. Moses, Baltimore, Md.)

ical symptoms suggestive of stroke.[59] Both dynamic and static brain scans have been utilized to great advantage in this clinical problem.[18] Moses et al.[72] found that in 38 patients with acute strokes, the radionuclide cerebral blood flow study was abnormal in 22, while corresponding brain scans were abnormal in only 13. The dynamic study was usually performed in the vertex position (Fig. 11-10) and showed diminished radioactivity in the arterial phase of the study with increased radioactivity on the side of the abnormality in the later phases ("flip"). A number of other authors have advocated radiopertechnetate cerebral angiography in the anterior position with particular attention to the radioactivity in the carotid artery[25] (Fig. 11-11). Although the combination of unilaterally decreased hemispheric perfusion and a normal static scan has been said to be quite characteristic of recent infarction, these findings may also occur in normal patients and in those with nonfocal neurologic disorders.[88] Thus careful clinical correlation is required in the interpretation of these studies.

Whether or not a cerebral artery occlusion is seen on the radionuclide study depends upon its size, location, and the interval between the insult and performance of the scan.[39,85,99] Lesions of major branches of the middle cerebral artery are much more likely to yield positive results in studies than are occlusions of the anterior or posterior cerebral arteries.[18] Hemorrhagic infarcts produce positive results more often than ischemic ones. Molinari et al.,[70] in utilizing serial brain scans in patients with cerebral infarction, reported

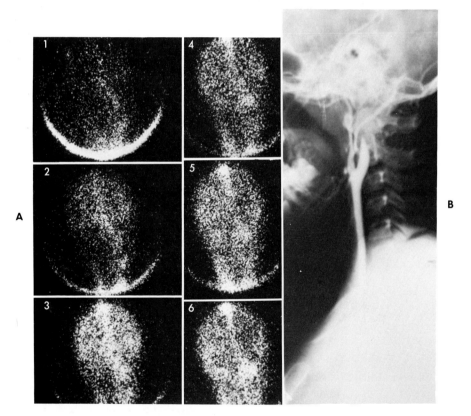

Fig. 11-11. Internal carotid artery obstruction. **A,** Intravenous radionuclide angiograms in anterior projection, including both neck and head. Lack of flow in right internal carotid artery is best seen in early arterial phase and early venous phase, *1* to *3*. **B,** Lateral view of carotid angiogram with complete occlusion of right internal carotid artery.

that these studies are often negative for several days to a week (Fig. 11-12). By the second to third week, the scans of 70% to 80% of his patients were abnormal; these returned to normal in 60 to 80 days. Glascow et al.[36] found that within 8 to 28 days after infarction, the scans of 86% of the patients were abnormal. Scans of patients with transient ischemic attacks will not usually be abnormal,[72] and in our experience such patients also have normal dynamic cerebral transit studies.

Regional cerebral blood flow may be reflected by studies employing both diffusible and nondiffusible indicators.[74,75] These dynamic studies do increase the sensitivity in detecting strokes. In utilizing dynamic studies to examine 72 patients, Rossler[91] reported 100% accuracy in detecting an abnormality. Occasionally areas of infarction remain avascular, and delayed scans performed at long time intervals after radiopharmaceutical injection can increase accuracy.

Subarachnoid hemorrhages do not usually produce abnormal brain scans unless they are accompanied by intracerebral hematomas or cerebral infarction secondary to vascular spasm. Berry aneurysms and arteriovenous malformations (Fig. 11-13), unless they are larger than 1 to 2 cm or associated with bleeding, are not detected by brain scans. However, following a subarachnoid hemorrhage a patient may be seen in the emergency treatment area with signs and symptoms of hydrocephalus.[5,20] In 21 patients evaluated for communicating hydrocephalus by cisternography following subarachnoid hemorrhage,

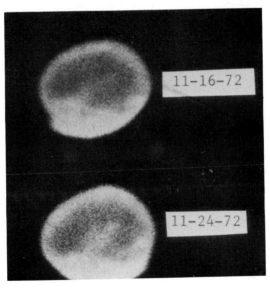

Fig. 11-12. Evolving infarct. Left lateral views of brain scans performed 1 day and 9 days after sudden onset of right hemiplegia. Initial scan is normal, but second study shows increased radioactivity in left temporoparietal region. Cerebral angiography demonstrated branch occlusions in left middle cerebral artery.

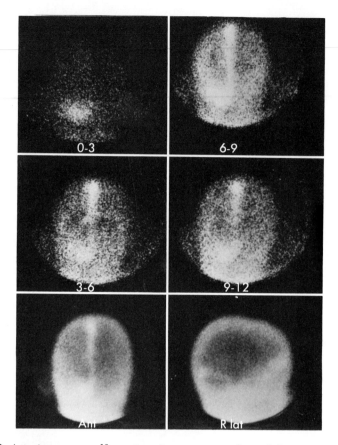

Fig. 11-13. Arteriovenous malformation. Intravenous radionuclide angiogram in anterior projection and static anterior and right lateral views. Dynamic study shows area of early increased activity in right subfrontal region, in which activity subsequently decreases. Static views again demonstrate increased activity in same region. Cerebral angiogram confirmed presence of arteriovenous malformation.

results of 10 studies were positive.[115] Eight patients underwent surgery to create cerebrospinal fluid diversionary shunts, and all but one experienced dramatic neurologic improvement. Rudd et al.[92] examined 9 patients who had suffered subarachnoid hemorrhages from 3 to 26 weeks earlier; all had abnormal cisternograms. These studies suggest that cerebrospinal fluid imaging studies should be considered for a patient presenting to the emergency treatment area with signs and symptoms of acute hydrocephalus.[52,56]

Rapidly growing neoplasms often produce seizurelike episodes or apoplectic onset of symptoms that are difficult to differentiate clinically from strokes. Combined dynamic and static brain scans can often make this differentiation. If a lesion initially shows increased activity on the dynamic study, it is much more likely to be a neoplasm than a cerebral infarction (Fig. 11-14). Neoplasms

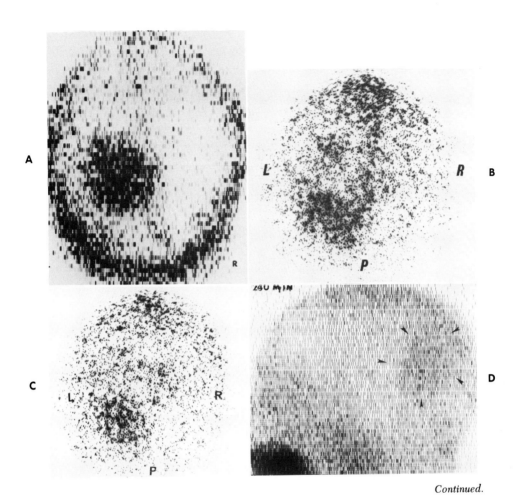

Continued.

Fig. 11-14. Glioblastoma multiforme. **A,** Vertex view of static brain scan with large abnormal area of radioactivity in left posterior parietal area. Intravenous radionuclide angiograms done in vertex position show both early, **B,** and late, **C,** accumulation of radioactivity within lesion noted on static scan. **D,** Four-hour delayed left lateral image shows persistent activity in same area seen on both early static and dynamic studies. **E,** Anterior cerebral angiogram showing inferior and medial displacement of middle cerebral artery with shift of anterior cerebral vessels. **F,** Subtraction study of left lateral cerebral angiogram showing definite tumor stain corresponding in size and location to abnormality noted on radionuclide studies. Branches of external carotid artery (arrows) give blood supply to lesion. (Modified from James, A. E., and Squires, L. F.: Nuclear radiology, Philadelphia, 1973, W. B. Saunders Co.)

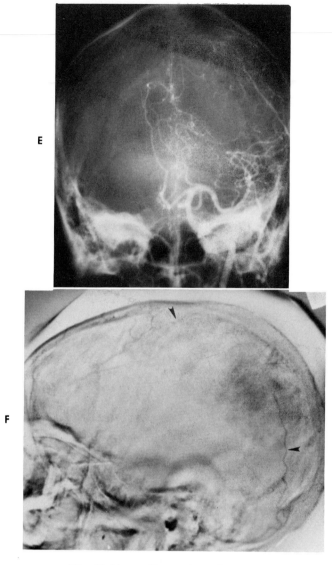

Fig. 11-14, cont'd. For legend see p. 279.

very rarely present as avascular areas on the dynamic brain scan. In addition, positive static scans obtained shortly after the onset of symptoms support a diagnosis of cerebral neoplasm.

Seizure episodes are often the reason that patients are brought to an emergency care center. Seizures whose onset occurs in adulthood are much more often associated with focal brain scan abnormalities than those beginning in childhood. This is especially true if localizing neurologic signs are also present.

In our experience, generalized seizures in adults and children and temporal lobe seizures in children are not often associated with abnormal brain scans.

Brain abscess is much more often a diagnostic problem than textbook descriptions would suggest. Patients are often comatose with only minimal signs of infection. Jordan et al.[58] described several patients in their series that were examined in a hospital for several months before the correct diagnosis of brain abscess was made (Fig. 11-15). In comparing brain scans and angiograms in 20 patients in their series, the brain scan was more sensitive in detecting an area of inflammation. Brain scans have detected abscesses in nearly all cases in several reported series.[16,102] As a word of caution, areas of cerebritis will also produce an abnormality on the brain scan[16] (Fig. 11-16). Therefore a contrast angiogram should be obtained prior to surgical removal or drainage of an abscess. In vivo detection of cerebral edema remains a problem but appears to be an important area for future development.[81]

A potential pathway for bacterial infection of the meninges exists in cerebrospinal fluid rhinorrhea or otorrhea. Accurate localization of the tear in the brain coverings is necessary prior to definitive surgery; this may be difficult to accomplish by means of physical examination or injection of dyes. The injection of small amounts of a radiopharmaceutical into the subarachnoid space and imaging (Fig. 11-17) as well as counting appropriately placed swabs

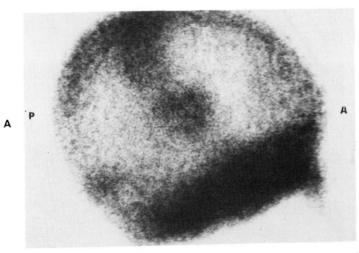

A   P   A

Continued.

Fig. 11-15. Cerebral abscess. **A,** Right lateral view of brain scan with large accumulation of radioactivity in parietal region. Patient had ventricular septal defect and multiple episodes of lethargy and disorientation. Previous studies had been normal. **B** and **C,** Anterior and right lateral views of cerebral angiogram from early arterial and capillary phases of study show both mass effect of abscess as well as vascular stain and partial "rim sign." (Courtesy Dr. Charles M. Jordan, Baltimore, Md.)

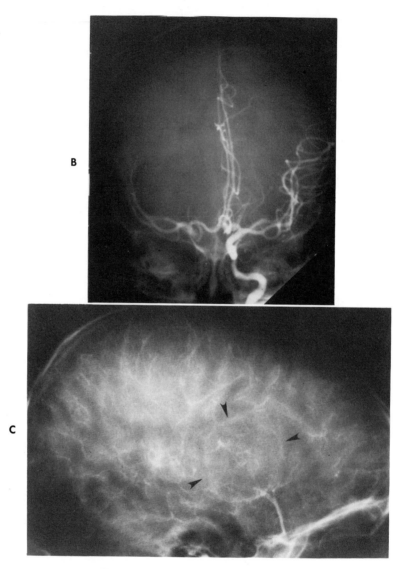

Fig. 11-15, cont'd. For legend see p. 281.

is a sensitive and accurate method of diagnosing cerebrospinal fluid fistulas and leaks. Certain technical modifications of routine cisternographic procedures have been described and should be employed in order to avoid inaccurate diagnoses.[19,20]

Encephalitis due to herpes simplex will often produce abnormal results in a scan.[16,83] The abnormality in most cases is in the temporal lobes, but increased activity in areas of the frontal or parietal lobes can be seen. Encephalitis due to other viruses usually is more diffuse and produces no abnormalities on the brain scan.

The brain scans of patients with meningitis usually are normal or exhibit minimal superficial areas of increased activity. However, subdural effusions associated with meningitis in pediatric patients may be detected by dynamic or static imaging. Tuberculous meningitis, which has mainly basilar involvement, presents on static images with increased activity in the suprasellar region.[63]

Brain death can be determined by injecting a bolus of ^{99m}Tc-pertechnetate and obtaining rapid sequential images or by using a scintillation probe. With cerebral death there is no evidence of cerebral perfusion by imaging and no bolus effect on the probe tracing from the head.[10] The exact role this procedure has in diagnosing cerebral death has not been fully determined, but with flat electroencephalograms over a period of time, they should be diagnostic of cerebral death.[10]

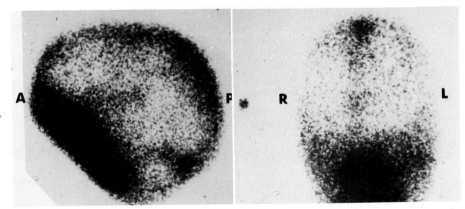

Continued.

Fig. 11-16. Cerebritis. **A,** Left lateral and anterior brain scans with diffuse increase in radioactivity in left hemisphere most marked in posterior parietal region peripherally. **B,** PA and lateral views of cerebral angiogram arterial phase with no displacement of vasculature. **C,** PA and lateral views of cerebral angiogram capillary and early venous phases with early venous filling but no definite stain. Findings are not specific and are felt to represent cerebritis phase of inflammation in acutely ill child with definite inflammatory process. (Courtesy Dr. Charles M. Jordan, Baltimore, Md.)

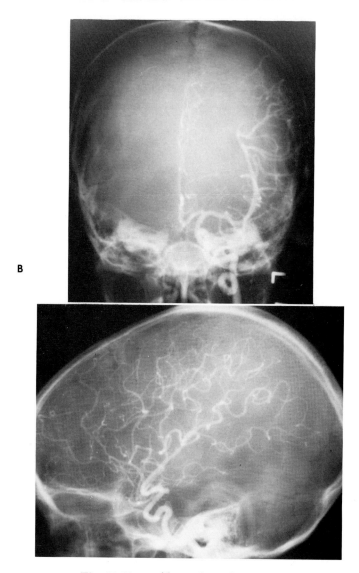

B

Fig. 11-16, cont'd. For legend see p. 283.

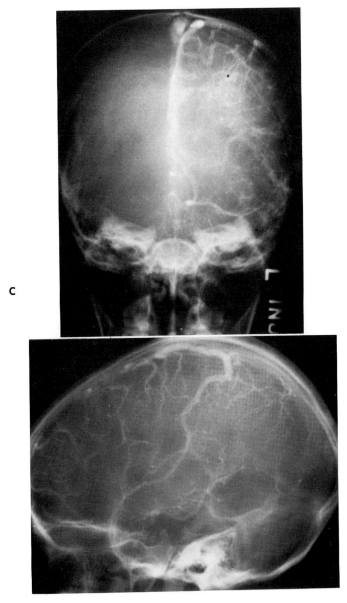

C

Fig. 11-16, cont'd. For legend see p. 283.

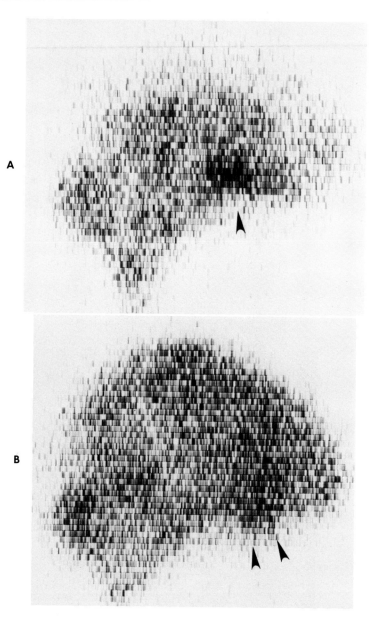

Fig. 11-17. Cerebrospinal fluid fistula. **A,** Right lateral image of cisternogram obtained 2 hours after lumbar subarachnoid injection of ^{111}In-DTPA shows abnormal accumulation of radioactivity in middle cranial fossa. **B,** Right lateral view at 24 hours shows extension of radioactivity inferiorly from middle cranial fossa in manner characteristic of CSF extravasation in that area.

Thus nuclear medicine studies appear appropriate in patients following trauma if an underlying dural fluid collection is suspected and in patients with focal seizures or signs suggesting a stroke, intracranial space–occupying lesion, or inflammatory disease. Their use should be considered in any comatose patient when the cause is unknown and in patients with cerebrospinal fluid draining from the nose or ear.

CARDIAC PROCEDURES

The use of nuclear medicine procedures to evaluate cardiac disease in an acute clinical situation has been largely confined to the detection of increased pericardial fluid. However, newer radiopharmaceutical agents that image cardiac musculature, improved instrumentation both for imaging and for quantitation, and the application of tracer principles for physiologic measurements have allowed present and future extension of our horizons in this area.

Pericardial effusion can be detected by the use of a radionuclide label that remains confined to the blood pool. On the anterior view in pericardial effusion, the radioactivity in the heart will be separated from that in the lungs, the hilar regions (pulmonary vessels) will appear elevated, and liver radioactivity will be separated from that in the right heart by a clear zone (Fig. 11-18, *A*). Separation of activity in the right heart from the right lung is the single most reliable sign of pericardial effusion. A thickened left ventricular muscle will separate the left ventricular cavity from the left lung. Left anterior oblique views will aid in this differential diagnosis, for the intraventricular septum may be widened with muscular hypertrophy. Blood pool scanning is an atraumatic but rather insensitive method of detecting pericardial fluid. As large a volume as 50 to 100 ml of pericardial fluid can go undetected by this technique.[37] Utilization of ultrasound and contrast angiography (with carbon dioxide as the contrast medium are more sensitive and probably more specific diagnostic methods (Fig. 11-18, *B*). Injection of technetium pertechnetate for radionuclide angiocardiography has been advocated by some as a means of detecting pericardial effusion. The pertechnetate is an intravascular label on the first passage through the circulatory system but rapidly equilibrates with the extracellular fluid and may be present in the pericardial fluid. Failure to consider this property of pertechnetate ion has resulted in false negative diagnoses on delayed static images.

Chest pain is a frequent symptom of patients arriving at the emergency care area. The problems of clinically identifying those patients with pulmonary thromboembolism have been discussed previously. Often it is equally difficult to distinguish patients with aortic dissection from those suffering from myocardial infarction and angina pectoris. The diagnosis of aortic dissection rests upon accurate delineation of anatomic detail and contrast angiographic studies are required; nuclear medicine procedures do not provide the precise structural representation necessary.

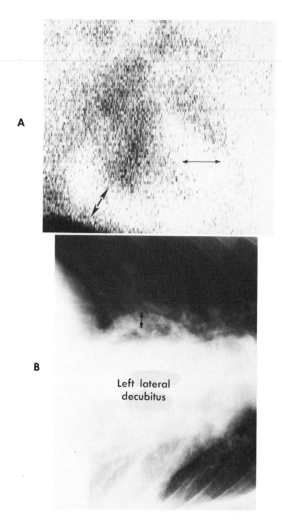

Fig. 11-18. Pericardial effusion. **A,** 99mTechnetium serum albumin blood pool study showing large area devoid of radioactivity surrounding heart, with elevation of pulmonary vasculature and separation of cardiac and hepatic blood pools. These are findings characteristic of large pericardial effusion. **B,** Carbon dioxide study obtained with patient lying on his left side. Soft tissue density between carbon dioxide in right atrium and interface with right lung is greater than 5 mm (upper limits of normal). This confirms presence of pericardial effusion. (Modified from James, A. E., and Squire, L. F.: Nuclear radiology, Philadelphia, 1973, W. B. Saunders Co.)

The use of radiopharmaceuticals that accumulate in myocardial muscle as a means of detecting myocardial infarction is in its infancy, but greatly increased utilization of this technique is anticipated. Many radiopharmaceuticals, including ^{43}KCl, $^{129}CsCl$, ^{131}I-labeled fatty acids, and $^{13}NH_3$, have been most commonly employed. These radiopharmaceuticals are accumulated

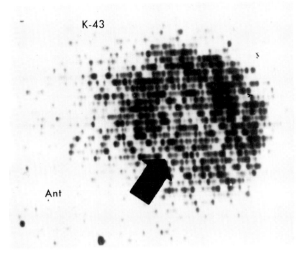

Fig. 11-19. Myocardial infarction. Myocardial scan using ^{43}KCl with an inferomedial defect on anterior view. Electrocardiogram confirmed occurrence of myocardial infarction.

in myocardial muscle, and areas of infarction or scar formation are manifest on scans as negative defects[13] (Fig. 11-19). More recently, ^{99m}Tc-tetracycline and other agents have been shown to localize in areas of recent infarction. The sensitivity and specificity of these techniques have not been determined, nor have comparative studies with electrocardiographic results been made. The simplicity of directly imaging the infarcted myocardium is very appealing and offers future promise in the emergency diagnosis and care of cardiac problems.

Even though a diagnosis of myocardial infarction has been established, the questions raised in terms of immediate care are often complex. Treatment decisions are often based upon assumptions regarding the amount of extravascular pulmonary water or the status of the left ventricular function (reflected by the cardiac ejection fraction, or output). Accurate measurements of these parameters can be obtained by the use of nuclear medicine techniques. The studies, however, are often complex and time consuming, or they present logistical problems that, for the present, preclude their routine use in emergency situations. Some coronary care units now employ gamma cameras with the ability to do ejection fractions on a routine basis. Adequate assessment of left ventricular function is necessary, since aggressive therapy is now being applied earlier in acute myocardial infarction.

Infants with respiratory distress and cyanosis present a particularly difficult diagnostic problem.[47] Whether the cyanosis is of central nervous system, pulmonary, or cardiac origin should be immediately established. Radionuclide angiocardiography is reported to be valuable in this differentiation. Results of isotope angiocardiograms performed on infants with cyanosis of pulmonary origin will usually be normal.[47,113] Rarely, the pulmonary resistance is severe enough to effect an intracardiac right-to-left shunt through a patent foramen ovale.[46] In a series of 30 infants with cyanotic congenital heart disease, Hurley et al.[47] were able to correctly detect intracardiac right-to-left shunts in all. In the 46 patients studied by radionuclide angiocardiography without intracardiac shunts, three were incorrectly suspected of having shunts. Utilizing techniques to monitor the recirculation of radioactivity through the lungs, Alazaraki et al.[1] have studied 93 patients. Fifty patients were thought to have left-to-right shunts that were later confirmed by other studies. Of the 44 patients in whom intracardiac shunts were not demonstrated by this technique, eight subsequently underwent cardiac catheterization, and no shunt was found.

In cyanotic infants with congenital heart disease, certain abnormalities can be identified by radionuclide angiocardiography and shunt determination.[47] Transposition of the great vessels can often be diagnosed by this technique, but in certain patients it is difficult to differentiate this condition from truncus arteriosus and the tetralogy of Fallot. Pulmonary atresia with intact ventricular septum has been successfully diagnosed, but other causes of a small right ventricle continue to present problems in differential diagnosis. In infants with certain types of left heart syndrome, catheterization should be avoided because no effective mode of therapy exists. The radionuclide angiocardiogram shows persistence of the radiopharmaceutical in the right heart and poor delineation of the left ventricle and aorta. The abnormalities that are identified may eliminate the need for some cardiac catheterization procedures and can assist in more appropriate planning of the catheterization and shorten the time of the procedure. Ultrasound appears to offer promise in the diagnosis of left heart syndrome, transposition of the great vessels, and other types of congenital heart disease and thus may limit the use of radionuclide angiocardiography as the screening procedure for examination of structural detail.

GASTROINTESTINAL PROCEDURES

Nuclear medicine studies to diagnose acute intra-abdominal diseases that require emergency therapy employ many different principles and will therefore be described separately.

Trauma to the solid organs of the abdomen often presents a diagnostic problem.[21,67,111] The abdominal wall, because of its nonrigid character, allows organs such as the liver and spleen to receive almost direct force at impact. Fractures, contusions, hematomas, and subcapsular extravasations of blood result; these may be successfully diagnosed by liver and spleen scans. Through the use of radioactively labeled colloids, the liver and spleen are normally delineated as areas of increased radioactivity with fairly homogeneous distribution. Trauma to these organs will result in areas of absent reticuloendothelial

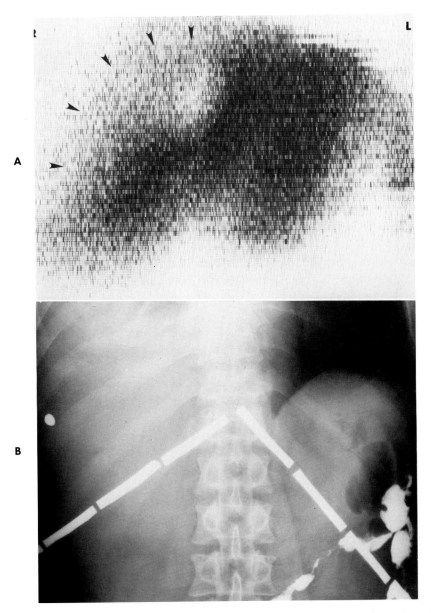

Fig. 11-20. Hepatic trauma. **A,** Liver scan with ^{99m}Tc-sulfur colloid shows large left lobe and defect in superlateral portion of right lobe. Patient had gunshot wound of right lower chest and abdomen. **B,** Abdominal radiograph shows bullet fragment in this area as well as pleural effusion and elevation of right hemidiaphragm. (Modified from James, A. E., and Squire, L. F.: Nuclear radiology, Philadelphia, 1973, W. B. Saunders Co.)

cell function that will be manifest as "negative defects" in a field of radioactivity (Fig. 11-20). Concomitant abdominal radiographs with appropriate markers for orientation of the scans will aid in localization of the abnormality. They may also assist in differential diagnosis if metallic foreign bodies are present or a gas-distended bowel is displaced.[29]

Gunshot wounds many times are characterized by an unpredictable course of the metallic foreign object within the abdomen because the path has been altered by dense structures such as the lumbar spine. Such patients may present an acute diagnostic problem due to a declining hematocrit, which suggests intra-abdominal bleeding. Successful exploratory laparotomy can be aided by liver, spleen, or renal scans that localize the area of trauma and provide data regarding the function of these organs (Fig. 11-21).

Patients with sickle cell disease can present with acute abdominal pain. During periods of sickle cell crisis, functional asplenia has been reported.[77] Splenic infarcts and ruptures following silent subcapsular hematomas have been diagnosed by scans.[27,49,73,106,119] However, no single series can provide sufficient data for inferring the accuracy or sensitivity of this procedure.

Assessment of polygonal cell function by ^{131}I rose bengal scanning is useful in differentiating obstructive from other types of jaundice.[87] The use of disappearance curves of radioactivity from the intravascular compartment and accumulation of radioactivity in the liver provides a rapid method for quantifying hepatic physiology. Rapid disappearance of the radiopharmaceutical from the blood and its early appearance and accumulation in the liver is characteristic of extrahepatic biliary obstruction. Extrahepatic biliary obstruction can also be suggested on colloid scans of the liver by a characteristic central branching area devoid of radioactivity due to dilated bile ducts.[42] Intravenous cholangiography is a more appropriate diagnostic method for this purpose. One of the very complex problems is the differentiation of patients with intrahepatic jaundice from those with extrahepatic jaundice because in a short period of time biliary stasis will cause abnormalities in polygonal cell function. Children with biliary atresia often develop biliary cirrhosis.

Patients with symptoms of acute pain in the right upper quadrant of the abdomen and suspected cholecystitis are currently evaluated by gallbladder series or intravenous cholangiography. In many patients, "faint visualization" of the gallbladder occurs in contrast studies. Radiopharmaceuticals now being tested may allow accurate quantification of gallbladder function and more sensitive identification of patients with acute or subacute cholecystitis.[24]

Patients with abdominal pain and sepsis may harbor perihepatic or splenic abscesses.[62] Several investigators have emphasized that, with the current liberal use of antibiotics, the signs and symptoms of intra-abdominal septic abnormalities may be masked.[76,94] In a study of 50 patients by Sanders et al.,[94] results of liver scans were only 60% accurate in detecting an abnormality in

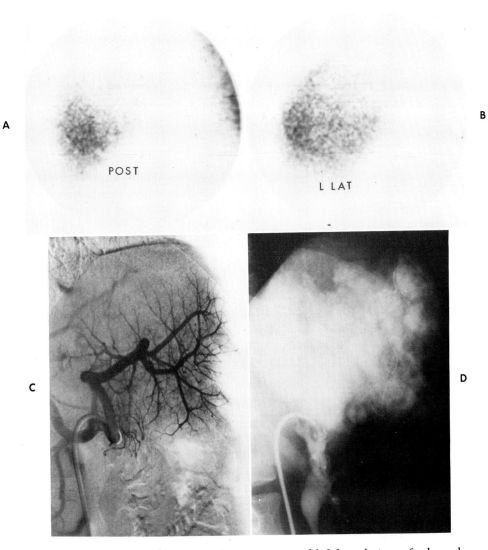

Fig. 11-21. Splenic hematoma. **A** and **B,** Posterior and left lateral views of spleen obtained with ⁹⁹ᵐTc-sulfur colloid. There is a superior intrasplenic defect. Patient fell from a horse and sustained blunt trauma to left upper quadrant without rib fracture. **C,** Selective splenic angiogram shows displacement of splenic vessels and lack of filling in superior portion of spleen. **D,** Splenogram shows failure of opacification of superior area of spleen. This was found to be splenic hematoma. (Courtesy Dr. Robert I. White, Baltimore, Md.)

perihepatic sepsis. Intrahepatic abscesses cause discrete negative defects on the liver scan[15] (Fig. 11-22). Employing dynamic studies (rapid sequential images after a bolus injection), Waxman et al.[108] found that abscesses showed diminished activity throughout the study, whereas vascular neoplasms demonstrated focal increase in radioactivity on the early images. Good-quality radiographs will aid in differential diagnosis as intrahepatic gas is sometimes present; nonbowel gas is present in about one third of patients with subphrenic abscesses. The use of ^{67}Ga citrate imaging to localize abdominal abscesses is still under investigation but appears to be quite promising.

On liver images, subphrenic abscesses are characteristically seen as diffuse areas of diminished radioactivity of the superior border. Many articles have emphasized the value of combined liver-lung scans in the detection of subphrenic abscesses.[11,17] However, if there is consolidation of the right lower lobe of the lung or a significant pleural effusion on the right side, an area devoid of radioactivity will be present, not because of subphrenic abscess but due to disease above the diaphragm.[31] Specific attention should be directed to the superior border of the liver. If its contour is smooth, the disease process is more likely to have its locus above the diaphragm. Again, correlation with chest and abdominal radiographs (with appropriate markers) and fluoroscopic examination will assist in avoiding these pitfalls.[94]

Subhepatic abscesses are difficult to detect on liver images and are manifested as irregular areas of diminished radioactivity along the lower border or the liver. Since a decrease in tissue volume is normally present inferiorly, the presence of a subhepatic abscess can only be inferred from liver scans. Lesser sac abscesses must be diagnosed by plain radiographs, barium studies, ultrasound, or exploratory laparotomy; a liver scan is helpful only in eliminating subphrenic and intrahepatic abscesses.

Acute hepatitis cannot be specifically diagnosed by liver scans. Generalized diminished uptake of the radiopharmaceutical agent by the reticuloendothelial or polygonal cells is usually seen. The size of the liver and spleen can be measured, and this data may provide a valuable baseline for subsequent evaluation. The use of rapid sequential liver imaging to assess hepatic blood flow in the emergency evaluation of candidates for portal-caval shunt surgery has been attempted but is not clinically employed at present.[89] Quantification of the separate contribution of the portal vein and the hepatic artery by radionuclide methods would be advantageous in presurgical evaluation.

Pancreatic scanning was initially greeted with great enthusiasm that was shortly replaced by skepticism to the extent of cynicism and rejection.[97] Recently there has been renewed interest in this procedure, even though its use remains limited by a radiopharmaceutical agent with a number of undesirable characteristics.[23] Hatchette et al.[41] found that in 12 cases of pancreatitis, 10 studies were positive. Characteristically, there is diffusely poor uptake of ^{75}Se-selenomethionine or there is failure to visualize the pancreas altogether. Pseu-

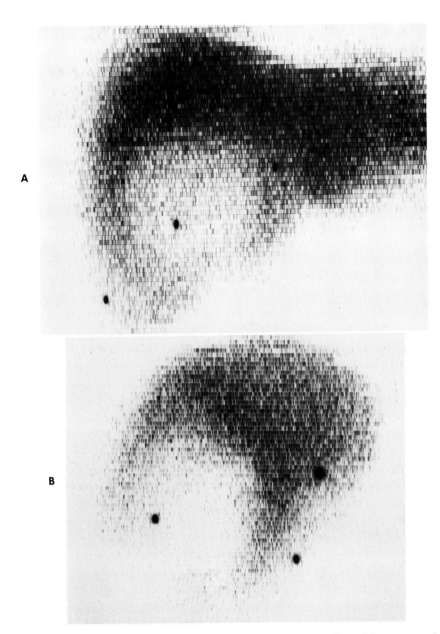

Fig. 11-22. Intrahepatic abcess. **A** and **B,** Anterior and right lateral liver scans show large defect posteriorly involving midportion of right lobe. Patient had intrahepatic abscess due to previous appendiceal perforation. Defect is surrounded by radioactivity on anterior view and margins curve inward on right lateral view, suggesting intrahepatic nature of process. This appearance is different from that seen with invasion or compression by adjacent retroperitoneal abnormality. (Courtesy Dr. R. C. Sanders and Dr. Wendy North, Baltimore, Md.)

docysts of the pancreas may present in the emergency care area as abdominal masses. These can be diagnosed by pancreatic scans, but abdominal sonography or upper gastrointestinal series are more appropriate initial studies.[61] Abdominal sonography has also been advocated for the diagnosis of pancreatitis.[103] Pancreatic scanning, until the development of a better radiopharmaceutical agent, appears to be of limited utility in the evaluation of acutely ill patients.

Abnormalities of bowel blood flow are particularly difficult diagnostic problems. A number of plain film radiographic signs have been described, but these are suggestive and not specific, and no prospective study testing the sensitivity or accuracy of these manifestations is available. The angiographic diagnosis of intestinal ischemia or infarction is also difficult. In most emergencies in which a compromised intestinal blood flow is suspected, an immediate exploratory laparotomy is performed. Radionuclide techniques utilizing intravascular labels have been only moderately successful in experimental animals, and no clinical trials have been attempted. The development of portable imaging and probe devices will probably facilitate the use of radionuclide techniques on an emergency basis in the operating room to determine the extent of the resection to be performed on an infarcted intestine or during revascularization procedures[118] (Fig. 11-23).

Radionuclide scans have been reported to be successful in the diagnosis of intussusception and Meckel's diverticulum. The area of intussusception is seen as an area in the abdomen that accumulates increased radioactivity (^{99m}Tc-pertechnetate) after intravenous injection. Duszynski and Anthone[22] believe that the localized concentration of the radiopharmaceutical is due to the presence of marked edema and hyperemia of the bowel wall and is associated with pertechnetate accumulation in the interstitial fluid. However, we have encountered increased amounts of the radiopharmaceutical in intestinal loops proximal to an experimental mechanical obstruction in animals. The increased level of radiopharmaceutical was present to the greatest extent in the intraluminal fluid, although increased amounts were encountered also in the intestinal wall proximal to the obstruction.

Meckel's diverticula are present in 1.5% of the population. Nearly half of these diverticula contain ectopic gastric mucosa. Meckel's diverticulum as a cause of acute gastrointestinal bleeding or small bowel obstruction in children may be diagnosed by abdominal scans (Fig. 11-24). Rosenthall et al.[90] studied 10 patients with Meckel's diverticula (8 of which were subsequently found to contain gastric mucosa) and the abdominal scans of 4 were positive after injection of ^{99m}Tc-pertechnetate. This may represent an alternative study following abdominal radiographs and barium studies in acute gastrointestinal hemorrhage in children.

Nuclear medicine studies have thus been successfully employed in the diagnosis of emergency gastrointestinal disorders. The ability to quantify blood

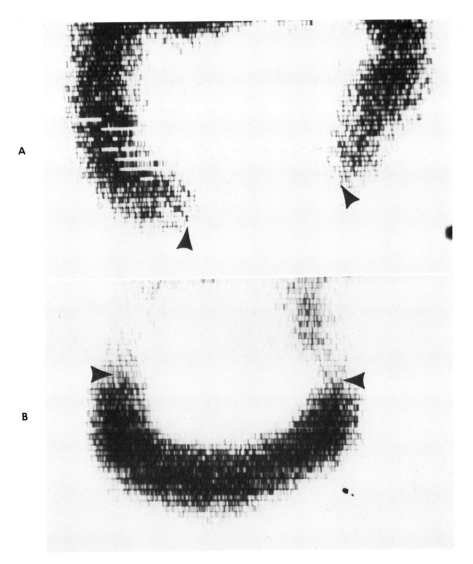

Fig. 11-23. Mesenteric infarction. **A,** ^{99m}Tc-microsphere injection into superior mesenteric artery in animal with experimental segmental mesenteric infarction. Normal bowel shows perfusion, but area supplied by occluded vessel does not. In surgery this bowel was found to be nonviable and necrotic. **B,** Scan of animal with similarly induced vascular lesion with area of bowel with occluded vessel showing reactive hyperemia. At surgery, segment appeared viable. Absence or presence of reactive hyperemia following experimental vascular injury was found to be an excellent predictor of survival of bowel segment. It also may prove clinically useful in distinguishing between necrotic and viable bowel. (Courtesy Dr. Christopher Zarins, Ann Arbor, Mich.)

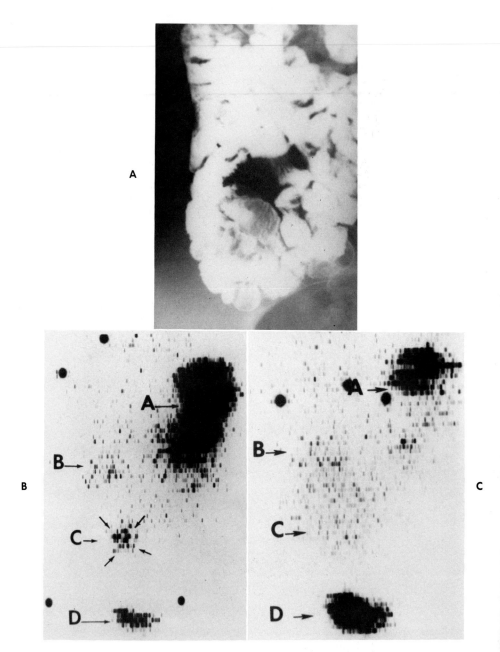

Fig. 11-24. Meckel's diverticulum. **A,** Small bowel series in man with rectal bleeding shows mass effect in area of terminal ileum and iliocecal valve. **B,** ^{99m}Tc-pertechnetate abdominal scan shows abnormal accumulation of radioactivity, *C,* in right lower quadrant. Pertechnetate is also present in stomach, *A;* duodenum, *B;* and bladder, *D.* **C,** Postoperative abdominal scan showing disappearance of abnormal area of radioactivity following removal of Meckel's diverticulum. (Courtesy Dr. K. S. Oh, Baltimore, Md.)

flow offers future promise in an area in which we presently have no suitable diagnostic test.

GENITOURINARY PROCEDURES

Renal scans and renograms are noninvasive methods of exploring altered kidney function in a rapid, simple manner.[84] However, the anatomic detail derived from these studies is often insufficient as a basis for selecting the appropriate therapy, and other diagnostic modalities must also be employed Following renal trauma, intravenous urograms will sometimes fail to show abnormalities or displacement and distortion of the calyces during the nephrographic phase. Scans will often delineate subcapsular hematomas or contusions, as they have the ability to demonstrate localized areas of tubular or glomerular dysfunction that can be further evaluated by contrast angiography (Fig. 11-25).

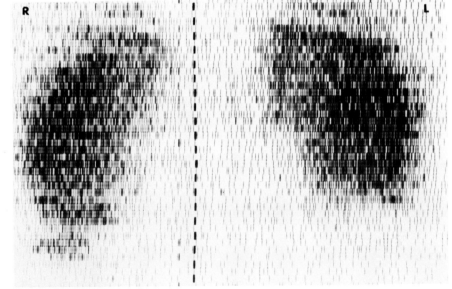

Continued.

Fig. 11-25. Renal trauma with lower pole infarct. **A,** Renal scan (^{197}Hg-chlormerodrin) of young woman after automobile accident with trauma to left side of abdomen. Scan was obtained because of dropping hematocrit and shows difference in size of kidneys with failure of radiopharmaceutical to concentrate in left lower pole. **B,** Abdominal angiogram shows irregularity of origin of accessory vessel to lower pole of left kidney due to hematoma within vessel wall. **C,** Nephrogram of lower portion of kidney is irregular and corresponds to defect noted on renal scan. At surgery this patient was found to have hematoma of accessory vessel to left kidney with resultant lower pole infarction. (Modified from James, A. E., and Squire, L. F.: Nuclear radiology, Philadelphia, 1973, W. B. Saunders Co.)

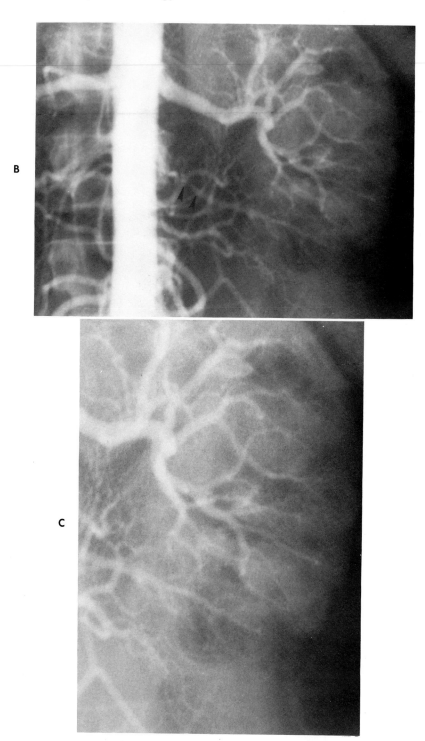

Fig. 11-25, cont'd. For legend see p. 299.

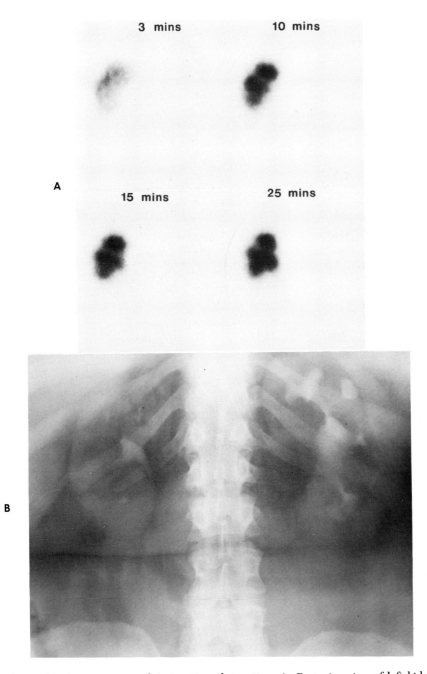

Fig. 11-26. Acute ureteropelvic junction obstruction. **A,** Posterior view of left kidney as dynamic renal study (^{99m}Tc-DTPA). Lobulated appearance of radioactivity is characteristic of that seen with dilatation of renal calyces. **B,** Intravenous urogram shows dilatation of collecting system on left side due to acute obstruction at ureteropelvic junction. (Courtesy Dr. Peter Kirchner, Bethesda, Md.)

Obstructive uropathy can be detected by nephrograms and dynamic renal scans; however, localization of the obstruction is desirable before initiation of therapy, and urograms with delayed exposures offer a greater likelihood of providing this necessary data (Fig. 11-26). In patients with elevated levels of serum urea nitrogen, radionuclide renal studies may provide structural detail when contrast urograms fail to do so. Whether or not there is a kidney present and its size as well as the status of the ureters can be evaluated.[60] Ultrasonography also offers a rapid, noninvasive, and accurate technique for evaluating renal size and location as well as in diagnosing hydronephrosis.[6]

Radionuclide evaluation of the kidneys of patients with acute renal failure can predict the ultimate outcome of renal function.[98] If good renal visualization with ^{131}I-hippuran is obtained, there is a high probability of recovery of renal function sufficient to sustain life without the need for dialysis or transplantation. However, if the kidneys are not visualized within 30 minutes, the patient will generally require either transplantation or dialysis.

Dynamic renal studies have been utilized to diagnose acute renal failure due to embolism[40] and to evaluate the patency of major renal vascular pathways.[30] The value of these studies appears to be as a screening procedure for renal angiography. Several articles have reported the use of dynamic renal scans in evaluation of renal masses. Hypernephromas have been characteristically described as areas of increased radioactivity in the earlier phases of the dynamic study. Cysts, because of their avascular nature and lack of function, present as negative defects. In our experience most renal neoplasms show diminished radioactivity during all phases of dynamic renal study, and we have found these studies of limited use in evaluating renal masses.

In hospitals with active renal transplant programs, radionuclide renal studies are often requested in emergency circumstances to determine whether transplant failure has occurred for technical reasons or due to rejection (Fig. 11-27). Vascular compromise and hydronephrosis have been reported to mimic

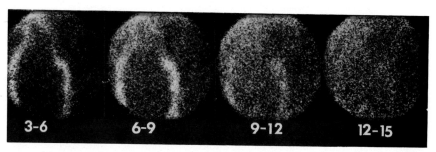

Fig. 11-27. Infarcted renal transplant. Rapid sequence study using ^{99m}Tc-DTPA with absence of perfusion in region of transplanted kidney. Negative defect is secondary to displacement of normal vasculature by infarcted kidney. Finding was confirmed through angiography and surgery.

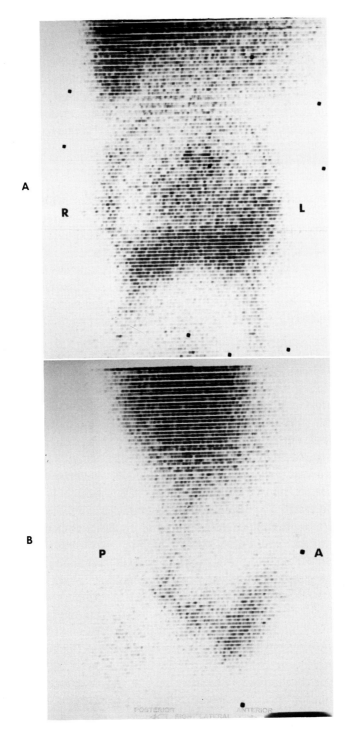

Fig. 11-28. Blood pool images with ^{113m}In-transferrin demonstrates anteroinferior location of placenta that overlies internal cervical os. **A,** Anterior view. **B,** Right lateral view.

transplant rejection and may be successfully differentiated by radionuclide studies.[112] Renograms and dynamic renal scans are more sensitive than intravenous urograms and contrast angiography in detecting the earliest phases of transport rejection.

Radionuclide placentography is a method of directly localizing the placenta by imaging the placental blood pool[51] (Fig. 11-28). In a series of 84 patients studied in this manner with either ^{99m}Tc-albumin or [113m]In-transferrin, the placenta was correctly localized in all but one instance of marginal placenta previa. Ultrasonography can localize the placenta with the same order of accuracy and, in addition, provides information regarding intrauterine contents (number of fetuses, fetal head size, orientation of the fetus, and so on). We have found a decrease in the number of placentograms performed, and an increased use of sonography in this circumstance.

Thus the use of nuclear medicine procedures for evaluation of acute genitourinary disease is limited to specific areas. Further development of techniques to rapidly evaluate renal function will probably be the area of future development for emergency care of renal problems.

VASCULAR STUDIES OF EXTREMITIES

Patients are often seen following trauma or with extremity pain in which there is diagnostic uncertainty regarding the peripheral arterial blood supply and perfusion to the extremities. Utilizing labeled microspheres, one can assess the capillary blood flow as well as perfusion to large muscle groups. Angiographic techniques will very accurately depict the large vessels but do not fully assess the functional significance of collateral circulation or the adequacy of blood flow in the microcirculation.[38]

Following intra-arterial injection of microspheres, the scans that are obtained normally show a homogeneous distribution of the radioactive substance to large muscle groups, with diminished radioactivity seen only in the relatively avascular areas of the joints (Fig. 11-29). In patients with emboli involving major vessels or interruption of blood flow due to obstruction, spasm, or compression from trauma, localized areas of soft tissue supplied by the involved vessel will be seen as specific areas of diminished radioactivity (Fig. 11-30).

Recently, perfusion extremity scans have been correlated with angiograms and clinical histories to demonstrate the utility of this technique.[32] Preliminary data also suggest that perfusion studies may be utilized in determining which superficial ulcers of the distal extremities may be treated by conservative means and which are best treated by surgical excision or amputation of the involved area.[114]

Nuclear medicine techniques have been utilized to visualize intravascular thrombi by Webber et al.[109] Labeled streptokinase, urokinase, fibrinogen, and albumin macroaggregates have been employed to detect venous thrombi

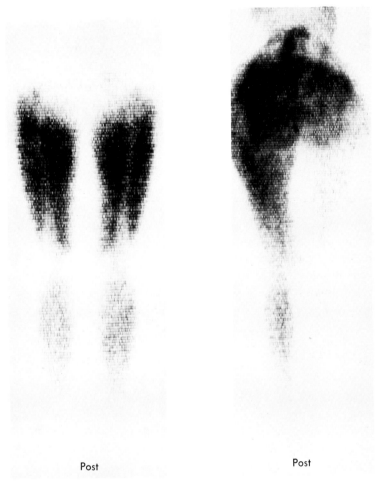

Post   Post

Fig. 11-29   Fig. 11-30

Fig. 11-29. Perfusion scan of lower extremities obtained with ^{99m}Tc-microspheres demonstrates normal perfusion pattern. There is good visualization of major muscle distributions. (Courtesy Dr. Frank Giargiana and Dr. M. E. Siegel, Baltimore, Md.)

Fig. 11-30. Arteriosclerosis. Perfusion scan in patient with claudication in right leg shows lack of perfusion to whole right lower extremity. (Courtesy Dr. Frank Giargiana and Dr. M. E. Siegel, Baltimore, Md.)

as the origin of significant pulmonary emboli. The clinical utility of these procedures is still not known.

OSSEOUS STUDIES

Patients are often seen in emergency rooms with extremity pains that are only vaguely related to some antecedent trauma. In such cases the pain might be due to infection or neoplasm. Plain radiographs often fail to identify osteomyelitis during the first 7 to 10 days after onset. During this period of time, osseous scans may show increased accumulations of radionuclide. Reticulo-endothelial scans of the bone marrow will show diminished uptake of the radio-colloid in the same area due to diminished function of the reticuloendothelial system. Experimental studies with staphylococcal osteomyelitis in rabbit femurs have demonstrated that diminished reticuloendothelial function is present before radiographic changes are manifest on good quality radiographs.[26] Thus it appears that although they are not clinically employed at present, osseous and reticuloendothelial scans to visualize bone and bone marrow may be useful in the early detection of osteomyelitis. Occult fractures are probably best diagnosed by plain radiographs, and nuclear medicine procedures do not appear to offer significant help in diagnosing in bone trauma.

We have occasionally obtained reticuloendothelial scans to assess the distribution of the bone marrow prior to biopsy. This is a rarely performed procedure, and very few osseous or bone marrow scans are obtained as emergency studies at present for any reason. Whether or not the improved anatomic resolution from the ^{99m}Tc-labeled bone agents (such as pyrophosphate, diphosphonate, and polyphosphate) will result in increased utilization in emergency care has not yet been determined.

IN VITRO STUDIES

Development of immunoassay techniques has great implications for improved clinical care at all levels. These studies are not employed at present as emergency procedures. However, the principles of immunoassay are particularly suited to accurate measurement of minute concentrations of various substances in the blood and will soon be widely employed in such common disorders as digoxin overdosage as well as other forms of drug intoxication. At present these techniques are uncommonly employed in emergency care, but as they become generally available, the number of immunoassays done both on a routine and emergency basis will predictably increase. Occasionally patients are seen with acute thyrotoxicosis or "thyroid storm," and emergency radioactive iodine uptake studies are performed to confirm the diagnosis.

Automated detection of bacterial growth using radioactive techniques is accurate and rapid and requires minimal patient cooperation. These techniques are being improved and have great future potential in patients with infection.[17]

In treatment of patients with many disorders including acute blood loss, congestive heart failure, and dehydration, accurate determination of blood volume is extremely useful in deciding upon an appropriate therapy. Other indicators of blood volume such as central venous pressure monitoring have been found as useful in the clinical circumstances, thus decreasing the number of radionuclide studies requested at present.

In summary, there are many indications for nuclear medicine procedures in emergency health care. These should be considered with regard to other diagnostic modalities, which may or may not provide the same information. One should also determine the degree of structural detail necessary to select the most appropriate therapy. In those instances in which nuclear medicine procedures will not provide the necessary information, they should not be employed solely because they are simple, easy to perform, and require very little in the way of patient cooperation.

In the treatment of emergencies it is becoming apparent that assessment of physiologic alterations is mandatory. The utilization of minute amounts of radioactivity to make these determinations as well as the added ability to correlate these with anatomic images make nuclear medicine techniques useful. At present the greatest limitation to the use of nuclear medicine procedures in emergency care areas is a logistical one; the laboratory is removed from the emergency facility. Continued improvement of radiopharmaceutical agents and the development of more advanced instruments and diagnostic techniques will result in increased utilization.

Acknowledgments

We wish to express our appreciation to Drs. Paul Hoffer, John Dorst, Wendy North, Robert I. White, Henry Wagner, and Richard C. Reba for their helpful suggestions and assistance in the preparation of the manuscript.

References

1. Alazaraki, N. P., et al.: Detection of left-to right cardiac shunts with scintillation camera pulmonary dilution curve, J. Nucl. Med. **13:**142, 1972.
2. Alderson, P. O., Secker-Walker, R. H., and Forrest, J. V.: Detection of obstructive pulmonary disease: relative sensitivity of ventilation-perfusion studies and chest radiography, Radiology **111:**643, 1974.
3. Apau, R. L., Saenz, R. and Siemsen, J. K.: Bloodless lung due to bronchial obstruction, J. Nucl. Med. **13:**561, 1972.
4. Applebaum, R. I., Newman, S. A., and Zingesser, L. H.: Dynamics of technetium scanning in subdural hematomas, Invest. Radiol. **102:**646, 1965.
5. Bagley, C.: Functional and organic alterations following introduction of blood into the cerebrospinal fluid, Res. Publ. Assoc. Res. Nerv. Men. Dis. **8:**214, 1929.
6. Bearman, S.: Personal communication, 1973.
7. Blahd, W. H., editor: Nuclear medicine, New York, 1971, McGraw-Hill Book Co.
8. Bonte, F. J., and Williams, J. R.: The roentgenological aspect of nonpenetrating chest injuries, Springfield, Ill., 1961, Charles C Thomas, Publisher.
9. Bookstein, J. J., and Voegeli, E.: A critical analysis of magnification radiography: laboratory investigation, Radiology **98:**23, 1971.
10. Braunstein, P., et al.: Cerebral death: rapid and reliable diagnostic adjunct using radioisotopes, J. Nucl. Med. **14:**122, 1973.
11. Brown, D. W.: Combined lung-liver radioisotope scans in the diagnosis of subdiaphragmatic abscess, Am. J. Surg. **109:**521, 1965.
12. Conway, J. J., and Vollert, J. M.: The accuracy of radionuclide imaging in detecting pediatric dural fluid collections, Radiology **105:**77, 1972.

13. Cooper, M., et al.: [43]KCl: a new radiopharmaceutical for imaging the heart, J. Nucl. Med. **12**:516, 1971.

14. Cowan, R. J., Maynard, C. D., and Lassitev, K. R.: Technetium [99m]pertechnetate brain scans in the detection of subdural hematomas: a study of the age of the lesion as related to the development of a positive scan, J. Neurosurg. **32**:30, 1970.

15. Curron, A., and Gordon, F.: Liver scanning: analysis of 2,500 cases of amebic hepatic abscesses, J. Nucl. Med. **11**:435, 1970.

16. Davis, D. O., and Potchen, E. J.: Brain scanning and intracranial inflammatory disease, Radiology **95**:345, 1970.

17. DeBlanc, H., Jr., Deland, F., and Wagner, H. N., Jr.: Automated radiometric detection of bacteria in 2967 blood cultures, Appl. Microbiol. **22**:846, 1971.

18. Deland, F. H.: Brain scanning in cerebral vascular disease, Semin. Nucl. Med. **1**:31, 1971.

19. DiChiro, G.: Movement of cerebrospinal fluid in human beings, Nature **204**:290, 1964.

20. DiChiro, G., and Ashburn, W. L.: Radioisotope cisternography, ventriculography, and myelography. In Blahd, W. H., editor: Nuclear medicine, New York, 1971, McGraw-Hill Book Co.

21. Drum, D. E., and Christacopoulos, J. S.: Hepatic scintigraphy in clinical decision making, J. Nucl. Med. **13**:908, 1972.

22. Duszynski, D. O., and Anthone, R.: Jejunal intussusception demonstrated by ^{99}Tc-pertechnetate and abdominal scanning, Am. J. Roentgenol. **109**:729, 1970.

23. Eaton, S. B., et al.: Comparison of current radiologic approaches to the diagnosis of pancreatic disease, N. Engl. J. Med. **279**:389, 1968.

24. Eikman, E. A., et al.: Radioactive tracer techniques in the diagnosis of acute cholecystitis, J. Nucl. Med. **14**:393, 1973. (Abstract.)

25. Farrar, P. A., Roghair, G., and Steinhacker, R.: Radiopertechnetate cerebral angiography in the early diagnosis and detection of strokes, J. Nucl. Med. **10**:401, 1969.

26. Feigin, D.: Personal communication, 1974.

27. Fink, D. W.: Scintiphotographic demonstration of rupture of an accessary spleen, J. Nucl. Med. **13**:333, 1972.

28. Freeman, L. M., and Johnson, P. M.: Clinical scintillation scanning, New York, 1969, Harper & Row, Publishers.

29. Freeman, L. M., et al.: False positive liver scans caused by disease processes in adjacent structures, Br. J. Radiol. **42**:651, 1969.

30. Freeman, L. M., et al.: Patency of major renal vascular pathways demonstrated by rapid blood flow scintiphotography, J. Urol. **105**:473, 1971.

31. Genant, H. K., and Hoffer, P. B.: False positive liver scan due to lung abscess, J. Nucl. Med. **13**:945, 1972.

32. Giargiana, F., et al.: The complementary roles of arteriography and perfusion scanning in assessment of peripheral vascular disease, Radiology **108**:619, 1973.

33. Gilday, D., and James, A. E.: Perfusion lung scan patterns in patients with pulmonary embolism, emphysema and pulmonary edema, CRC Crit. Rev. Radiol. Sci. **3**:321, 1972.

34. Gilday, D. L., Coates, G., and Goldenberg, D.: Subdural hematoma—what is the role of brain scanning in its diagnosis? J. Nucl. Med. **14**:283, 1973.

35. Gilson, A. J., and Gargano, F. P.: Correlation of brain scans and angiography in intracranial trauma, Am. J. Roentgenol. **94**:819, 1965.

36. Glascow, J. L., et al.: Brain scans at varied intervals following C.V.A., J. Nucl. Med. **6**:902, 1965.

37. Goldenberg, D., and Brogdon, B. G.: A comparison of venous angiography and radioisotope heart scanning in the diagnosis of pericardial effusion, Am. J. Roentgenol. **102**:320, 1968.
38. Greyson, N. D., et al.: Absence of anatomic arteriovenous shunts in Paget's disease of bones, N. Engl. J. Med. **287**:686, 1972.
39. Handa, J.: Dynamic aspects of brain scanning, Tokyo, 1972, Igaku Shoin, Ltd.
40. Hartenbower, D. L., et al.: Scintillation camera in embolic acute renal failure, J. Urol. **104**:799, 1970.
41. Hatchette, J. B., Shuler, S. E., and Murison, P. J.: Scintiphotos of the pancreas: analysis of 135 studies, J. Nucl. Med. **13**:51, 1972.
42. Heck, L. L., and Gottschalk, A.: The appearance of intrahepatic biliary duct dilatation on the liver scan, Radiology **99**:517, 1970.
43. Holloway, W., El Gammal, T., and Pool, W. H., Jr.: Doughnut sign in subdural hematomas, J. Nucl. Med. **13**:630, 1972.
44. Hopkins, G. B., and Kristensen, K. A. B.: Rapid sequential scintiphotography in the radionuclide detection of subdural hematomas, J. Nucl. Med. **14**:288, 1973.
45. Hurley, P. J.: Effect of craniotomy on the brain scan related to time elapsed after surgery, J. Nucl. Med. **13**:156, 1972.
46. Hurley, P. J.: Patent foramen ovale demonstrated by lung scanning, J. Nucl. Med. **13**:177, 1972.
47. Hurley, P. J., Wesselhoeft, H., and James, A. E., Jr.: Use of nuclear imaging in the evaluation of pediatric cardiac disease, Semin. Nucl. Med. **2**:353, 1972.
48. Isawa, T., Wasserman, K., and Taplin, G. V.: Variability of lung scans following pulmonary embolization: a concept of regional pulmonary ischemia of functional origin, Am. Rev. Respir. Dis. **101**:207, 1970.
49. Jackson, G. L., and Albright, D.: Splenic rupture: application of radioisotopic techniques in diagnosis, J.A.M.A. **204**:930, 1968.
50. James, A. E., Jr., and Wagner, H. N., Jr.: Nuclear medicine procedures in evaluation of cancer patients. In Deely, T., Modern trends in radiotherapy, London, 1972, Butterworth & Co. (Publishers), Ltd.
51. James, A. E., Jr., White, R. I., and Cooper, M.: Comparison of interstitial and alveolar patterns of pulmonary edema on chest radiographs with patterns on perfusion lung scans, Radiol. Clin. Biol. **41**:14, 1972.
52. James, A. E., Jr., et al.: Normal pressure hydrocephalus: role of cisternography in diagnosis, J.A.M.A. **213**:1615, 1970.
53. James, A. E., Jr., et al.: Scintigraphic patterns of large and small pulmonary emboli, J. Nucl. Med. **11**:214, 1970.
54. James, A. E., Jr., et al.: Perfusion changes on lung scans in patients with congestive heart failure, Radiology **100**:99, 1971.
55. James, A. E., Jr., et al.: The fissure sign: its multiple causes, Am. J. Roentgenol. **111**:492, 1971.
56. James, A. E., Jr., et al.: A cisternographic classification of hydrocephalus, Am. J. Roentgenol. **115**:39, 1972.
57. James, A. E., et al.: Placental imaging with ^{99m}Tc serum albumin and [113]In transferrin, J. Obstet. Gynecol. **37**:602, 1971.
58. Jordan, C. E., James, A. E., Jr., and Hodges, F. J.: Comparison of the cerebral angiogram and the brain radionuclide image in brain abscess, Radiology **104**:327, 1972.
59. Kilgore, B. B., and Bonte, F. J.: Scintigraphic demonstration of cerebral infarction in a "watershed" distribution, J. Nucl. Med. **12**:756, 1971.
60. Kirchner, P.: Personal communication, 1973.

61. Leopold, G. R.: Pancreatic echography: a new dimension in the diagnosis of pseudocyst, Radiology **104:**365, 1972.

62. LePage, J. R., et al.: Diagnosis of splenic abscess by radionuclide scanning and selective arteriography, J. Nucl. Med. **13:**331, 1972.

63. Maroon, J. C., Jones, R., and Mishkin, F. S.: Tuberculous meningitis diagnosed by brain scan, Radiology **104:**333, 1972.

64. Maynard, C. D.: Clinical nuclear medicine, Philadelphia, 1969, Lea & Febiger.

65. Maynard, C. D., Hanner, T. G., and Witcofski, R. L.: Positive brain scans due to lesion of the skull, Arch. Neurol. **18:**93, 1968.

66. McIntyre, K. V., and Sasahara, A. A.: Hemodynamic alterations related to extent of lung scan perfusion defect in pulmonary embolism, J. Nucl. Med. **12:**166, 1971.

67. McRae, J., Stening, G. F., and Volk, P. E.: Use of scintiphotography to outline abdominal masses, J. Nucl. Med. **13:**219, 1972.

68. Mishkin, F. S., and Mealey, J.: Use and interpretation of the brain scan, Springfield, Ill., 1969, Charles C Thomas, Publisher.

69. Mishkin, K. M., and Brashear, R. E.: An experimental study of the effect of free pleural fluid on the lung scan, Radiology **97:**283, 1970.

70. Molinari, G. F., Pircher, F., and Heyman, A.: Serial brain scanning using technetium ^{99m} in patients with cerebral infarction, Neurology **17:**627, 1967.

71. Moser, K. M., et al.: Assessment of pulmonary photoscanning and angiography in experimental pulmonary embolism, Circulation **39:**663, 1969.

72. Moses, D. C., et al.: Regional cerebral blood flow estimation in the diagnosis of cerebrovascular disease, J. Nucl. Med. **13:**135, 1972.

73. Nelp, W. B., and Kuhn, I. N.: Splenic infarction diagnosed preoperatively by photoscanning, J.A.M.A. **197:**368, 1966.

74. Ojemann, R. G., et al.: Extracranial measurement of regional cerebral circulation, J. Nucl. Med. **12:**532, 1971.

75. Oldendorf, W. H.: Distribution of various classes of radiolabelled tracers in plasma, scalp and brain, J. Nucl. Med. **13:**681, 1972.

76. Pai, S. T., and Bakk, Y. W.: Radioisotope scanning in the diagnosis of liver abscesses, Am. J. Surg. **119:**330, 1970.

77. Pearson, H. A., Spencer, R. P., and Cornelius, E. A.: Functional asplenia in sickle cell anemia, N. Engl. J. Med. **281:**923, 1969.

78. Perkerson, R. B., Jr., Smith, C. D., and Weller, W. F.: The rim sign of subdural hematoma, J. Nucl. Med. **13:**637, 1972.

79. Pirker, E.: Dynamics of bilateral intracranial hematoma, Fortschr. Rontgenstr. **102:**646, 1965.

80. Potchen, E. J., and Evens, R. G.: The physiologic factors affecting regional ventilation and perfusion, Semin. Nucl. Med. **1:**153, 1971.

81. Prockop, L. D., and Fishman, R. A.: Experimental pneumococcal meningitis: permeability changes influencing the concentration of sugars and macromolecules in CSF, Arch. Neurol. **19:**449, 1968.

82. Quinn, J. L., III, and Head, L.: Radioisotope scanning in pulmonary disease, J. Nucl. Med. **7:**1, 1966.

83. Radcliffe, W. B., et al.: Herpes simplex encephalitis: a radiologic-pathologic study of 4 cases, Am. J. Roentgenol. Radium Ther. Nucl. Med. **12:**263, 1971.

84. Raynaud, C., et al.: Use of renal uptake of ^{197}Hg as a method for testing the functional value of each kidney, J. Nucl. Med. **11:**125, 1970.

85. Rhoton, A. L., et al.: Brain scanning in ischemic cerebrovascular disease, Arch. Neurol. **14:**506, 1966.

86. Rinaldi, I., Harris, W. O., and DiChiro, G.: Radionuclide cisternography in subdural hematomas, Radiology **105**:597, 1972.
87. Rosenthall, L.: The application of radioiodinated rose bengal and colloidal radiogold in the detection of hepatobiliary disease, St. Louis, 1969, Warren H. Green, Inc.
88. Rosenthall, L.: Intravenous dynamic nucleography of the brain. In Croll, M. N., et al., editors: Clinical dynamic function studies with radionuclides, New York, 1972, Appleton-Century-Crofts.
89. Rosenthall, L., et al.: A liver trapping index of radiocolloid as an estimation of perfusion, Radiology **100**:363, 1971.
90. Rosenthall, L., et al.: Radiopertechnetate imaging of the Meckel's diverticulum, Radiology **105**:371, 1972.
91. Rosler, H., Huber, P., and Hesse, M.: Serienszintigraphische befunde beim Schlaganfall, Schweiz. Med. Wochenschr. **100**:1401, 1970.
92. Rudd, T. G., O'Neal, J. T., and Nelp, W. B.: Cerebrospinal fluid circulation following subarachnoid hemorrhage, J. Nucl. Med. **12**:61, 1971.
93. Rutherford, R., Hurley, P. J., and Strauss, H. W.: Unpublished observations.
94. Sanders, R. C., James, A. E., Jr., and Fischer, K.: Correlation of liver scans and images with abdominal radiographs in perihepatic sepsis, Am. J. Surg. **124**:346, 1972.
95. Smoak, W. M., and Gilson, A. J.: Scintillation visualization of a vascular rim in subdural hematoma, J. Nucl. Med. **11**:695, 1970.
96. Sobel, B. E.: Serum enzymes and the diagnosis of pulmonary embolism. In Moser, E. M., and Stein, M., editors: Pulmonary thromboembolism, Chicago, 1973, Year Book Medical Publishers, Inc.
97. Sodee, D. B.: Radioisotope scanning of the pancreas with selenomethionine (^{75}Se), Radiology **83**:910, 1964.
98. Staab, E. V., et al.: The use of radionuclide studies in the prediction of function in renal failure, Radiology **106**:141, 1973.
99. Stebner, F. C., Wilner, H. I., and Eyler, W. R.: Correlation of pathologic and radiologic findings in brain infarction, Radiology **91**:280, 1968.
100. Stein, M., et al.: Airway responses to pulmonary embolism-pharmacologic aspects. In Moser, E. M., and Stein, M., editors: Pulmonary thromboembolism, Chicago, 1973, Year Book Medical Publishers, Inc.
101. Suwanwela, C. H., Poshyachinda, V., and Poshyachinda, M.: Brain scanning in the diagnosis of intracranial abscess, Acta Neurochir. **25**:165, 1971.
102. Szucs, M. M., et al.: Diagnostic sensitivity of laboratory findings in acute pulmonary embolism, Ann. Intern. Med. **74**:161, 1971.
103. Templeton, A. W., and Stuber, J. L.: Abdominal retroperitoneal sonography, Am. J. Roentgenol. **113**:741, 1972.
104. Tetalman, M. R., et al.: Efficacy of emergency lung scans, J. Nucl. Med. **14**:460, 1973. (Abstract.)
105. Tow, D. E., Wagner, H. N., Jr.: Effect of pleural fluid on the appearance of the lung scan, J. Nucl. Med. **11**:138, 1970.
106. Vagenakis, A. G., Abreau, C. M., and Braverman, L. E.: Splenic infarction diagnosed by photoscanning, J. Nucl. Med. **13**:563, 1972.
107. Wagner, H. N., Jr., editor: Principles of nuclear medicine, Philadelphia, 1968, W. B. Saunders Co.
108. Waxman, A. D., Apau, R., and Siemsen, J. K.: Rapid sequential liver imaging, J. Nucl. Med. **13**:522, 1972.

109. Webber, M. M., et al.: Thrombosis demonstrated by scintiscanning, J. Nucl. Med. **10**:379, 1969.
110. Webster, J. R., Jr., et al.: Wheezing due to pulmonary embolism—treatment with heparin, N. Engl. J. Med. **274**:931, 1966.
111. Weiner, J., and Boyd, C. O.: Splenic scintiscanning in the preoperative diagnosis of subcapsular hematoma, N. Engl. J. Med. **277**:35, 1967.
112. Weiss, E. R., et al.: Ureteral kinking and hydronephrosis in a transplanted kidney mimicking the rejection phenomenon, J. Nucl. Med. **12**:43, 1971.
113. Wesselhoeft, H., et al.: Nuclear angiocardiography in the diagnosis of congenital heart disease in infants, Circulation **45**:77, 1972.
114. Williams, G. M., et al.: The clinical usefulness of leg scanning with radioactive microspheres in arterial insufficiency, Surg. Forum **23**:247, 1972.
115. Williams, J. P., et al.: Isotope cisternography in the evaluation of patients with subarachnoid hemorrhage, J. Nucl. Med. **11**:592, 1970.
116. Wilson, A. F., et al.: The significance of regional pulmonary function changes in bronchial asthma, Am. J. Med. **48**:416, 1970.
117. Yeh, E. L., Rutz, P. P., and Meade, R. C.: Separation of liver-lung scintiphotos due to ascites—a false positive test for subdiaphragmatic abscess, J. Nucl. Med. **13**:249, 1972.
118. Zarins, C., et al.: Bowel scans for revascularization procedures, Surg. Forum **24**:416, 1973.
119. Zook, E. G., Bolivar, J. C., and Epstein, L. I.: The value of scintiscans in the diagnosis of splenic abscess, Surg. Gynecol. Obstet. **131**:1125, 1970.

Index